MW01258106

Neurogerontology

James F. Willott, PhD, received his doctorate in psychobiology from the University of California, Davis in 1976. He took a position in behavioral neuroscience at Northern Illinois University and presently holds the rank of Distinguished Research Professor. He has been engaged in research on aging, specializing in the auditory system, since the early 1980s. Willott has published more than 80 research articles and chapters dealing with anatomical, neurophysiological, and behavioral aspects of aging and has produced two books, including *Aging and the Auditory System*, published in 1991. The National Institute on Aging has supported his research since 1982 and continues to do so. He received an NIA MERIT Award in 1988 and a Research Career Development Award in 1983.

Neurogerontology

Aging and the Nervous System

James F. Willott, PhD

Springer Publishing Company

Springer Publishing Company, Inc.
536 Broadway
New York, NY 10012-3955

Acquisitions Editor: Bill Tucker
Production Editor: Jean Hurkin-Torres
Cover design by Janet Joachim

99 00 01 02 03 / 5 4 3 2 1

Library of Congress Cataloging-in-Publication Data

Willott, James F.
     Neurogerontology: aging and the nervous system / by James F. Willott.
         p.   cm.
     Includes bibliographical references and index.
     ISBN 0-8261-1259-5 (hardcover)
     1. Nervous system—Aging.   2. Geriatric neurology.
3. Neuropsychology.   I. Title.
     [DNLM: 1. Nervous System Physiology—in old age.   2. Aging—physiology.   3. Behavior—in old age.   4. Aged—psychology.
WL 102 W739w 1999]
QP356.25.V55   1999
612.8—dc21
DNLM/DLC
for Library of Congress   98-43500
                                                                            CIP

Printed in the United States of America

Contents

List of Figures

To Niki and growing old together

Preface

"I've never heard of this Willott fellow, so where does he get off writing a book on neurogerontology?" I'm sure many gerontologists and neuroscientists will ask this question, even though I've published scores of journal articles and chapters on neurogerontological issues, written a book on aging and the auditory system, and have had my research supported by the National Institute on Aging since 1982, including receiving one of the NIA's 10-year MERIT awards. But that's okay, and indeed inevitable, because the field of neurogerontology is so diverse, specialized, compartmentalized, and comprised of many hundreds of scientists doing their own thing, often intellectually isolated from one another. In fact, this is the reason I decided to accept an offer by Dr. Ursula Springer to write this book. It is a broad overview of the field (as I see it), designed to bridge many gaps and provide the diverse neurogerontological community with an idea of what the folks in the lab down the hall are doing.

Writing a book of this nature presents a number of problems, the foremost being the target audience and what level of sophistication to expect or require of the reader. Obviously, many students and others with an interest in gerontology will have little sophistication in neuroscience; likewise, most neuroscientists don't know much about the gerontological literature. There are also topics of experimental psychology such as learning, memory, and emotion that are unfamiliar to some readers. So, if one is to have a book that is accessible to a wide audience, it is necessary to provide some review and tutorial material on basic neuroscience, gerontology, and behavioral science in conjunction with discussions of aging and the nervous system. Because I wanted an accessible book, I decided to go that route and include basic reviews of topics in neuroscience, gerontology, and psychology where applicable. Indeed, all chapters contain basic background information.

On the other hand, the specialization/compartmentalization within the neurogerontological research community, referred to earlier, cries out for a book that reaches a level of timeliness and sophistication appropriate for advanced students and professional researchers who wish to broaden their gerontological horizons. I wanted a book like this as well, so I also included an up-to-date (albeit not exhaustive) review of the literature in various areas of neurogerontology. For example, there are more than 700 references cited, with well over 300 of these published between 1995 and 1997. It is my hope that my review of the literature, as well as the way I have organized the discussion of the nervous system, will be fresh and informative for readers who possess an advanced knowledge of neuroscience and/or gerontology.

I am well aware of the risk in this venture. A graduate student in neuroscience will find some of the discussions to be overly elementary, whereas a novice neuroscientist may have trouble with some of the more technical issues. Indeed, a reviewer of the book manuscript, who is a prominent biological gerontologist, was troubled by this very issue. Although I was happy to make some changes along the line he suggested, I do not see a serious problem here. Readers with little background in neuroscience should be able to understand and digest 80% of the material without difficulty, and neuro-sophisticated readers who are concerned about being talked down to need only skip over about 20% of the text. Because we are all nonexperts in many areas of neurogerontology, both novice and expert will find that there is lots to learn. In this regard, I made an attempt to cite recent reviews of several levels of difficulty for each topic discussed.

It is my belief that this sort of compromise between introductory and advanced levels of neuroscience and gerontology will make this a useful and flexible textbook for courses in either discipline (not to mention the discipline of neurogerontology per se). It should also be a readable reference book for professionals who wish to see what is going on in other areas of research. I have written the book largely from a behavioral neuroscience perspective, focusing on structural and functional relationships between the nervous system and psychological phenomena such as perception, emotions, arousal, learning, cognition, and motor behavior, as well as maintenance of homeostasis. The emphasis is on healthy aging, but dementia and other pathological conditions are discussed when relevant.

I believe the book provides an overview of the field that not only presents many empirical findings but also makes it clear that there are many disagreements and contradictions in the literature. This generated the second concern of the reviewer of the book manuscript: Would undergraduates or nonscientists be confused by the lack of consensus? Perhaps, but I think most can (and should) be able to handle it. We are used to hearing about contradictory scientific findings in the news media, and this is a characteristic of science in general. This book presents a way of thinking about the science of neurogerontology, and part of this is being cautious about accepting findings as fact, while considering a variety of often disparate viewpoints.

I would like to acknowledge the contributions of various individuals to the writing of this book. My wife, Niki, read the entire manuscript from the nonscientist's perspective and made many helpful comments. Other colleagues provided input on their areas of expertise, including Drs. Stephanie Carlson, Gary Coover, Jim Corwin, Don Caspary, John Disterhoft, Bill Falls, Martin Farlow (who provided an unpublished review on pharmacological treatments in dementia), Ken Ferraro, Bob Helfert, and Jeremy Turner. My research associate, Lori Bross, provided excellent technical assistance and has been an invaluable sounding board. I am also grateful to Dr. Judy Finkelstein, Dr. Andrew Monjan, and others at the National Institute on Aging for their long-term support of my gerontological career, without which this book would never have been written.

I frequently browsed excellent neuroscience textbooks that I have used in the classroom to get current views on basic "conventional wisdom" issues and how they are best explained; these included Kalat's *Biological Psychology*; Kandel, Schwartz, and Jessell's *Essentials of Neural Science and Behavior*; and Rosenzweig, Leiman, and Breedlove's *Biological Psychology*. In reviewing the gerontological literature, I relied on my own extensive reprint collection and on the direction provided by various reviews, especially the *Handbook of the Biology and Aging* and *Handbook of the Psychology of Aging* series. Other important books were Mann's *Sense and Senility: The Neuropathology of the Aged Human Brain*, *The Encyclopedia of Gerontology*, Kausler's *Learning and Memory in Normal Aging*, Khatchaturian and Radenbaugh's *Alzheimer's Disease: Cause(s), Diagnosis, Treatment, and Care*, and the *Handbook of Neuropsychology of Aging*. I made extensive use of *Medline* to identify recent articles as well.

Finally, I apologize to those researchers whose works could have been cited but were not. This book was not meant to be an exhaustive review of the literature, and it was simply not possible to include all of the good articles (or to exclude some that may turn out to be not so good). If your deserving article was not mentioned, there is no implication whatsoever concerning its quality or value.

1
Introduction

Neurogerontology is a hybrid of the disciplines of neuroscience and gerontology, two rapidly growing, diverse fields with multifaceted basic scientific and clinical dimensions. An appreciation of the methods, principles, theories, and substance of both parental fields is a prerequisite if they are to be fused and integrated into a comprehensive discipline of neurogerontology. Because few people have substantial training in both fields, a book on neurogerontology must begin at basic levels in both disciplines (obviously, the knowledgeable reader can skip the introductory-level material). Thus, we first address the question What is aging? followed by a discussion of the complexity of nervous systems, why they evolved, and what they do. Then we will be ready to move on to other neurogerontological issues.

WHAT IS AGING?

In his recent book on aging, Hayflick (1996) points out what many people have found if they have tried to define aging: We know it when we see it, but a simple definition of aging is elusive. Aging of humans and other animals cannot be satisfactorily characterized by the passage of time alone (chronological age); rather, it is more germane to consider it as the manifestation of biological and ecological events that occur over some span of time. What makes characterizations of aging so difficult is that the effects of biological and other factors (e.g., environment, experience) vary greatly within the chronological time frame. We are often surprised by individuals who seem to be in their 60s but are actually much older (and vice versa). Furthermore, various abilities can age at different rates; by one standard a person can still be "young," and by another standard, "old." Despite some thorny issues in defining aging, most would agree that aging represents *changes* in structure and function that occur after maturation to the peak age of physiological vigor and reproductive capability (i.e., young adulthood). Whereas it could be argued that one begins to age from the moment of birth or before (and chronologically this is true), the changes occurring as adulthood progresses are qualitatively different from those that occur during maturation. The brain and other parts of the body continue to grow and accrue new fundamental capabilities during the first two decades of life, and it is not productive to view this as aging in the gerontological sense.

The inevitable end point of aging is death, and this implies that the net effect of the biological changes associated with age is a negative one. However, it is also implicit here that some of the changes can be positive ones, and we shall see that this is indeed often the case. It is now becoming possible to impede the inevitable declines and to greatly enrich the quality of life as people age.

A number of theories have attempted to account for aging, and a discussion of these is beyond the scope of this book (see Hayflick, 1996). One of the most prominent is the free radical theory of aging, and this can serve as one frame of reference to think about how and why deleterious changes can occur in cells as organisms live on. Oxygen is the major culprit. It is highly reactive chemically and tends to combine with atoms and molecules and, therefore, change their properties. Assuming that original (preoxidized) properties are beneficial, the oxidized product is likely to be inferior. Thus, when oxygen reacts with iron, it produces rust, and rusty metal is weaker and less stable. In living cells, oxidation is associated with the production of molecules with an unpaired electron, free radicals, that readily react with and damage proteins, lipids (fats), and DNA (genetic material), causing them to malfunction. Fortunately, organisms have a number of defenses to counteract the reactive proclivities of free radicals, such as antioxidants and enzymes that neutralize free radicals. As long as these defenses hold up, they can presumably help to stave off aging. However, over time the damage may slowly accumulate and the defenses may weaken, bringing about age-related declines in function.

Brain cells may be particularly vulnerable to free radical damage over extended periods of time. Brain cells do not turn over (i.e., die and be replaced by new cells, like skin cells, for example), so they must last a lifetime. The mechanisms that protect them from free radical damage may not be able to keep up, and damage and resulting mini-malfunctions within the cells can accumulate. The nervous system also has a very high level of metabolic activity (i.e., uses a great deal of oxygen), which could also put it at risk for free radical damage.

Although free radical damage may not be the overarching mechanism of aging, the notion is conceptually valuable as we attempt to understand aging and the nervous system in the chapters that follow. Because the general effects of oxidation are familiar, the free radical theory provides an intuitive heuristic with which to understand why age-related changes should occur in the cells of the nervous system. Aging, however, is not as simple as the mere gradual demise of cellular function. Many variables enter into the equation to complicate matters, conferring a great deal of variability upon the process.

Let us use a favorite analogy of gerontologists, the automobile. How long does it take for a new car to "age" to the point where it needs to be towed to the junkyard? Of course, all cars are subject to oxidation and wear and tear of their parts, and, given enough time, key parts will cease to function normally (in this analogy, the car's engine—like the human body—must be running at all times, and some parts—like brain cells— cannot be replaced). But the actual rate of aging will be determined by various factors: how expensive and well built it was to begin with (its constitutional endowment); the quality of maintenance it was given (oil changes, etc.); the quality of mechanical treatments when problems arose; exposure to corrosive salts or damp climates (the external environment); how often, how far, and how well it was driven. Also complicating matters is the fact that the car's constituent parts are not equally vulnerable to aging, and they do not play an equal role in automotive "physiology." For example, the parts on the car's underside are particularly vulnerable to rust and corrosion, and a failed cooling system can result in widespread damage to other parts. Finally, malfunction of a system that controls the car's "behavior" (e.g., steering, braking) might result in an erroneous operation that could spell the end.

It is apparent from this analogy that aging is a multifaceted and compli- cated process, even in a relatively simple device like an automobile, whose operation is fully understood. An animal's body (in particular, its nervous system) is infinitely more complex and less well understood than an automobile, and the challenge of neurogerontology to unravel the myster- ies of aging and the nervous system is a daunting one, particularly when one considers just how complex nervous systems are.

THE COMPLEXITY OF NERVOUS SYSTEMS

A nervous system consists of numerous cells, the most important of which are neurons. Collectively, the neurons that make up our own nervous system have features that are difficult for the human brain itself to fathom. First is their vast number—about 100 billion packed into the human brain. Imagine filling a large room chest-high with kernels of corn (a compelling metaphor, as I write in DeKalb, Illinois). Then, imagine 600 of such corn-filled rooms. The number of kernels here approximates the number of neurons in the human brain. More difficult to fathom is the fact that these 100 billion cells have intricate, precise connections to many other cells. Each neuron has a wirelike axon or nerve fiber that leaves its cell body (*soma*; plural: *somata*), and in most cases the axon branches, again and again as it makes its way through the brain. Electrical impulses (action potentials) are generated by neurons and travel down these axons, and through this branching process one neuron's axon can send impulse messages to hundreds or even thousands of other neurons. Considering the fact that billions of neurons are multiplying their axonal targets through branching, the number of connections made by neural circuits is truly astronomical.

Obviously, if axons branch repeatedly, neurons must receive inputs from many other neurons, even as they themselves send their output to numerous target neurons. If neurons were simple cornlike ovoids, the number of contacts they could receive from other neurons would be limited by their surface area. This limitation is overcome by having an array of branches (dendrites) emanating from the neuron's cell body. The shape neurons take is largely described by the dendritic trees they give rise to, often in the form of elaborate arbors with thousands of branches upon branches, each of which is contacted by the terminals of axons from other neurons. The evolution of extensive dendritic trees, coupled with branching axons, permits neurons to participate in neural circuits of enormous complexity. However, it is important to note that, despite their complexity, the circuits conform closely to the overall grand wiring diagram dictated by genetic instructions during development.

As if the baffling complexity conferred by the anatomical organization of nervous systems were not enough, there is yet another variable to consider: properties of synapses, the sites at which neurons influence one another ("communicate"), for the most part by chemical neurotransmitter systems. Synapses add another layer of complexity to the functioning of the nervous system (discussed in more detail in chapter 4). For example, a variety of different neurotransmitters are used by the nervous system. Which transmitter is used at a particular synapse is not haphazard, but is specified by genetic instructions. Thus, to understand various aspects of neural operations (e.g., drug effects), it is necessary to know which chemical neurotransmitter systems are involved in various circuit components. In addition, neurotransmitters affect postsynaptic neurons in different ways and over different time courses (see chapter 4).

In order to understand how the brain works—and how it fares with aging—we must ultimately learn how neurons work, the pathways their axons follow throughout the nervous system, where their synaptic inputs come from, what transmitters are used, what happens at various synapses, how all of this is affected by nature and nurture, and a host of other issues.

WHY A BRAIN?

Consider any animal (human or otherwise) you encounter. How is it that it exists today? Obviously, at some time in the past its constituent body components had to be assembled, and this had to be done well, so that the resulting individual would do what was necessary to stay alive. This construction job was accomplished using a set of genetic instructions that designed and automatically assembled a viable individual from available material such as protein, fat, carbohydrates, minerals, and water (this occurred both during fetal development and after birth). The same set of instructions also directed various physiological operations within the animal's body to maintain and operate the animal effectively. In two respects, however, the animal's survival is also indebted to its parents' genetic instructions. First, the set of building/operating instructions was inherited from its parents (some genes from each); without the existence of parents, there would be no genetic blueprints to make offspring. Second, the parents' own genetic instructions had to build them in such a way that they would survive to adulthood, be compelled to engage in reproductive behavior (and get it right), then perform whatever parental behaviors were required for the offspring to survive (this, of course, depended on their parents' genes and behavior, ad infinitum).

Because all animals have a limited life span, the continued existence of a species requires the unceasing production of new, well-designed individuals to replace the ones that die. Purveyors of genetic instructions (parents) must be available in adequate numbers to produce sufficient additional carriers of gene sets (offspring, who in turn become parents), or the species will cease to exist when all of its current members grow old and die. If genetic instructions for the species are no longer available, the species will disappear forever. Thus, it is absolutely essential that the genes make individuals who will age to sexual maturity and produce offspring who in turn will carry these same genes for their species.

All extant species of plants and animals possess a strategy by which this is accomplished. In many species of animals, a key element of the survival strategy is the formation of a nervous system whose major command center is a concentration of neurons, the brain. In such animals (all vertebrates and many invertebrates), virtually everything the brain does seems to be designed to contribute in some way to their genetic success.

A genetic-evolutionary view of the nervous system such as this provides a unifying framework to understand and evaluate what nervous systems do for us and other species, and how these functions are affected when aging occurs. For virtually all animals, nervous systems have seven basic functions.

WHAT NERVOUS SYSTEMS DO

1. Maintain vital functions.   The most fundamental function of a nervous system is to maintain our bodies in proper working condition, keeping us alive and well. It is the nervous system that governs the cardiovascular and respiratory systems, regulates the body's temperature, evaluates fuel intake and use, and controls numerous other biological activities at their optimal levels (i.e., maintain homeostasis). As discussed in chapter 6, a decline in the nervous system's ability to operate the body at suitable physiological levels can be responsible for many of the unpleasant aspects of aging, not to mention the ultimate end point.

2. Obtain information.   It is essential for animals to obtain information about themselves and the outside world. An animal cannot exist without a constant stream of information (visual, auditory, chemical, etc.) about its self and its surroundings. This ranges from information about the other organisms with which it needs to interact (predators, prey, enemies, friends, and mates) to the condition of its own body (Is it too hot or too cold? Is it injured or feeling good? Are there sufficient nutrients and oxygen in the blood?). The sensory systems are primarily responsible for obtaining and processing this input, but there is far more going on than an information conduit from body and outside world to brain. The brain interprets and elaborates the information (perception), and our very consciousness is formed and framed by sensory experiences. As we shall see in chapter 7, both the ability of the sense organs to deliver accurate input to the brain and the brain's ability to process the input can change as animals age, with significant consequences.

3. Store information. An organism that can learn from its mistakes, successes, or other experiences is at a great advantage over one that does not. Animals that can learn are more likely to survive, find mates and reproduce, and in the process, pass on the genes that confer the ability to learn. Thus, it should not be surprising that even very simple animals are capable of some form of learning. Nervous systems provide the "machinery" for learning, with the brain being the ultimate learning machine. The brain is also the place where learned information is stored as memory, and a highly developed brain has greater capacity for learning and memory. The rather large brain possessed by our own species seems to have bestowed upon us learning and memory capacities that, compared to other animals, are impressive (to us, at least). Indeed, in the evolution of *Homo sapiens* the ability to learn and remember has been central to our strategy for survival and competition with other species. It will become clear in chapter 8 that learning and memory often decline with age, a decline that can be especially troublesome, given the importance of these processes for our species.

4. Produce behavior. All animals behave in some fashion; it does an animal little good to receive and store information if it cannot do anything about it. Thus, nervous systems must produce behavioral output, namely all movement, locomotion, and communicative behavior (activation of glands and organs also constitute output; these are addressed in chapter 6). Movement is generated by numerous nerve fibers that emanate from the brain stem and spinal cord, make their way to muscles, and cause groups of muscle fibers to contract. Contraction of the muscle fibers must occur in a complicated, precisely organized and timed sequence in order for effective behavior to occur. A great amount of brain tissue and circuitry are devoted to motor behavior, and much of this is vulnerable to age-related change (see chapter 9).

5. Modulate the overall activity of the system (emotion, arousal). When chess champion Garry Kasparov lost a highly publicized match to the IBM computer Deep Blue, a key difference between the human nervous system and the computer became quite evident: Mr. Kasparov displayed an emotional response (frustration?), and the performance of his nervous system was modulated negatively with respect to completing the chess match. The brain's limbic and autonomic nervous systems, using chemical and hormonal mechanisms, are constantly altering and coloring the way the nervous system responds, spawning a variety of emotions ranging from fear, anxiety, and depression to pleasure, contentment, and elation. The nervous system also modulates its own levels of arousal, which range from periods of agitation to deep sleep. Age-related changes in emotions are difficult to understand and often inconsistent, but chapter 10 will attempt to make sense of these. It will also be seen that sleep and arousal become altered with age.

6. Integrate information and behavior. The brain must tie incoming, stored, and emotional data together to make "decisions" about appropriate behaviors. Integration can range from simple sensory-motor behaviors to complex cognitive processes such as "intelligence," language, and making judgments. In addition to sensory and learned information stemming from the environment, the decisions made by the brain are often guided or constrained by built-in neural circuits. Even complex integrative processes such as the use of language by humans often have a strong or dominant built-in, biological component. The brain mechanisms involved in complex integration (cognition) can be slowed or otherwise affected when organisms age, and are devastated by Alzheimer's disease, as discussed in chapter 11.

7. Carry out the genetic mandate (pass on the genes). Because the transmission of genes is of such elemental importance, the other six functions of nervous systems are, ultimately, subservient to this end. However, it is also necessary that certain brain mechanisms and circuits are specifically designed to produce behaviors that ensure the production and survival of offspring. These include sex, reproductive behavior, and parenting. As discussed in chapter 12, and later in this chapter, these behaviors have a special relationship to aging because they are largely carried out prior to old age. Thus, gerontological discussions tend to center on the decline of reproductive behavior with age. However, there are many exceptions, especially with respect to human aging and the onslaught of advances in medical and reproductive technology.

It will become evident in later chapters that each of these basic nervous system functions—and the behaviors that go with them—changes in one way or another, for better or for worse, as aging ensues.

Behaviors—and how they change with age—often involve all seven basic neural functions. A 20-year-old unmarried man and his 85-year-old grandfather, 10 years a widower, are sitting together at a family wedding reception, the band playing a dance tune. The young man asks an attractive young woman to dance, but the grandfather does not. To understand the behavior of each man, we must consider the seven basic neural functions outlined above. What possesses the grandson to act? He is aware that the young woman possesses the visual features and other sensory stimuli he finds attractive because his sensory systems provide that information. His brain calls up stored information (she's not going out with one of his friends, her clothes suggest similar social interests, he hasn't had a date in a while, etc.), all of which are compatible with asking her to dance. Several systems in his brain cause him to experience emotional reactions that both encourage him (e.g., lust, pleasure) and discourage him (e.g., fear of rejection), but the former are stronger (learned information stored in the brain also influences the emotions, e.g., the degree of fear will be determined by his knowledge of how much past success he's had in his social relations with women or how good a dancer he is). Given all this, his brain makes a decision to act and engages the appropriate motor systems to walk over to her, talk to her, and ultimately dance with her. The behavior is further encouraged by the possibility of eventual sex (the ultimate genetic mandate). Of course, his vital bodily functions are maintained through all of this (to his relief). In summary, all of the basic functions of the nervous system contribute to his behavior.

Why did the grandfather's brain *not* make the decision to engage in this behavior? Here is a short list of possibilities: His eyes are failing somewhat, and he cannot evaluate the young woman's good looks; he sees her quite well, but the stored knowledge in his brain suggests that she would not be the most appropriate social match for him; information about dance steps, once stored in his brain, is now forgotten; he had trouble sleeping last night and is too tired to dance; his sexual motivation is reduced; he can't move smoothly on the dance floor because his motor coordination is not what it once was or his arthritis is acting up; the possibility of being "unfaithful" to his departed wife conjures up the emotional response of guilt; he believes such behavior would not be socially acceptable for a man of his age; he knows that intense physical activity would overtax his cardiovascular system. All of these variables would tend to interfere with asking the young woman to dance. Gerontologists trying to explain which aspect of aging was responsible for the difference between his behavior and that of his grandson would have no way of knowing, on casual observation, which factors are in play here.

Even a trivial act such as this demonstrates how involvement of all the basic neural functions conspire to make it difficult to understand behavior and the nervous system, let alone their roles in aging. Many changes in behavior that accompany aging can be influenced by a variety of factors, often in very subtle and/or complex ways.

The seven basic functions can affect one another, particularly in the context of aging.   The task of understanding the relationship between aging and the seven functions is further complicated by *interactions* among them. An interaction occurs when the effects of one neural function are influenced by age-related changes in another function. That is, age-related changes in one function cannot be fully explained without knowing how another function has fared. For example, recognizing a new person requires first, that our sensory systems provide key information about the person (e.g., what he or she looks like) and second, that certain brain processes store this information in our memory. Either poor vision or a poor memory would make this more difficult.

Let us consider situations where both vision and memory are reduced in effectiveness for this task by 25%: A person with poor vision but good memory would have a 25% loss, as would a person with good vision but poor memory. If a person with both poor vision and poor memory had a 50% loss, this would be a simple summation of the main effects of vision and memory. An interaction occurs when the person with poor vision and memory exhibits a loss of more than 50%. The likely cause of such an interaction is that the person's impaired memory needs as much information as it can get (normal vision), just to function at a 25% loss; with a reduction in the quality of visual information, the impaired memory system simply fails.

Thus, if a person's sensory and memory systems are both affected with age, their interaction might make things even worse. In gerontological terms, the same visual deficit may have a greater effect in an old person than in a young person if the older person has additional age-related deficits (in this example, memory). Theoretically, age-related changes in any or all of the seven basic functions have the potential to interact.

NATURE-NURTURE: IMPLICATIONS FOR AGING

The particulars of the seven basic neural functions are influenced to one extent or another by both built-in ("prewired," species-specific, instinctive) processes and experience (learning, exposure to the environment). Nature and nurture interact to determine the properties of virtually all behavior. Some activities of the nervous system are less influenced by experience than others. For example, animals do not have to "learn" to control the rate at which the heart beats in order to provide ample blood supply to various parts of the body; this task is automatic (controlled by built-in neural circuitry) and is exhibited by all members of a species (assuming they are not ill). Yet the heart rate is also significantly affected by events ranging from learned fears (which may speed it up) to Zen Buddhist techniques (which may slow it down). Other aspects of behavior are more strongly influenced by an individual's experience and the unique things he or she has learned. For example, courtship practices among humans vary dramatically across cultures; socially acceptable, effective behaviors are learned and shaped by experience. However, young lovers do not have to "learn" to have a sexual yen; such motivators of behavior are built in to our species (and others that use sex to reproduce).

The ubiquity of nature-nurture interactions makes the task of understanding age-related changes in the nervous system that much more challenging. Except for identical twins, no two people have the same combination of the thousands of genes that define us genetically (our genotype). Because each of us is constructed and operated by a different set of genetic instructions, we each go through life with a unique biological identity. Our uniqueness can be manifested in everything from the properties of enzymes and chemical constituents of our cells to the outward appearance our body takes on. By nature we are different from one another right from the start of life. Thus, the starting point upon which age-related changes accrue are different for each of us, producing a huge source of biological variation among individuals as they age. Furthermore, some of the genetically mandated differences in anatomy (form) and physiology (functional properties) appear to determine how our cells, tissues, organs, and bodies fare as aging occurs. That is, the rate and magnitude of age-related biological changes can vary greatly from person to person because of differences in the gene actions that affect the condition of cells and tissues over time (to take a benign example, mechanisms by which graying of the hair and/or baldness occur have substantial hereditary components). Even if it were possible to provide two people with the exact same experiences from the time of fertilization on, they would age in different ways because their genotypes are different.

Of course, none of us (even identical twins) have the same life experiences. Even genetically identical individuals, such as inbred mice, will not age in an identical fashion or all live to the same age, presumably because of differences in their environment and experiences. Perhaps the most dramatic (and familiar) effects of experience on individuals as they go through life are manifested by the brain and many of the behaviors it produces. Obvious examples are the skills and information people obtain and store, the things one grows to like or dislike, the effects various people have on one's life, etc. Each of these contributes to our uniqueness as individuals, irrespective of our biological constitution. And, of course, the longer one lives, the more distinctive experiences one accumulates. Changes in thoughts and behaviors go hand in hand with changes in the brain, and many of those changes last a lifetime (e.g., learning a new bit of information that is never forgotten).

It is not surprising that one of the hallmarks of human aging is the occurrence of individual differences, and that this is especially true when it comes to the brain and behavior. Each person is a unique biological entity, with different genetic propensities for biological changes across time, modulated by a lifetime of experiences and environmental events that are very different for each of us. Throughout this book an attempt will be made to find generalities with respect to aging and the nervous system. However, superimposed on any generalities that can be discerned is a huge degree of variation from person to person.

CAUSE AND EFFECT IN AGING: LOGIC AND SEMANTICS

As the discussion of nature and nurture suggests, it is often difficult to identify the causes of changes in the brain or behavior that accompany aging. Indeed, there can be confusion with respect to whether or when aging per se can be a cause of something. For example, one often encounters phrases in the literature, such as "This [behavioral or biological change] was *caused by aging.*" Such statements may or may not be appropriate, depending on the context and use of the word *aging.* If one is referring to aging in the general or global sense (becoming or having become old), it does not make sense to view it as a cause of behavioral or biological change. In most neurogerontological contexts, behavioral and biological changes are the definitive aspects of aging, so the latter statement would be tantamount to saying, "Aging causes aging," or "That person is acting old because she has aged," tautologies that get us nowhere. This problem is not necessarily solved by viewing aging as the result or outcome of biological changes. Whereas it makes sense to say, "That person has aged and is behaving like an old person because of changes in the nervous system," this begs the question of what caused those changes in the nervous system. Perhaps it was damage to DNA or other intracellular components that caused the changes in the neurons. But this simply continues the question begging: What caused the cellular changes?

Despite this reductionistic spiral, it is often valid to use the term *aging* as an active player in the causal chain. This is easy to do in sociological or political contexts, as in "Aging of the citizenry has caused a crisis in health care." With respect to neurogerontological issues, an example would be "Aging of the visual system causes a number of other problems in elderly people" (of course, something had first caused the changes in the visual system). Some semantic issues are subtle. The commonly used phrase "the effect of age on [whatever]" implies causality and, therefore, should be used with appropriate care. However, used as a noun, the term *age effect* does not necessarily imply causality. An age effect is an inferential statistical concept that refers to a difference between measured entities for which the age of the subjects turns out to be a significant variable. For example, in comparing two age groups, one can find a significant age effect, meaning the two groups differed as a function of age.

We will often take the easy way out of potential semantic dilemmas by using terms like *age-related change, changes associated with age,* and *changes that accompany aging.* Such terminology is scientifically conservative and avoids misidentifying causes and effects. However, when a particular variable or event is clearly the cause of another, it is appropriate to say so. For example, "A loss of neurons caused [this behavior] to change." Furthermore, cause-effect-neutral and cause-effect terminologies can be used together when applicable: "An age-related loss of neurons caused . . . "

The Brain May Modulate Its Own Aging

Most neurogerontological research has focused on both the causes and effects of age-related biological changes in neurons and other tissue—changes in the nervous system that are part and parcel of aging. This focus is most certainly reflected by the bulk of research and ideas reviewed in this book. However, several hypotheses have attributed a direct, causative modulatory role to the nervous system with respect to aging. These do not rely on some degenerative or age-related change first occurring in neurons to begin a cascade of effects. Rather, they suggest ways the brain's normal activity might contribute to or regulate its own aging, either speeding up or slowing down the process.

Neuroendocrine systems as a cause of aging.   The endocrine system (comprised of various glands that secrete hormones into the bloodstream, such as the testes, ovaries, adrenal gland, and thyroid) is under the intimate control of the nervous system (see chapter 6). It has been hypothesized (Landfield, 1980; Sapolsky, 1992) that the very necessary activity of the neuroendocrine system may, ironically, be a cause of aging. The notion is that a "use-it-*and*-lose-it" mechanism associated with normal endocrine function causes age-related declines. By this view, then, the persistent effects of normal exposure to hormones may render the body less able to maintain various biological functions and, therefore, be a cause of aging. In particular, it is thought that elevated levels of glucocorticoids secreted by the adrenal glands are, over time, toxic to neural brain tissue in certain parts of the brain (hippocampus). This in turn may be associated with other physiological changes associated with aging.

Brain size and longevity.   Hakeem, Sandoval, Jones, and Allman (1996) note that there is a positive correlation between brain size and longevity. Longer-lived animals tend to have larger brains. They argue that the brain acts as a buffer against environmental variations that might be deleterious to survival: Having a large brain that can store large amounts of information goes hand in hand with a long life. The relationship is quite strong in primates, whose brain size and life span range greatly (with humans at the top in both respects).

Intellect and aging. Another way the brain may directly influence the aging process may be unique to humans. Our ability to acquire, retain, and transmit knowledge has made it possible for us to increase our longevity dramatically during the last century. The intellect and creativity arising from our brain's neural activity has made medical science possible, and this has enabled us to conquer a number of diseases, increasing life expectancy by decades.

The human intellect may also give rise to another very unusual situation in the animal kingdom: a contribution of postreproductive individuals to the evolutionary fitness of the species. As discussed earlier in this chapter, the engine that drives both evolution and our continued existence is successful propagation of genes. A huge amount of biological energy is directed at producing offspring and seeing that they survive to sexual maturity. In most species, when old individuals cease to reproduce and their offspring have achieved reproductive maturity, their biological job is done. For many species (familiar examples being salmon and short-lived insects), the individuals die shortly after they reproduce. In species in which individuals may continue to live beyond sexual productivity, their contribution is limited or nil. Humans (and perhaps some other primates and sea mammals) may provide an exception to this rule because elders often continue to make contributions that enhance the chances that their relatives (who share many of their genes) will survive. These contributions come from the application of acquired knowledge and skill ("wisdom") that continues into old age. The wisdom and teaching of elders has no doubt contributed to success in agriculture, warfare, predator control, health maintenance, and so on of younger kin. Many genes can presumably contribute to longevity (see Smith, 1995), and some of these, operative after the individual has reached his or her reproductive prime, would be maintained in any offspring, who would be more likely to survive because of the presence of elders. If this were the case, the brain's influence on aging would extend to the evolutionary domain.

SUMMARY AND IMPLICATIONS

Nervous systems perform seven basic functions, and these depend to some extent on one another. Even with this simple conceptual scheme, the immense complexity of the nervous system reveals itself, as does the daunting challenge to neurogerontology. The challenge is made even tougher when one contemplates the limitless number of interconnections among neurons that form the substrate for the brain's activity, not to mention the inaccessibility of the neurons themselves. What is more, the brain is not a passive entity in the aging process, but can influence and alter the course of its own aging, further complicating the story. Fortunately, modern neuroscience has an impressive arsenal of research tools at hand (as discussed in detail in chapter 2), and the following chapters will demonstrate that much has been learned about aging and the nervous system. Unfortunately, it will also become clear that the tools remain woefully inadequate to fully meet the challenge, and most of our neurogerontological knowledge lies ahead of us.

In the chapters that follow, an attempt will be made to provide solid, useful information and insights into aging and the nervous system. However, many of the discussions will, by necessity, end with unanswered questions, possibilities, issues that need to be addressed, and speculations, all of which should keep neurogerontologists busy for a long time.

2
The Research Methods
of Neurogerontology

As an interdisciplinary field, neurogerontology draws on methodological approaches from neuroscience, psychology, gerontology, and a number of other areas. This chapter reviews the basics.

STRATEGIES FOR STUDYING THE AGING BRAIN

Given that there are many millions of microscopic-sized cells in circuits of Gordian complexity, performing a myriad of functions, and housed in a rather compact space protected by a thick skull, research on the brain is challenging, to say the least. Neuroscientists are meeting the challenge, but neuroscience research has generally progressed in small steps, with thousands of neuroscientists each working on a relatively circumscribed part of the grand puzzle. The fruits of this labor are found in thousands of scientific research articles, convention papers, chapters, and books produced at an accelerating rate. Neuroscience is a techniques-driven discipline, and new approaches come onto the research scene all the time, opening up possibilities for new insights about the brain. When appropriate, various methodologies are discussed in more detail in later chapters.

The Use of Animal Models

Many of the methods to be described must be used on nonhuman animals— animal models of the human condition. The reasons for using animal models are ethical, scientific, and practical. Ethically, methods such as intentionally altering a part of the brain, invasive techniques, or control of diet and environment during aging cannot be employed with human subjects, so animals must be studied in their stead. This is not to say that anything goes in animal research. Indeed, no experimentation on animals can be performed unless strict guidelines for animal welfare, care, and use are met, and the use of animal subjects is justified. Animal experimentation is regulated by laws and institutional committees in virtually all countries where research is performed, with the goal of minimizing pain or discomfort (of course, one point of view is that the ethical line between the treatment of human and nonhuman animals is blurred or nonexistent). Scientifically, there can be many reasons for studying nonhuman animals. For example, genetic lines of animals reliably exhibit certain traits (or lack thereof) that are important to the aging process (see Jucker & Ingram, 1997), and an aging animal's environment can be controlled to help distinguish nature and nurture. One such animal model, developed in Japan, is the *senescence accelerated mouse* (SAM). These mice exhibit aging-like changes in the brain (Shimada, Hosokawa, Ohta, Akiguchi, & Takeda, 1994) and other systems at a much more rapid rate than normal. Determining the causes of the accelerated rate of aging may provide unique insights into normal aging. Practically, rodents and other animals have a relatively short life span, so aging processes are compressed in time, making them easier to study.

It is always the case that research findings from other species may not be fully generalizable to humans. Nevertheless, animal models show us what kinds of anatomical and physiological phenomena can and do occur in nervous systems that are in many respects similar to our own. Indeed, when comparing, for example, mice and humans with regard to their physiological responses to aging, drugs, and so on, it is common to find close similarities rather than striking differences.

Basic Neuroanatomy and Histology

Perhaps the most basic approach to determining how the brain changes with age is to compare anatomical features of old versus young brains. This can be done at different levels of resolution ranging from gross (macroscopic) anatomy to light microscopy to electron-microscopy. Gross anatomy has been used to evaluate general changes in the size and form of the brain (see chapter 3). Basic histological evaluations of brain tissue sections using light microscopy rely on various histological stains that reveal the structure of neurons. Two commonly used stains in neurogerontological work are *Nissl* stains and *Golgi* stains. The former stains reveal Nissl substance, found in the cytoplasm of neurons, and can be used as a general marker for all types of neurons in a thin tissue section (see Figure 2.1A). Thus, Nissl stains (often in combination with another stain for axons) are commonly used to count the number of neurons in sections obtained from various regions of the brain. Nissl stains, however, do not show dendrites and other morphological details of neurons very well. The Golgi methods use relatively thick tissue sections but stain only a few neurons; however, the dendrites, axon, and soma surface are all stained in full detail. A major use of Golgi stains (see Figure 2.1E) is to determine how dendrites change with age. Electron microscopy reveals the ultrastructure of neurons in very thin sections (see Figure 3.5). This method can be used to evaluate age-related changes in synapses, intracellular organelles, and other fine features of neurons. Each method has its advantages and disadvantages, and these are discussed when appropriate.

Revealing the Wiring Diagrams of the Brain

The nervous system relies on an elaborate, complex, yet precise assortment of neural circuits. Modern anatomical methods for tracing neural connections have revealed the details of many neural circuits, and neural tract-tracing techniques can expand our knowledge of aging and the nervous system. Tract-tracing methods typically involve the injection of a *tracer* substance into a small region of the brain. Tracers can be fluorescent dyes or enzymes that are incorporated by neurons and transported by the axon. The tracers are given some period of time to allow transport (e.g., one or more days), and the brain is prepared for microscopic viewing of brain tissue slices. By looking at the location of the injection of tracer into the brain and those parts of the brain that are labeled by transported tracer, one can conclude that the injection site and labeled sites are connected by axons. Tracers are of two types. *Retrograde* tracers are taken up by axon terminals and transported back to the neuron's cell body and dendrites. *Anterograde* tracers are transported toward the axon terminal. Retrograde

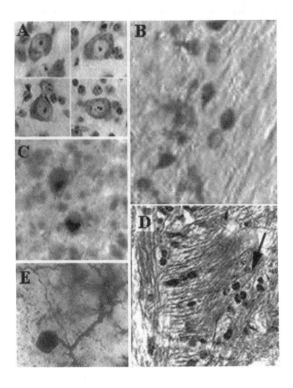

FIGURE 2.1 Several views of the cochlear nucleus of the mouse brain using different histological stains. A. Four small panels each contain a neuron stained with the Nissl stain, cresyl violet. The pale nucleus with small dark nucleolus is visible, surrounded by the soma, whose cytoplasm stains for Nissl substance. The small, darkly stained structures surrounding the neurons are glial cells. B. Several neurons are darkly labeled with the retrograde tracer, horseradish peroxidase-wheat germ agglutinin. This was injected into the inferior colliculus, to which the cochlear nucleus sends axons, and was transported back into the cell somata. C. Two neurons immunolabeled for the neurotransmitter glycine. Other nonglycinergic neurons did not stain. D. The Hirano-Zimmerman stain for axons shows patterns of axons going vertically (left side of the panel), horizontally (middle), and obliquely (right side). The small dark ovals (arrow) are glial cells. E. A neuron stained with a Golgi method. The round soma has one large dendrite extending to the right and branching. A thin axon from another neuron is seen going from the upper left to lower middle of the panel.

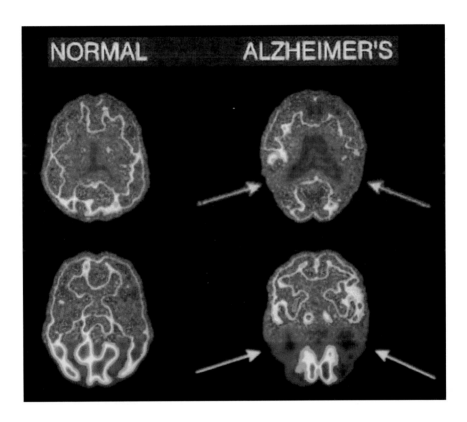

FIGURE 2.2   A PET scan showing glucose metabolism of the brain of a normal 68-year-old and that of a 65-year-old Alzheimer's patient. High metabolic rate is in red with progressively lower values in orange, yellow, green, blue, and purple. The arrows point out the metabolic deficits that are the hallmark of Alzheimer's disease as seen in PET (see chapter 11). Courtesy of Gary W. Small, MD, Department of Psychiatry and Biobehavioral Sciences, and Department of Molecular and Medical Pharmacology, Crump Institute for Biological Imaging, UCLA.

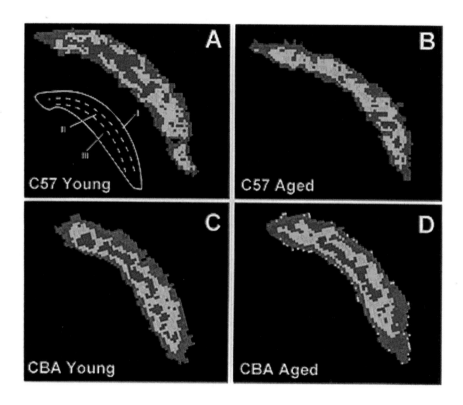

FIGURE 2.3   Glycine receptor binding in young and old mice of two strains (red/yellow = high density; blue/purple = low density). Aging C57 mice exhibit a loss of strychnine-sensitive glycine receptors, but CBA mice do not. From Willott, J. F., Milbrandt, J. C., Bross, L. S., & Caspary, D. M. (1997). Glycine immunoreactivity and receptor binding in the cochlear nucleus of C57BL/6J and CBA/CaJ mice: Effects of cochlear impairment and aging. *Journal of Comparative Neurology, 385,* 405–414. With permission from Wiley-Liss, Inc.

tracers show us which neurons project their axons into the injection site; anterograde tracers show the brain sites to which neurons in the injection site project. Neural tract tracing is a very important tool for determining if neural circuits are stable, degenerate, or change as animals age. An example of retrograde transport is shown in Figure 2.1B.

Revealing the Brain's Properties with Immunocytochemistry and Other Methods

A variety of techniques that provide information about neurotransmitter systems have been added recently to the neuroscientist's arsenal. *Immunocytochemical* methods take advantage of the immune system of animals, which combats foreign substances invading the body. If a substance (an antigen) is introduced into an animal's body, the immune system produces antibodies that attach or bind specifically to that antigen. Once specific antibodies are produced, they can be extracted from blood drawn from the animal. This antibody is purified and applied to brain or other tissue, where it will attach specifically to sites where that particular antigen is found. The antibodies are treated in a way that makes them visible (e.g., by attaching a fluorescent chemical tag), so the places where the antigens are found are "immunolabeled."

Antibodies can be made for a variety of substances, including neurotransmitters or chemical compounds associated with them. For example, by using a neurotransmitter such as the amino acid glutamate as an antigen, glutamate antibody can be produced in an animal, extracted and purified, tagged for visualization, and applied to slices of brain tissue from another species of animal. The glutamate antibody will attach to (immunolabel) neurons that contain glutamate (the antigen), allowing us to see what neurons contain this neurotransmitter. One might compare the number or distribution of labeled neurons in young and old animals for any number of neurotransmitters or other important compounds. Examples of immunolabeling are shown in Figure 2.1C.

Neuroimaging Techniques

The development of computer technology in recent years has seen the emergence of modern imaging techniques. These allow us to visualize anatomical features in the living brain and get a glimpse of correlates of the physiological activity of the human brain at work. These methods are particularly exciting because they allow specific regions of the brain to be viewed with a degree of resolution that is already remarkable, yet always being improved upon with advances in technology.

The *CT scan* (computerized tomography) was the first modern imaging technique to be developed. The head is placed in a kind of X-ray tube, and X-rays are passed through to a detector on the other side. The amount of X-ray activity that gets through is measured, scanning the entire head, producing pictures of "sections" through the head, identifying tumors, blood clots, and degenerative diseases. *MRI* (magnetic resonance imaging) can provide a detailed picture of the brain by using a strong magnetic field passed through the subject's head, affecting different molecules in various ways. *Functional MRI* (fMRI) takes the technique even further, allowing the brain's physiological activity to be viewed as well. *PET* (positron emission tomography) and *SPECT* (single-photon emission computed tomography) assess metabolic activity in parts of the brain using radioactive forms of substances (e.g., glucose analogues or neurotransmitter-related compounds) that are used by the brain when it is physiologically active. The radioactive material is injected into the bloodstream, where it finds its way to the brain and emits positrons that are detected and shown graphically on a computer monitor. The highest concentrations of radioactivity/positron emissions indicate the most active brain regions. Regional cerebral blood flow can also be measured with PET by detecting oxygen concentrations.

Neuroimaging techniques are proving to be valuable in gerontological work. Anatomical imaging, such as CT scans and MRI, are well suited to reveal age-related changes in the size and morphology of brain regions (see chapter 11). It used to be the case that morphological measurements on the human brain had to await autopsy. With imaging, this is no longer so. PET and other techniques that measure ongoing physiological activity allow comparison of young and old brains as they perform any number of sensory or cognitive tasks. Imaging should also become a key diagnostic and research tool for working with Alzheimer's and other neurodegenerative diseases that can accompany aging. An example is shown in Figure 2.2 (see colorplate following page 20).

The Lesion Method

This approach also evaluates the living brain, but in a much different way from imaging. The lesion method asks what the damaged (lesioned) brain can tell us about the normal brain. Brain lesions can be studied in humans when they occur as a result of accidents, warfare, surgery, or disease, or they can be intentionally and more precisely made in experimental animals. The basic logic is to compare behavior or some aspect of neural function in subjects whose brains are intact and subjects whose brains have a specific locus of damage. If differences are observed between the lesioned and intact groups, it can be inferred that the brain damage is in some way associated with this difference. Although the logic is seemingly straightforward, interpretation of lesion effects can be tricky. If, for example, a particular change in behavior follows damage to brain structure X, it does not necessarily mean that structure X plays a direct role in that behavior. Damage to structure X might have an influence on structure Y, which really controls the behavior; damage to structure X might alter another brain function that indirectly influences the behavior (e.g., changing motivation or arousal); or damage to structure X might have some generalized effect that alters many behaviors. An old joke makes the point: A scientist wished to study jumping behavior in the frog. He put the frog on the floor and said, "Jump, frog, jump!" He observed the behavior and wrote in his notes, "Frog has two legs, frog jumps 20 inches." He then removed one of the frog's jumping legs (the lesion method, here applied to the leg rather than the brain) and repeated, "Jump, frog, jump!" And wrote, "Frog has one leg, frog jumps 10 inches." Next, he removed the second jumping leg. "Jump, frog, jump!" The frog did not jump any distance at all. His conclusion, "Frog is deaf."

It will become evident in later chapters that aging can be associated with degenerative changes in certain parts of the brain and the diminution of certain physiological operations. In this sense, the aging process acts as a natural lesion-maker. Thus, one might be able to compare the behavior of young subjects given a specific brain lesion to old "age-lesioned" subjects and make inferences about the relationship between the brain structure and age-related changes and behavior. For example, if the two groups of "lesioned" subjects were behaviorally similar (and both were different from intact young subjects), this would be consistent with a hypothesized age-related change in the damaged structure. Such conclusions must be tempered with caution, however. Because many neural functions may change concurrently during aging, unknown "lesions" might actually be responsible. Furthermore, the effects of an acute lesion (e.g., experimental or traumatic) can be quite different from one that comes on gradually during aging. Thus, it would be difficult to attribute a behavioral age effect to changes in a particular brain structure that happens to accompany aging. Nonetheless, one can ask whether age-related changes in brain function (age lesions) are at least consistent with what would be expected from lesions in young adults.

Experimental lesion studies on animals can be particularly useful in neurogerontological research on the ability of the brain to recover from damage. For example, one might compare behavioral recovery in young and old animals that have received comparable brain damage.

The Stimulation Method

A logical complement to the lesion method is to stimulate parts of the brain using electricity or chemicals and determine the effect on behavior or neural function. The amount of tissue stimulated can vary from relatively large areas to individual neurons. In the latter case, minute amounts of drug can be ejected from the tip of a fine micropipet using *iontophoresis*. As a neurogerontological research method, one might establish the effects of stimulating certain neural circuits in young subjects and compare these results with those obtained from old subjects. For example, one could stimulate axon bundles (nerve fiber tracts) that activate muscles and measure how long it takes for the muscles to contract. If it took longer for this to happen in older subjects, an age effect on axon conduction speed (and/or synaptic activation of the muscle fibers) could be inferred. Or, one might apply drugs iontophoretically to individual neurons and compare the response in young versus old animals. Stimulation methods can also be used to study more complex neural functions and behaviors and how they might be affected during aging.

Electrophysiological Methods

Because the brain operates on the basis of electrical activity (action potentials and synaptic currents), one can eavesdrop on neurons at work by measuring the voltage changes in the nervous system (voltage being easier to measure than current or resistance, which are all in an interrelated state of flux). Two basic categories of electrophysiological techniques have been widely used: measuring action and synaptic potentials from individual neurons (often referred to as "single units") and measuring the electrical activity produced simultaneously by large populations (thousands/millions) of neurons. The ongoing electrical activity of large populations is referred to as an *electroencephalogram* (EEG).

Single-unit recordings are obtained by introducing a fine-tipped wire (microelectrode) or electrolyte-filled glass micropipet into the brain; when the microelectrode tip is positioned very close to a neuron, its action potentials can be detected by a sophisticated amplifier/voltmeter connected to the microelectrode. When action potentials are measured from an electrode tip near—but outside of—a neuron, they are called *extracellular* recordings. In some applications, a fine glass microelectrode tip can actually be used to puncture and enter a neuron, obtaining *intracellular* recordings of synaptic events.

EEGs are obtained using a relatively large disk electrode or needle contacting the scalp. As in the case of single-unit recordings, the EEG electrode is hooked up to an elaborate voltmeter. The EEG is used to monitor rather general brain activity, such as the stages of sleep or abnormal (epileptic) neural activity, although an array of many electrodes can localize EEG activity to certain regions of the brain. Some consistent changes in EEG patterns have been found to accompany aging in healthy subjects, perhaps related to cognitive and other behavioral changes (Dustman, Shearer, & Emmerson, 1993).

When specific sensory, cognitive, or electrical stimuli are used with the EEG, in conjunction with computer averaging, *event-related potentials* (ERPs) can be recorded from the scalp. ERPs are voltage changes associated with neural activity evoked by specific stimuli (computer averaging is usually used to eliminate the EEG waves that are not time locked to the stimulus). A variety of ERPs can be used to study the aging brain. The simplest are evoked potentials in response to simple sensory stimuli. Evoked potentials can be used, for example, to determine if the brain's sensory systems are being effectively engaged by sensory stimuli. Thus, they provide a means by which to evaluate age-related changes in sensory systems. Other ERPs are sensitive to more complex ongoing cognitive processes. Examples are the P300 (positive wave occurring about 300 msec after the stimulus) and N400 (negative wave occurring at about 400 msec), which can reflect the processing of information by the brain under certain circumstances. Such ERPs can be used to study age-related changes in cognitive processes.

By combining single-unit, EEG, and ERP techniques, it is possible to get various perspectives of brain activity. Let us use the analogy of

Martians trying to understand a large Earth city by studying the general activity of thousands of Earthlings at once (lots of them enter the city in the morning; lots leave in the evening) or interviewing a limited number of individuals. Both approaches provide valuable, complementary information of different types. The former would be analogous to the EEG (general patterns of activity by a population); the latter analogous to single-unit recordings (varied characteristics of individuals embedded in the population's activity). An example of an ERP analog would be the occurrence of a severe snowstorm (the event) and how it affected the movement and activity of the people.

In Vitro Techniques

The physiological methods discussed thus far have involved intact organisms, with measurements taken from within the living body, or *in vivo*. It is also possible to maintain living nervous system tissue "in a dish" (*in vitro*). Two widely used methods are *tissue or cell culture* and *slice preparations*. When provided with appropriate nutrients and conditions, neurons and other types of cells will survive in a tissue culture. The cells can be viewed under a microscope, and physiological and other properties can be studied directly. Of course, the normal microenvironment, anatomy, and circuitry will be absent from tissue cultures. Nevertheless, they are very useful for evaluating membrane properties, biochemical reactions, and other physiological activities.

For slice preparations, slabs of brain are physically removed and kept alive. Because the slab is essentially a piece of brain (albeit without the inputs and outputs it would normally have), individual neurons and portions of neural circuits can be directly stimulated with electricity or drugs and responses can be recorded intracellularly from other neurons. The access one has to the circuits provides great advantages for studying circumscribed neural circuits.

Cognitive Neuroscience

People's thoughts and experiences can tell us much about the brain. For example, the reaction time—how long it takes for the nervous system and muscles to perform a particular operation—depends on factors such as the complexity of the brain circuitry involved and the properties of neurons in the circuits (e.g., how fast axons conduct action potentials). Simple behaviors, such as tapping a key in response to seeing a particular visual stimulus, occur very rapidly because the circuitry is relatively simple. In contrast, performing mental arithmetic takes considerably longer because the task (and underlying neural processes) are more complicated. As more is learned about how the brain supports various cognitive processes and behaviors, increasingly sophisticated cognitive experiments can be designed to gain insights into the underlying neural processes. Cognitive neuroscience has been very useful in suggesting how or where changes in the brain and changes in behavior are related.

Behavior Genetics

Issues related to the interaction of genetic and environmental influences on behavior constitute the focus of behavior genetics. In the context of gerontology, the techniques of behavior genetics can be used to unravel the factors that underlie the formidable individual differences in aging, as discussed in chapter 1. A central issue in behavior genetics is determining what portions of the variance among individuals can be attributed to genetic and environmental factors. For example, aging patterns of identical twins (whose genetic makeup is virtually identical) reared apart (and therefore having a different environmental history) can be compared. As noted by Pedersen (1996) in a review of the current state of the art, a large body of behavioral genetic data (much of it from ongoing twin studies) is now becoming available. Among the interesting gerontological questions being investigated is the relative contributions to variance as a function of aging: How do these factors determine whether certain behaviors remain stable across the life span or change as people grow older?

Molecular Biological Methods

A rapidly developing area of neuroscience makes use of molecular biology, scrutinizing the brain in the minutest of detail (e.g., see Gold, 1996). The tools of molecular biology can be used (at least potentially) to elucidate age-related changes in synaptic receptors, membrane channels through which ions pass to generate action potentials, the structure of proteins in neurons, how genes are expressed during aging, and myriad other details of the nervous system. Figure 2.3 (see colorplate following page 20) presents an example of the receptor binding method. A radioactive strychnine ligand (which binds to the glycine receptor) is allowed to bind with brain tissue sections. Because the ligand is specific for this receptor, the radioactive sites can be measured and visualized using radioactive-sensitive film. Figure 2.3 shows that aging was associated with a reduction in glycine receptors for the C57 mouse strain, but not for CBA. The C57 mice had severe age-related hearing impairment, suggesting that aging plus hearing loss resulted in a loss of glycine receptors (see Willott, Milbrandt, Bross, & Caspary, 1997).

Molecular biological tools can also be used in an active fashion to change experimental subjects. Specific genes can be altered at the molecular level to produce *transgenic* mice, which possess a particular trait, or *knockout* mice, which lack a trait. The creation of *antisense oligonucleotides* is another tool that can be used to inhibit the expression of specific genes. The ability to introduce new genes or inactivate certain genes provides potential new tools to investigate the aging nervous system. For example, genetic engineering can create young adult mice with learning deficits. This might provide clues about how learning processes change with age. Or, it might be instructive to determine how learning that is genetically impaired in young adults is further modified during aging.

SPECIAL METHODOLOGICAL ISSUES IN GERONTOLOGICAL RESEARCH

As the literature on aging and the nervous system is reviewed, it will become evident that research findings are sometimes inconsistent or contradictory. This situation exists in virtually all walks of scientific research, with the variance arising from many sources. Some factors are particularly relevant to gerontological research, particularly when human subjects are involved.

Subject Selection

To perform research on aging, subjects must first be selected, and this is often not done with consistency. First, the definition of *old* and *young* can differ significantly among studies, so that *old* may mean the 50s in one study, in the 70s in another. Second, the criteria used to choose subjects for experiments or surveys differ and are sometimes not clearly stated. Subjects are typically screened in some way with respect to medical histories, health status, or other factors, and this can vary across studies. Third, the comparability of "normal" old and young subjects can be problematic. For example, in research on hearing, older subjects typically have greater hearing loss than young subjects, even when they fall within a normal range or are "normal for their age." Nevertheless, the assumption is often made that the use of "normal-hearing" subjects controls for the effects of hearing loss—an assumption that is often not valid. Fourth, factors such as *period* or *cohort effects* can influence cross-sectional studies of aging, which make up the vast majority of the research studies. Depending on the occurrence of wars, industrialization, medical advances, dietary practices, and so on, different-aged people being tested at the same time may have rather different histories (cohort effects); by the same token, comparison of like-aged subjects by studies conducted in different decades or different geographical regions may be confounded (period effects).

It should be noted here that one cannot obtain direct information about age-related changes from cross-sectional experiments because subjects are not tested repeatedly. However, if cohort effects or other confounds are assumed to be minimal, it is a reasonable assumption that properties of older subject groups do reflect changes that have occurred in the individuals comprising these groups. Because it is both prosaically smoother and reflective of likely reality to describe differences between age groups as age-related changes, we plead guilty in advance to frequent commissions of this semantic transgression, with apologies to semantic purists.

Neurogerontological Changes in "Oldest Old" Versus "Young Old"

Where should a researcher stop in defining the "old" subjects in a study? This is often a difficult question scientifically as well as practically and ethically. The scientific implications stem from observations that some changes in the nervous system appear only very late in life, or accelerate greatly as the end of life approaches. In the latter instances, age effects can be much larger if "oldest old" subjects are included. This has been observed in our own anatomical studies of the aging mouse brain, as shown in Figure 2.4. Mice age 2 years can be considered old (around the median life span); those 2.5 years of age can be considered the oldest old and near the end of life. A reduction in size (volume) of some brain structures (DCN I and OCA) but not others (DCN II and DCN III) accelerates as the terminal period of life approaches (see Figure 2.4 for definitions of abbreviations). Clearly, both the definition of *old* and the brain structure studied influence the magnitude of age effects.

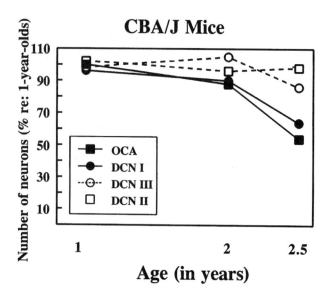

FIGURE 2.4   Terminal decline can occur in some brain regions but not in others. There is little or no shrinkage (loss of volume) for dorsal cochlear nucleus layers II and III (DCN II and DCN III) into old age (2.5 years). However, dorsal cochlear nucleus layer I (DCN I) and the octopus cell areas (OCA) exhibit a precipitous loss of volume after the median life span of 2 years.

Older Subjects Can Respond Differently to the Tests Used to Measure Aging

The performance of older people may differ from that of other age groups in ways that can influence test results. For example, compared to young subjects, some older subjects tend to be intimidated by computers used in psychological testing or by a high-tech laboratory setting. They may be more conservative in their responses to test items, anxious, or distracted. Thus, there is a potential for age differences that are being measured to be confounded by unmeasured age differences that bias test performance.

The "Resolution" of Aging in Gerontological Studies

Cross-sectional research studies vary a great deal in the number and spacing of age groups, or the resolution of time. This can make a difference in the results of a study if the variable being examined changes rapidly or slowly with age. In general, it is valuable to have a minimum of three age groups in gerontological studies, in order to produce an aging function.

Biological Rhythms

Resolution within shorter time intervals can be a concern as well. Many neural, hormonal, and behavioral functions vary in a rhythmic fashion, which can be annual or seasonal, monthly (lunar), daily (circadian), or shorter than daily (ultradian). As discussed in chapter 10, some circadian rhythms are known to become attenuated with age. This would mean that daily variations in the levels of a hormone, for example, might be greater in young subjects. Depending on the time of day measurements were obtained, levels could be especially high or low in the young subjects but more consistent in the old; however, the average daily levels might be the same. Furthermore, the timing or phase of circadian rhythms may change with age. Thus, if measurements were made at the same time of day in young and old subjects (a reasonable thing to do), the researcher could be sampling each age group at different parts of the circadian cycle. Clearly, age effects—or lack thereof—could be confounded by differences in circadian rhythms. It would probably behoove many gerontologists studying phenomena with biological rhythms to determine how rhythmic changes in their various age groups compare.

Aging Is an Extended Process

Many neurophysiological and behavioral deficits in elderly people take a long time to develop; they do not suddenly emerge at age 65. The decline in athletic ability provides a good example. For most sports, peak performance occurs in the 20s, after which the athlete may be described as old. Even professional athletes under the best of conditions cannot maintain adequate performance levels beyond about age 35 in most sports. Whereas the gradual decline in physical ability may not interfere with normal activity until decades later, the aging process clearly begins relatively early when it comes to athletics and many other endeavors. When trying to understand age effects in the nervous system (or other systems), it may be necessary to study young and middle-aged adults as well. This can be particularly important with respect to research on the amelioration of age-related changes.

Attributing Age Effects to Aging or Exposure to the Environment

As indicated in chapter 1, both nature and nurture determine how the brain changes with age. Gerontological researchers sometimes attempt to differentiate between "pure" age effects and age effects that are "contaminated" by exogenous influences. This is often reasonable and doable as, for example, ruling out pathology or physiological changes caused by past or present diseases or in tissue culture experiments where the environment can be held stable. However, it can also be frustrating and perhaps counterproductive, particularly when the brain and behavior of individuals are involved. For example, imagine trying to identify "pure" effects of the brain's biological aging on an elderly person's memory. One would have to rule out the lifelong influences of variables that affect performance on memory tests such as education, profession, general health, diet, socioeconomic status, exercise, motivation, and intelligence. However, it is likely that any or all of these variables would affect memory in ways that would contribute to (and interact with) biological changes in the brain over time.

In the real world, aging does not occur independently of the organism's environment, and many environmental variables strongly affect the course of aging. Thus, it often makes sense to view the phenomenon of aging as encompassing aspects that are both endogenous (accumulated biological changes in cells) and exogenous (accumulated changes in cells and neural circuits due to inevitable environmental variables). This does not imply that toxic events, disease, specific genetic syndromes, or other etiologies are not often primary causes of deficits in older people; they are often significant and should be distinguished from age effects whenever possible. However, "ordinary" environmental and genetic factors are inevitable components of normal, or healthy, aging—terms used to describe aging that has not been marred by debilitating trauma, dementia, or disease.

Multiple Sources of Neural Age Effects

A related issue stems from the fact that many nonneural physiological and biochemical processes affect the way the nervous system functions. The nervous system is integrated with the body's other systems. Therefore, even in the absence of disease, age-associated changes known to occur in cardiovascular function, blood chemistry, immune responses, and myriad other bodily processes might indirectly influence neural physiology. Furthermore, age effects occurring in one part of the nervous system often influence neurons in another part. In 1994 I was asked to discuss aging and homeostasis (physiological stability) of the inner ear at a symposium. In preparation for this task, a brainstorming session produced a list of factors that could conceivably affect the inner ear as people age. As seen in Figure 2.5, quite a few variables emerged, and this was just for the inner ear, a minuscule component of the nervous system. The details of Figure 2.5 (or for that matter, their validity) need not concern us here. The point is, an older individual's general physiological condition is likely to differ from that of young adults; this has the potential to influence neurogerontological findings in ways that may be unsuspected or subtle. This is something to keep in mind as we focus on the nervous system per se.

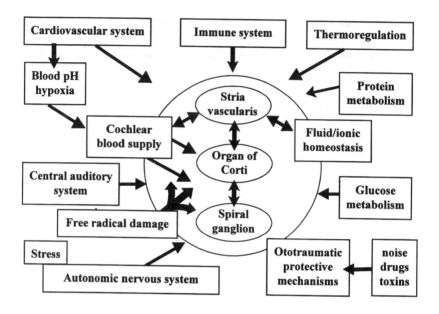

FIGURE 2.5   Some variables that could affect aging of the cochlea of the inner ear. Within the cochlea itself (circle), changes in each component (the stria vascularis, organ of corti, and spiral ganglion) have the potential to affect each other. Also directly affecting the cochlea are the local blood supply and maintenance of fluid and ionic homeostasis within the cochlea. Cochlear physiology is also beholden to a variety of physiological systems and events, each of which can become altered with age under some circumstances. From Willott, J. F. (1994). Homeostasis of the inner ear across the life span. *Homeostatic mechanisms of the inner ear.* Symposium conducted at the meeting of the Association for Research in Otolaryngology, St. Petersberg Beach, FL.

SUMMARY AND IMPLICATIONS

It is obvious that a broad range of tools and approaches are available to study the aging brain. Each has its advantages and limitations. Together, they can provide an incredibly rich and comprehensive description and understanding of the aging nervous system. Many of the newer techniques have barely begun to be applied to neurogerontological research, so the most exciting times lie ahead. However, a caveat accompanies the recruitment of new approaches: The methodological issues and pitfalls attendant to gerontological research must be appreciated by those of us performing and evaluating research in neurogerontology.

3

Some Basics of Neuroanatomy and Neurobiology and Their Neurogerontological Implications

Every neuron in the nervous system is an entity of exquisite anatomical and physiological complexity and sophistication. Although neuroscientists still have a huge amount to learn about the inner workings of neurons and how they communicate with one another, truly impressive scientific gains have been made. Of course, most neurobiological research is not performed under the aegis of gerontology, and neurogerontology lags well behind basic, mainstream neurobiology. Nevertheless, a good deal has been learned about the ways neurons are or are not affected as animals age, and new research questions are being asked and answered all the time. In this chapter we review a portion of this research, along with some basics of the neurobiology of neurons.

THE ANATOMICAL ORGANIZATION OF THE MAMMALIAN NERVOUS SYSTEM

We begin with a very basic outline of the nervous system anatomy.

The Peripheral Nervous System

For meaningful behavior to occur, data about the body and environment must gain entry into the central nervous system (CNS), comprised of the brain and spinal cord, and the CNS must be able to get instructions out to the muscles and glands so that the body can do things—two of the seven basic functions of nervous systems. The portion of the nervous system that interfaces between the CNS and the "outside" is the *peripheral nervous system*. It has two basic subsystems: the *somatic system* and the *autonomic system*.

The somatic system provides input to the brain via axons originating in the sensory organs (incoming axons are called *afferents*) and conveys action potentials outward through axons that synapse on skeletal muscles, causing them to contract to produce movements (outgoing axons are called *efferents*). The autonomic system is linked to emotion and arousal states. It activates glands (e.g., sweat glands), smooth muscles (e.g., controlling the pupils of the eyes, blood vessels, etc.), and the heart. The autonomic system contains two subsystems: The *sympathetic system* readies one for action (increases heart rate, dilates pupils), whereas the *parasympathetic system* has the opposite effect, restoring one toward a resting level when things have settled down. The activity of these systems is most obvious in situations in which emotions are running high. For example, a person might perspire, have a dry mouth, and feel his or her heart racing when under stress because the sympathetic system has kicked in. When the stress is over, the parasympathetic system brings things back to normal.

If the brain is to play its key role in interpreting and storing sensory information and directing the muscles and glands to act, there must be bidirectional communication between the brain and the peripheral systems. The transmission of neural data within the brain involves a dizzying array of incoming and outgoing action potentials and even more information exchange within the confines of the brain.

The Central Nervous System

The *spinal cord* is continuous with the brain, extending below it, encased by the vertebral bones of the neck and back. It is the spinal cord that receives the incoming action potentials from afferent somatic sensory nerves from the body (below the neck). The spinal cord also sends action potentials to activate synapses on the muscles and glands via outgoing efferents. Basically, sensory data are carried by nerves entering the back of the spinal cord, whereas output from the spinal cord's *motor neurons* exits at the front of the spinal cord to control muscles.

Although the motor neurons (and the movements they elicit) are primarily controlled by descending action potentials from the brain, the spinal cord itself contains an impressive assembly of neural circuitry. These circuits can perform a number of sensorimotor behaviors, such as withdrawal from a painful stimulus or generation of rhythmic movements associated with locomotion. However, even these intraspinal circuits can be modulated by action potentials descending from the brain, much as one of those toy cars that can be controlled with a cable: The car can move on its own, but it is modulated by electrical activity descending the cable.

If sensory data from the body are to be transformed into a conscious experience, they must be conveyed up the spinal cord by action potentials and into the brain for further processing. Thus, the spinal cord is, in part, an information highway bringing sensory data to the brain. Likewise, in order for the brain to send "instructions" to the muscles, action potentials must traverse pathways down the spinal cord and out to the muscles. For example, a paraplegic person cannot feel or move his or her lower extremities because the neural pathways to and from the brain have been interrupted.

A quick tour of the brain.   Merging with the spinal cord is the brainstem. Its basic subdivisions, from bottom to top, are the medulla, pons, and midbrain (see Figure 3.1). At the top of the brainstem is the thalamus. The neural traffic between the brain and spinal cord travels along axons through *fiber tracts* in the brainstem. In addition, sensory data (coded as action potentials) enter the brain through various cranial nerves, which also provide an exit route for action potentials to control muscles and glands.

Quite a bit of information processing takes place in the brainstem, without a necessary contribution from higher levels of the brain. For example, comparison of acoustic input from the two ears to compute the location of sounds in space and elicitation of startle responses by abrupt stimuli can be accomplished by the brainstem without help from above.

Behind the pons, near the base of the skull, is the cerebellum, looking like an appended mini-brain. Its neurons play key roles in coordinating movements, balance, and some types of learning. The cerebellum communicates extensively with other parts of the CNS via various axon pathways.

Above and around the brainstem and cerebellum is the forebrain. One prominent structure, the hippocampus, plays an important role in learning and memory and is also a component of the *limbic system* along with the

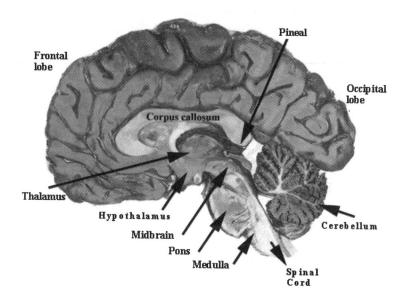

FIGURE 3.1   **A midsagittal section through the human brain. This is what would be seen if the brain were split into two halves, the right side rotated with the front to the left and viewed from the inside out.**

amygdala, olfactory bulb, cingulate gyrus, and other structures. The limbic system is the "emotional brain." Without it, people would probably be without emotions, more like rational computer-beings than people. The hypothalamus is another component of the limbic system, charged with a number of regulatory duties with respect to body temperature, biological rhythms, reproductive behavior and physiology, hormones, eating, and drinking.

Because movement is so important and so difficult to carry out smoothly, much of the brain is involved with the generation and control of behavior (see Figure 3.2). In addition to the cerebellum, the basal ganglia (caudate nucleus, putamen, globus pallidus, substantia nigra, subthalamic nucleus) are conspicuous parts of the brain, adjacent to the thalamus, that help to control movement (they play important roles in cognition, as well).

The human forebrain is dominated by two impressive *cerebral hemispheres* whose surface exhibits a tortuous pattern of folds (*gyri*) and creases (*sulci*) (see Figure 3.3). The folded surface is, in reality, a sheet

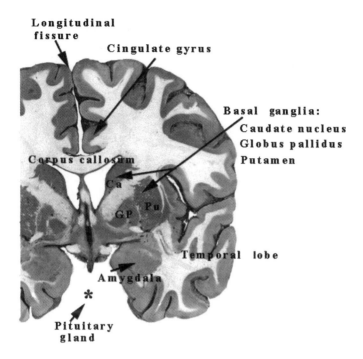

FIGURE 3.2 **A frontal section through the human brain. This is what would be seen if the brain were cut from left to right and viewed straight on. The gray and white matter are clearly delineated. Referring to Figure 3.1, this section cuts through the brain at the level of the *s* in *hypothalamus*.**

of neural tissue, the *cerebral cortex*. The cortical surface extends deep into the crevice separating the two hemispheres (the longitudinal fissure), resulting in distinct left and right hemispheres. By virtue of the surface pattern of gyri and sulci, the cerebral hemispheres can be subdivided into four major lobes: frontal (the front portion, dominated in humans by the prefrontal region), temporal (toward the sides), parietal (toward the top), and occipital (toward the back). The cerebral cortex, working in concert with the rest of the brain, is capable of incredible feats, most notably in humans, in which its size and complexity far exceed that of other species. Language, complex thoughts, logic, and many of our other "higher" functions are beholden to a highly advanced cerebral cortex.

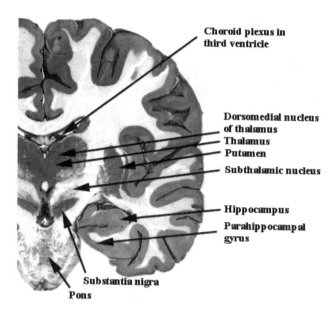

Choroid plexus in
third ventricle

Dorsomedial nucleus
of thalamus
Thalamus
Putamen
Subthalamic nucleus

Hippocampus
Parahippocampal
gyrus

Substantia nigra
Pons

FIGURE 3.3   A frontal section of the human brain slightly more posterior than that in Figure 3.2, cutting through the pons.

Two obvious properties of the brain's gross anatomy should be mentioned. First, regions of the brain that contain mostly fiber tracts are called *white matter* because they are insulated with *myelin,* a whitish insulating substance; the regions with a preponderance of cell somata and dendrites are called *gray matter.* Second, the interior of the brain has a system of interconnected cavities, the *ventricles*, which are filled with a clear watery fluid, *cerebrospinal fluid* (CSF). These are confluent with the spinal cord's *central canal* as well.

AGING AND CHANGES IN THE BRAIN

Given that some aspects of behavior and cognition can decline as people age, it is intuitively reasonable to expect that the brain will undergo degeneration as well. This is certainly true in many respects, but the story is not a simple one.

Gross Changes in the Aging Brain

The relationship between age and the brain's size and gross features (i.e., features that can be seen without the need of a microscope) have been well studied, since gross measurements can be readily obtained from postmortem material and from living humans using imaging techniques. Studies of autopsy material have reported a moderate (e.g., 6% to 11%) loss of brain weight in humans older than 80 years (Brody & Vijaya-shankar, 1977; Duara, London, & Rapoport, 1985; Mann, 1997). Several studies have determined that, after about age 50, brain weight typically decreases by 2% to 3% per decade (Mann, 1997). Atrophy of the gyri and expansion of the sulci of the cerebral surface and dilation of the ventricles within (see below) have also been observed by various researchers (Duara et al., 1985; T. L. Kemper, 1984, 1994; Scheibel, 1996).

Although this literature indicates that significant atrophy of the brain accompanies aging, the overall magnitude of the changes may have been overstated by various studies. One potential confound in studies of brain weights from autopsies stems from the fact that older people tend to be smaller than young people (a cohort effect; they were smaller when young). Because smaller people have smaller brains irrespective of age, values obtained for brain weight loss can be overestimated (Brody & Vijaya-shankar, 1977). Indications of gross atrophy can also be exaggerated if the studies inadvertently included older brains that were not completely free of pathology associated with neurodegenerative disease. Comprehensive premortem data on the mental condition of autopsied people are often impossible to come by, so dementia could have been present in some cases.

Such confounds are less problematic for studies using CT scans and MRI, which allow visualization of ventricle size, gyri and sulci, and relative amounts of white and gray matter in healthy subjects whose mental state can be directly evaluated. Imaging studies indicate that some loss of brain mass, white matter lesions, and expanded ventricles often accompany aging, but many older people are free of significant atrophy (see Coffey et al., 1992; Davis, Mirra, & Alazraki, 1994; Mann, 1997; Scheibel, 1996, for recent reviews). In short, despite the inevitable variability among individuals, atrophic changes (albeit often mild) typically accompany aging. As we are about to see, these sorts of gross changes could be symptomatic of any number of factors, ranging from atrophy and death of neurons to changes in nonneural tissue that supports and protects the neurons.

Aging and the Loss of Neurons

The total number of neurons in the adult brain can only change in one direction—down. Because they are *postmitotic* cells, once the maximum number of neurons is established prenatally, new neurons cannot be produced in most parts of the CNS (there are exceptions, such as certain neurons in the hippocampus, although the capacity for neurogenesis declines with age [Kuhn, Dickenson-Anson, & Gage, 1996]). Furthermore, the ability of CNS neurons to be repaired when damaged is quite limited. Given these properties, it seems likely that a loss of neurons would accompany aging. However, this is not such a clear-cut issue.

Are neurons lost during aging and if so, how many?   The answer to this question is elusive for several reasons. Some of the research showing a loss of neurons has had methodological flaws that plague studies counting neurons (see the appendix at the end of this chapter). Other methodological issues stem from the use of tissue obtained from human autopsy material. First, unless given special treatment not usually possible on autopsied brains (e.g., immediate fixation with formaldehyde or other fixative), brain tissue undergoes rapid *autolysis*, changes in the condition of the tissue that may make neurons look abnormal and therefore not counted. If older neurons had some morphological changes to begin with, such postmortem changes could be more severe. Second, there may be a difference in the premortem condition of young and old people who are autopsied. Older people are more likely to have died from chronic illnesses that could have resulted in neuron loss (e.g., cardiovascular disease), whereas more young deaths result from accidents or acute conditions that would not affect neurons prior to death. Thus, it is important to have some control over the sources of autopsy material when comparing brains of young and old subjects. Third, there may be an acceleration of neuron loss in the terminal phase of life (chapter 2), and this can be reflected in the cause of death from which autopsy material has been obtained (e.g., terminal cancer vs. a sudden heart attack).

The methodological problems attendant to human studies have probably resulted in overestimations of neuronal losses thought to be typical of healthy older people (see Mann, 1997; Scheibel, 1996; Wickelgren, 1996). One way of getting more accurate data is to turn to studies of animal models—particularly rodents—for which the methodological shortcomings of human studies can be largely overcome. Healthy rats or mice can be euthanized at various ages, and brain tissue can be properly prepared for histological procedures. Furthermore, rodent brains are small and structurally simpler than human brains, making it easier to count representative samples of neurons within specific brain regions. And, by using genetically uniform rodents raised in the same environment, individual differences can presumably be somewhat muted.

However, even with the use of animal models, it is impossible to answer the question How many neurons are lost during aging? For one, substantial species differences exist with respect to age changes, making it hard to generalize findings from one type of animal to another. And even within a species, significant differences can be found for different genetic strains (just as large differences can be found for genetically different humans). Further compounding the problem, different parts of the brain show different age changes, and even within a part of the brain, different types of neurons may fare differently with age. An example of some sources of variance from our own work is shown in Figure 3.4, which depicts the number of neurons in several brain regions of mice from two inbred strains. First, it is apparent that the number of neurons in several brain regions does not decrease with age, whereas neuron loss is observed in other regions. Second, in the case of the OCA (octopus cell area) of both strains, the loss of neurons accelerates in the oldest old; this does not occur for other regions. Third, there are strain differences in the pattern of cell loss for areas DCN I and DCN II (referring to layers of the dorsal cochlear nucleus); DCN I neurons are maintained in aging C57 mice but not in CBA mice; however, the opposite occurs for DCN III neurons. It is obvious that general statements about aging and neuron loss cannot be made.

What, then, can be concluded with respect to the impact of aging on the survival of neurons? It depends on whether one sees a glass as half full or half empty. The good news is, consistent loss of neurons often does not occur in many parts of the brain, and for many individuals losses may be minimal throughout much of the brain. The bad news is the exact converse of the previous statement: Neuron death often does occur in certain parts of the brain for many individuals. Given the variability in neuronal mortality, the topic is best dealt with in other chapters, in the context of specific brain regions and systems.

Mechanisms of Cell Death During Aging

Because a degree of neuronal loss often occurs in conjunction with normal aging and serious losses occur with neuropathological conditions, it is

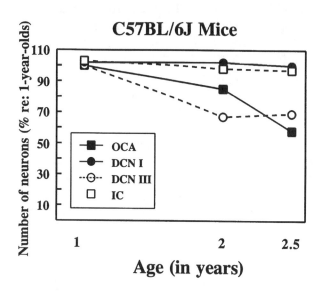

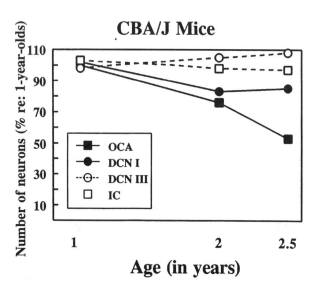

FIGURE 3.4   Aging and the loss of neurons in two inbred mouse strains. Neurons were counted in the octopus cell area (OCA) of the cochlear nucleus, layers I and III of the dorsal cochlear nucleus (DCN I, DCN III), and the inferior colliculus (IC) of the midbrain. Whether or not neurons were lost to aging depended on the brain region and strain. Furthermore, the rate of cell loss differed among regions. For example, in both strains there was an accelerating loss of OCA neurons after 2 years of age (median life span), but the DCN III of C57BL/6J mice was already reduced by more than 30% at 2 years of age. Data were taken from Willott and Bross (1990) and Willott, Bross, and McFadden (1992, 1994).

important to understand the processes that are responsible. Two mechanisms by which cells die are *necrosis* and *apoptosis*. Necrosis is a response to injury, certain diseases, drugs, or other pathological toxic processes that cause an "energy crisis." Apoptosis, also referred to as programmed cell death, is directed by genes and is very important during development, when it is normal for a portion of excess neurons to die off (see Johnson & Deckwerth, 1993). The biochemical and cellular changes are different for necrosis and apoptosis, and methods are available to distinguish the two in brain tissue. For example, in apoptosis, the cell's contents condense and break up, cells tend to shrink, and the DNA in the nucleus is damaged; in necrosis, cells swell, burst, and cause an inflammatory reaction. Whereas apoptosis and necrosis are different processes, they can apparently occur simultaneously under certain conditions that kill neurons (Portera-Cailliau, Hedreen, Price, & Koliatsos, 1995). Similarly, certain events (e.g., epileptic seizures, some toxic agents) apparently can kill neurons by either apoptosis or necrosis, depending on subtle variables (Ankarcrona et al., 1995; Sloviter, Dean, Sollas, & Goodman, 1996).

The occurrence of apoptosis appears to contribute to neuron death in normal aging, as well as in neurodegenerative diseases such as Alzheimer's and Parkinson's diseases. Research has suggested that, during aging, events may trigger apoptosis (by activating a so-called death signal or suicide switch). Such events might include the excessive influx of calcium into neurons (associated with certain excitatory neurotransmitters discussed later), reduced growth factors, loss of metabolic support, or oxidative processes. From cell to cell and within a given cell, a variety of genes can be implicated in the events leading to apoptosis (Smith & Osborne, 1997). Various events also trigger necrotic cell death (loss of oxygen and blood supply to brain tissue, seizures, and hypoglycemia; see Sapolsky, 1992). Thus, both mechanisms appear to contribute to neuronal death during aging via a variety of pathways.

Calcium: Too much of a good thing. The neurotoxic effects of alterations in the regulation of calcium ion (Ca^{++}) entry into neurons has received much attention from neurogerontologists. If the intracellular levels of Ca^{++} increase too much (by allowing excess calcium to enter and/or remain inside neurons) the neurons are damaged or killed. Evidence is building that the regulation of calcium is altered with aging, and this damages neurons or disrupts their physiology, not only in neurodegenerative diseases but also, to a lesser extent, in normal aging (Disterhoft,

Moyer, & Thompson, 1994; Khachaturian, 1989). Changes in calcium homeostasis can be associated with changes in neuronal membranes, calcium binding proteins (which capture free Ca^{++}), excitatory neurotransmission, neuroendocrine activity, and other factors, and these are discussed elsewhere as appropriate.

When neuron death does occur during aging, what are the consequences? This, of course, is the question that really matters. Unfortunately, there is no answer at this time, at least for nonpathological conditions (the consequences of severe neuronal loss in Alzheimer's or Parkinson's diseases, for example, are evident; see chapters 9 and 11). It is presently impossible to determine, in a living person, whether or not a significant loss of neurons has occurred in various parts of the brain and then correlate those losses with changes in behavior, cognition, and so on. And, because large individual differences occur in age-related changes in the brain, inferences about "average" degrees of neural loss for an age group cannot be made with any confidence. Perhaps we do not even know enough yet about how the brain works to address this question. A small focus of damage to the primary visual cortex (which processes visual stimuli) can result in a clear loss of function (a scotoma, or blind spot). On the other hand, people often recover dramatically from minor strokes or brain injury, suggesting that a significant loss of neurons need not be debilitating under certain circumstances. In Parkinson's disease patients, a loss of more than 50% of neurons in the substantia nigra is needed to produce significant clinical symptoms (Fearnley & Lees, 1991). Simply put, there is no simple equation to relate neuron loss to loss of function.

Then there is the huge number of neurons the nervous system has to begin with. As Scheibel (1996) reminds us, neuron death during early development is a normal aspect of maturation; indeed, most neuron death occurs during the early developmental period when unneeded or redundant neurons are programmed to be pruned back. Yet early development is a period of improvement of most functions, not decline. It is difficult to predict at what point (if any) the dying off of excess neurons would be transformed from a beneficial process to a detrimental one. Indeed, there is no a priori reason to conclude that some neuronal loss during adulthood is necessarily a bad thing. Downsized corporations often function more efficiently and/or use their resources more effectively with fewer employees. Might not "downsized" nervous systems do the same?

A final issue with respect to counting neurons in a particular brain region is *what those neurons are doing and whether this might have changed with age.* It is well established that sensory and motor deficits, learning, and other events can induce neural changes (plasticity) in the cerebral cortex and elsewhere (see chapters 7 and 13). Thus, the number of neurons participating in a particular task (their functional identity) might change with age, making it difficult to interpret the effects of neuron loss. For example, suppose adjacent brain areas A and B each contain 100 neurons in young adults. Area A processes information about stimulus I exclusively (100 neurons), and area B processes information only about stimulus II (100 neurons). With age, the ability to process stimulus II is lost due to damage in the peripheral sensory system, so area B no longer has anything to do. This triggers mechanisms of neural plasticity such that stimulus I "takes over" area B's territory, so that both areas A and B now are devoted solely to stimulus I (this sort of thing does indeed happen). In the mean time, 20% of the neurons in both areas A and B have been lost to aging. Despite this loss, however, there are now 160 neurons processing stimulus I (80% of 100 + 100), whereas there were only 100 neurons during young adulthood. The flip side of this example is that, despite only a 20% loss of neurons, there are now no neurons processing information about stimulus II. In this hypothetical example, the 20% loss of neurons has little meaning with respect to brain function.

The truth be told, our understanding of the relationship between the loss of neurons and the ultimate effects on behavior at this time remains fuzzy. Perhaps the rapidly advancing technology of neuroimaging can provide a way to directly assess the consequences of age-related changes in the number or physiology of neurons (or show us that this is the wrong question to be asking). Despite the uncertainty about the impact of neuron death in normal aging, however, there is no question that the impact is devastating in conditions such as Alzheimer's disease. Clearly, then, the loss of neurons can and does have consequences, *if the magnitude of loss is sufficiently great.* We simply do not yet have a good understanding of what "sufficiently great" is when it comes to the moderate declines in function commonly associated with healthy aging (refer to chapters 6 to 12).

NEURONAL AGING AT THE CELLULAR LEVEL

Neurons need not die in order for their contribution to the operation of the nervous system to be impaired. Indeed, diminished or altered physiological processes within still-viable neurons are proving to be far more important to the normal aging of the nervous system than cell death (e.g., Morrison & Hof, 1997). This section reviews some basics of cellular physiology and how these might become compromised with age.

The Neuron's Nucleus and Cell Body Perform Essential Functions

The neuron's cell body, or *soma*, is composed of the nucleus and surrounding cytoplasm, which is packed with mitochondria, ribosomes, and other organelles that provide for cellular metabolism and other physiological processes (see Figure 3.5). The genetic information of the cell is coded in the deoxyribonucleic acid (DNA) of the nucleus, and the expression (translation and manifestation) of these genes is accomplished using ribonucleic acid (RNA). The key products of gene expression are proteins, and these are employed in many roles, such as enzymes, membranes, internal structural components, and synaptic receptors. Neurons must synthesize very many different types of proteins in order to maintain their proper function across the life span. Changes in gene expression (e.g., changes in the protein products) would be expected to result from mutations in DNA that can accrue with age, and this is often mentioned as a basic mechanism of cellular aging. The various steps by which the genetic information is processed are also subject to age effects, and changes in the synthesis and degradation of both RNA and protein have been found to accompany aging in some cases (Finch & Morgan, 1990; Johnson & Finch, 1996). Such occurrences might be important in a variety of age effects in the nervous system. As reviewed by Johnson and Finch (1996) evidence is building rapidly for the importance of altered gene expression in age-related changes in the nervous system.

Many cellular physiological processes involve calcium. An effect of altered calcium homeostasis in the aging of the nervous system has been suggested in a variety of contexts including second messenger functions, activation of enzyme systems including kinases and phosphatases (important in various cellular activities), induction of genes, regulation of neuronal metabolic activity, dendritic growth, and synaptic plasticity (Disterhoft et al., 1994; Gibson & Peterson, 1987; Khachaturian, 1989; Landfield et al., 1992). As Khachaturian (1989) suggests, even minor alterations in one or more of these functions of calcium have the potential to create

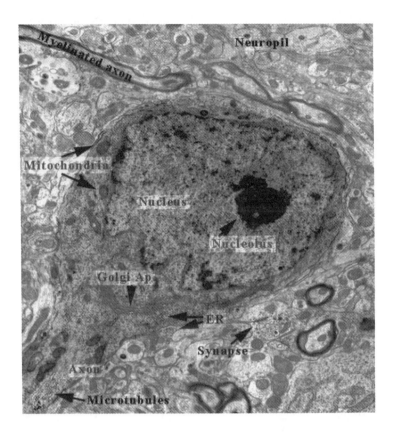

FIGURE 3.5 An electron micrograph figure showing various components of a neuron. Because of the way this section was cut, only a relatively small amount of cytoplasm surrounding the nucleus is seen compared to the typical neuron, and dendrites are not seen leaving the soma. The neuropil surrounding the neuron is packed with dendrites, glial processes, and darkly stained myelinated axons; many pale gray, oval mitochondria are present. The axon exits the neuron in the lower left, and microtubules can be seen inside the axon. The neuron's cytoplasm is filled with organelles (endoplasmic reticulum [ER], Golgi apparatus, and mitochondria). Micrograph courtesy of Jeremy Turner.

serious problems if they occur over an extended period of time, as would be the case with aging.

The complex molecular and biochemical activities taking place within neurons provide myriad potential targets for disruption by the aging process (not only in neurons but in all cells); neurogerontological research has begun to address these processes. However, a comprehensive discussion of cellular aging requires a level of biochemical and molecular biological sophistication that exceeds the scope and purpose of this book. Thus, the interested reader is urged to consult other sources (e.g., Danner & Holbrook, 1990; Finch & Morgan, 1990; Johnson & Finch, 1996; Khachaturian, 1989).

The Size of Neurons May Reflect Cellular Physiology

The size of neurons is a basic measure that may reflect cellular pathology or metabolic stress associated with aging. Therefore, many studies have measured neuron size as a function of age. The most commonly reported finding is a decrease in soma area, most frequently on the order of 10% to 20% (Flood & Coleman, 1988). Not unexpectedly, however, the scientific literature reveals no general pattern, as all three possible outcomes have been reported—increased, decreased, or unchanged sizes as a function of age (Duara et al., 1985; Finch, 1993; Flood & Coleman, 1988; Hinds & McNelly, 1977; T. L. Kemper, 1984; Peters & Vaughan, 1981). It seems that, like the loss of neurons with aging, changes in the size of neurons are not governed by a simple principle. This is not surprising, because as indicated earlier, different mechanisms of cell death (e.g., apoptosis, necrosis) are associated with different types of cellular change. Furthermore, various factors can influence cell size (see below).

To assess this body of research, one must ask two questions. First, Is the diversity of findings real or due to technical artifacts? Certainly, some variance in the literature may be accounted for by technical problems of fixation, postmortem change, and the like. It is also the case that different methods of measuring neuron size can lead to different outcomes. Furthermore, one wonders how many "no change" findings were discarded as unpublishable "negative" findings. Also, caution must be used in interpreting studies that either do not measure the number of neurons or that report a decrease in neuron number. In such studies, a smaller mean neuron size in old subjects could have resulted from a preferential loss of larger neurons (not shrinkage of neurons). What this would mean is, the smaller (surviving) neurons were actually the healthy neurons, the larger ones having died off. We can only rule out selective attrition and be confident that neurons have lost size in one of two ways: The total number of neurons in the region has not changed with age, or there are not many small neurons in the region to begin with (in young subjects). Fortunately, enough studies have been performed that are free from these potential pitfalls to indicate that diversity of age effects is a valid principle. Particularly compelling are studies that show different outcomes within the same animals (e.g., see Flood & Coleman, 1988). For example, a study performed in our laboratory (Willott, Jackson, & Hunter, 1987) measured the size of neurons in the anteroventral cochlear nucleus brain region of aging mice. One type of neuron decreased in size with aging, but another type of neuron in the same region increased in size. The size of Purkinje cells of the cerebellum did not change significantly. The size measurements were not systematically related cell loss, and obviously, fixation and other technical procedures did not vary for the same tissue sections.

The second question is, What are the neurogerontological implications of changes in neuron size? Like many other questions concerning functional significance, this one cannot be answered with confidence in the context of aging. Changes in neuron size may reflect physiological events that are informative and interesting, but this is difficult to demonstrate satisfactorily. A change in neuron size might be pathological shrinkage or swelling; however, neuron size can reflect changes in normal metabolic activity (up or down), as well (e.g., Warr, 1982). Given this, it is difficult to interpret size changes. For example, shrinkage of the soma could conceivably occur under the following scenarios: (1) the neuron's dendritic tree or axon branches have undergone some atrophy (a pathological change that reduces the metabolic demand but does not directly attack the soma); (2) there is age-related damage or dysfunction of the nucleus, neuronal membranes, or intracellular organelles (metabolic activity is reduced because of cellular pathology); (3) the neuron and its processes are perfectly intact, but it is not "being used" very much by the older animal (the metabolic demand is reduced in conjunction with normal changes in behavior, perception, etc.); (4) potentially, age-related changes in neuron size can be influenced by various "extracellular" factors. A partial list includes the effects of local toxins, levels of growth factors (see chapter 13), regional changes in blood supply, and changes in hormones or other systemic factors (Finch, 1993). Not only is it difficult or impossible to decide which scenario applies, we do not even know if a reduction in neuron size is a bad thing. It is certainly possible that a more compact neuron can still perform quite adequately.

Age-Associated Histological Structures May Affect Neural Functioning

A number of microscopic structures are observed with greater prevalence in and around neurons of aging brains. The human histopathological literature has recently been reviewed by Mann (1997). In most cases the origin and functional significance of these histological features is not clear. However, because most are more prevalent in brains of patients suffering from Alzheimer's or other degenerative diseases, they may be indicative of processes detrimental to cell function in healthy aging brains. The two most familiar are *senile plaques,* which represent foci of degenerating neural tissue containing amyloid protein, and *neurofibrillary tangles,* which appear as thick fibrils that occupy neurons. Both are characteristic of Alzheimer's disease and are discussed in chapter 11. Other structures also become increasingly evident with age in the absence of dementia, but typically to a much lesser extent than those suffering from neurodegenerative diseases. *Lewy bodies* are round inclusions within the cytoplasm, especially in neurons that are normally pigmented (substantia nigra and locus coeruleus in the brainstem). They contain fragmented neurofilaments and are characteristic of Parkinson's disease (chapter 9). *Hirano bodies* are typically found outside the pyramidal cells of the hippocampus and cerebellum, perhaps occupying dendrites. *Granulovacuolar degeneration* is characterized by clear, rounded vacuoles within neurons (usually hippocampal pyramidal neurons) that can displace the nucleus and distort the neuron's shape. *Intranuclear inclusions* called paracrystalline rodlets, spherical bodies, and Marinesco bodies can be seen within neuronal nuclei, and they may increase with age. *Intracytoplasmic inclusions* appear as clusters of granules in neurons of the substantia nigra, locus coeruleus, and elsewhere. *Polyglucosan bodies,* such as *corpora amylacea*, contain a glycogenlike substance and other components, located in astrocytes and neurons; they may play a positive role in response to neural degeneration.

The Risk of Oxidative Damage in Neurons

Of the various organelles, structures, and substances found with neuron cell bodies and subject to age-related alterations, those associated with oxidative damage (a likely mechanism of aging) deserve particular attention. *Mitochondria* are intracellular organelles where metabolic activities occur, providing energy for cellular activities. Mitochondria are inherited from the mother via the ovum and have a special type of DNA (mtDNA), which may be more vulnerable to damage than DNA found in the cell nuclei (Young, 1996). The mitochondria are a major generator of free radicals, and certain repair enzymes that exist in nuclei are not present in mitochondria. Thus, accumulation of damage to mtDNA may be especially important in aging, perhaps causing impairments of oxidative metabolism in brain cells associated with neurodegenerative diseases as well as normal aging (Blass, 1996; Fattoretti et al., 1996; Kadenbach, Munscher, Frank, Muller-Hocker, & Napiwotzki, 1995; Martinez, Hernandez, Martinez, & Ferrandiz, 1996).

A substance presumably related to oxidative damage is *lipofuscin*, a dark-pigmented substance that builds up within some neurons and other tissue as aging occurs. The accumulation of lipofuscin per se may not directly interfere with the ability of neurons to function normally. For instance, in one brain structure in humans, the inferior olive neurons can accumulate large amounts of lipofuscin yet survive (Monagle & Brody, 1974). However, lipofuscin is likely associated with lipid peroxidation, oxidative damage to lipid constituents of cells, and a possible mechanism of biological aging (Yin, 1996). Thus, it may be viewed as a marker of age-related stress on cells. Several studies suggest a negative relationship between lipofuscin content of neurons and normal physiology (Sharma, Maurya, & Singh, 1993; Sharma & Singh, 1996), and, even in young rats, stress (from a period of physical restraint) appears to induce the buildup of lipofuscin.

The Neuronal Cytoskeleton

Neurons have a cytoskeleton that gives them shape, structural support, and a conduit between cell soma and axon terminals. This "skeleton" is made up of minute proteinaceous microtubules and neurofilaments. These give the neuron its shape, move vital substances within the cell body and axons, and are important in the storage and release of chemical neurotransmitters. Several degenerative diseases that accompany aging seem to involve abnormalities in the neuronal cytoskeleton (Anderton et al., 1986; Morrison & Hof, 1997). One example is the neurofibrillary tangle of Alzheimer's disease, discussed in chapter 11. With respect to healthy elderly people, the extent to which more subtle age-related changes in neural function may involve the cytoskeleton (e.g., Benes, Majocha, & Marotta, 1988; Leterrier & Eyer, 1992) remains to be determined. However, there is evidence that the changes in the cytoskeleton may play a role in the degeneration in some neurons irrespective of Alzheimer's disease (Rao & Cohen, 1990; Vickers et al., 1994).

Axons use the cytoskeleton (microtubules in particular) to transport various substances to and from the neuron's cell body. The transport of substances by axons is presumably affected by changes in the cytoskeleton, and, indeed, axonal transport of various substances has been shown to slow in aging rats (Castel, Beaudet, & Laduron, 1994; Cooper, Lindholm, & Sofroniew, 1994; De Lacalle, Cooper, Svendsen, Dunnett, & Sofroniew, 1996; Fernandez & Hodges-Savola, 1994; Frolkis, Tanin, & Gorban, 1997; McQuarrie, Brady, & Lasek, 1989; Tashiro & Komiya, 1994). A decrease in proteins that produce neurofilaments appears to occur with aging, and this could result in fewer neurofilaments and thinner axons (Parhad et al., 1995). Thus, changes in the cytoskeleton may be linked to age-related decreases in axon diameter, which can slow the conduction speed of action potentials (chapter 4). It is evident that changes in the cytoskeleton are likely to have important effects on the aging nervous system, and these are probably not confined to neurodegenerative diseases.

MECHANISMS THAT PROTECT AND SUPPORT NEURONS AND HOW THEY ARE CHALLENGED BY AGING

Not surprisingly, various mechanisms have evolved that protect the brain from physical and chemical insults and ensure homeostasis for neurons. An important issue in neurogerontology is how well these mechanisms endure with age, and whether they contribute to physiological changes in the aging brain.

Cerebrospinal Fluid Cushions the Brain
on the Inside and Outside

As mentioned earlier, CSF fills the ventricles and spinal cord's central canal. It is also found near the surface of the brain, in the *subarachnoid space*. CSF is continually produced within these spaces by tissue called the *choroid plexus* and is, in turn, resorbed via blood vessels. CSF provides a cushion and support for the brain, contains substances important for normal brain functioning, and plays a role in the removal of physiological waste products. Assays of proteins and other substances in the CSF are used as clinical tests (e.g., spinal taps), so age-related changes in CSF have implications in this respect also.

There is little evidence that clinically important changes in the volume or pressure of CSF occur very often in healthy older people. Gideon, Thomsen, Stahlberg, and Henricksen (1994) used an MRI technique to measure the production of CSF and found no significant age effects (mean age of old subjects: 69 years). An earlier study found that the mean rate of CSF production was slower in subjects ages 67 to 84 years (May et al., 1990). That study concluded that the turnover (production and resorption) of CSF may be reduced in older people, especially since the size of the ventricles often increases with age, so more CSF is needed to fill them. Slower turnover does not necessarily alter the volume or pressure of CSF within the ventricles, but could result in higher concentrations of CSF constituents.

The size of ventricles is often a sign of brain pathology in conditions such as Alzheimer's disease. Degeneration and shrinkage of brain tissue allows the ventricles to expand because they can hold more CSF. These changes can be seen using methods such as CT scans or MRI. Other disorders that can afflict older people also involve changes in the ventricles associated with the flow of CSF, but the CSF change is a cause of the trouble, rather than a result of reduced brain mass. *Hydrocephalus* occurs when an abnormal amount of CSF accumulates in the ventricles due to an imbalance between the production and resorption of CSF, leading to an enlargement of the ventricles that encroach against the brain. A condition called normal pressure hydrocephalus (NPH) is not uncommon in geriatric patients. NPH might be caused by an obstruction of CSF flow and/or weakening of the ventricular walls that leads to their expansion. The expanded ventricular volume within a nonexpandable skull allows less space for brain tissue, with deleterious results. The symptoms of NPH include incontinence, movement disorders, and dementia (Krauss et al., 1997; St. Laurent, 1988), symptoms associated with a variety of other disorders that afflict older people (e.g., Parkinson's and Alzheimer's diseases). Hydrocephalus can often be corrected with a surgical shunt that allows the CSF to flow properly.

Although CSF production and resorption may remain relatively normal in healthy older people, it is possible that the role of CSF in aging is more important than it might seem. The fact that hydrocephalus (an abnormal condition) has serious consequences in afflicted older people begs this question: Might smaller ("normal") increases in CSF volume in some cases cause less severe but nevertheless bothersome changes in brain function? Also, if concentrations of proteins or other substances within the ventricles change with age, might the altered CSF affect neurons? For example, Takayama and colleagues (1992) found decreased concentrations of the inhibitory neurotransmitter GABA in the CSF of healthy aged subjects. Although this was presumably the result of changes in GABA metabolism by certain neurons, it is conceivable that the reduced GABA in the CSF per se could have secondary effects on other neurons. Also, a study on aging rats (Kvitnitskaya-Ryzhova, Shinkai, Ooka, & Ohtsuba, 1994) found evidence for a decrease in the ability of the choroid plexus to transport the hormone prolactin from the blood stream to the CSF (a route by which prolactin affects neurons).

The Blood-Brain Barrier Protects the Brain from Undesirable Substances and Transports Important Substances

The blood-brain barrier plays the role of chemical guardian for the brain, determining which substances can pass from the blood into the brain. This barrier is essentially a physical one, as endothelial cells packed tightly along the walls of capillaries prevent large molecules from leaving the bloodstream. Its integrity is critical to protect the brain from various toxic substances, and weakening of the barrier can potentially cause harm to neurons. Some substances (e.g., fat-soluble drugs like heroin or nicotine) normally pass through the barrier, but others are kept out unless the blood-brain barrier is not functioning properly. However, the blood-brain barrier also transports essential nutrients (e.g., glucose, vitamin C), hormones, and drugs from blood to brain and carries metabolic end products out of the CNS. Whether or not these carrier functions are diminished with age is still an open question, but one that is potentially important. Evidence indicates the ability to actively transport certain substances, including choline and glucose, may become diminished with age (Mooradian, 1988; Shah & Mooradian, 1997).

The blood-brain barrier can be compromised in geriatric patients suffering from certain neurological diseases (Mooradian, 1988), but what about healthy older people? The answer to this question is not clear. Some changes in the permeability of the blood-brain barrier have been found in studies of older humans (Edvinsson, MacKenzie, & McCulloch, 1993; Kleine, Hackler, & Zöfel, 1993) and rats (Mooradian, 1994; Saija, Princi, D'Amico, DePasquale, & Costa, 1990). Cardiovascular conditions such as hypertension may contribute to impairment of the blood-brain barrier as well. Changes observed in capillaries in the cortex of old monkeys (Burns, Kruckenberg, Comerford, & Buschmann, 1979, 1983) also suggest disruption of the blood-brain barrier, as do some structural changes observed in older human brains (Mooradian, 1988; Shah & Mooradian, 1997). Although clinically significant changes in the blood-brain barrier of healthy older people appear to be minimal in most cases (Garton, Keir, Lakshmi, & Thompson, 1991; Johnson & Finch, 1996), the cited studies taken together suggest increased risk of breaches in the blood-brain barrier under chemically stressful conditions.

Despite the Blood-Brain Barrier, Aging Neurons Are at Risk from Various Toxins

Because adults do not grow new neurons, the response of neurons to toxins can be different from that of cells that can replace themselves. In neurons, the effects of toxins can accumulate over a lifetime. Some types of neurons are more vulnerable to toxins than others. The vulnerability may be due to the properties of particular neurons vis-à-vis a specific toxin (see Young, 1996). For example, the neurotoxin 6-hydroxy-dopamine damages neurons that use as their transmitter dopamine, a closely related chemical. Kainic acid affects other neurons, those that possess the appropriate kainate receptors.

Some toxins are endogenous; that is, they are produced by the brain itself. Glutamate is a major excitatory transmitter in the CNS and neurons can possess different subtypes of glutamate receptors. A receptor that has been heavily studied is the NMDA receptor (named after N-methyl-D-aspartate, a substance that selectively activates this receptor). The NMDA receptors activate membrane channels that allow calcium to enter the neuron. Under certain conditions such as hypoxia or tissue damage, the effects of glutamate can become exaggerated, resulting in excessive entry of calcium into the neurons. This *excitotoxic* event can be very damaging to neurons. Another substance that activates NMDA receptors and may be neurotoxic is quinolinic acid, associated with the metabolism of the neurotransmitter serotonin.

There may be a number of other endogenous toxins as well, one example being free radicals, as discussed in chapter 1. Brain tissue is especially sensitive to free radical damage under pathological conditions, so it might be expected that oxidative stress would contribute to aging of the brain. The literature on this topic has been conflicting, but there is probably a significant contribution of free radical damage to normal brain aging (LeBel & Bondy, 1992). Whereas the role of endogenous neurotoxins in normal aging remains to be determined, they would appear to provide mechanisms by which damage to the brain could accrue over the years.

Genetics comes into play here, too. One's genetic endowment can influence the ability of certain liver enzymes to detoxify toxins (Young, 1996). Thus, to the extent that a certain toxin contributes to age-related changes, individuals may differ in their ability to withstand such challenges.

The Blood Provides Oxygen and Nourishment, and Neurons Require a Disproportionate Share of the Blood Supply

Neurons have a ravenous appetite for glucose and oxygen, and at least 15% of the body's blood is found in the brain at any time, supporting about 20% to 40% of the body's oxygen consumption (the brain typically amounts to about 2% of the total body weight). A drastic reduction in the supply of blood/oxygen to neurons results in rapid impairment, damage, or destruction, depending on the severity and duration of blood loss. Thus, any condition that reduces the brain's blood supply, such as atherosclerosis or diabetes (which are prevalent in older people) is a cause for concern. There is a bit of irony here. Oxygen in the guise of free radicals can damage neurons, albeit little by little over time, but so does the absence of oxygen.

Changes in the vascular system serving the brain can accompany aging even in the absence of diseases, and on average, there is a decline in cerebral blood flow and oxygen consumption with age (Dastur et al., 1963; Levine, Hanson, & Nickles, 1994; Meyer, Terayama, & Takashima, 1993). Martin, Evans, and Naylor (1994) used an imaging technique called transcranial color-coded sonography and found that the velocity of blood flow through cerebral blood vessels decreased with age and the resistance of vessels to blood flow increased. Related research has obtained some evidence for positive correlations between declines in blood circulation to specific regions of the human brain and cognitive impairment (Ivy, Petit, & Markus, 1992). Capillaries—the interface between the circulatory and nervous systems—can be affected also. For example, Casey and Feldman (1985) found a loss of vascularity in the brainstem of old rats, as revealed by a decline in the density of capillaries and large cavitations, or spaces in the capillary wall. As discussed earlier, changes in the blood-brain barrier might be associated with altered capillary structure and their transport function. There is also strong evidence showing that pathological capillaries and the resulting effects on energy metabolism play a key role in Alzheimer's disease (De la Torre, 1997). Although the picture is not clear at this time, it may turn out that relatively small decreases in cerebral circulation or capillary integrity in healthy older people can have significant effects on the brain's ability to function at optimum levels.

Another source of age-related change in cerebral blood flow may be secondary to changes in neurons, rather than blood vessels. Certain regions of the brain play a role in the regulation of cerebral blood supply, and if these were to degenerate with age, blood flow could be altered as well. The basal forebrain is one such area, and evidence for age effects on this regulatory function has been presented by Linville and Arneric (1991). When the basal forebrain of rats was electrically stimulated, cerebral blood flow was increased in various other brain regions. In aged rats, which are likely to exhibit declines in basal forebrain function, the same stimulation failed to produce increased blood flow in some of these regions (parietal cortex and caudate nucleus). These and other findings suggest that degenerative changes in the basal forebrain, which occur in Alzheimer's disease and often in normal aging, may contribute to diminished cerebral blood supply.

The most dramatic cause of blood loss to the brain is stroke. Stroke can involve infarctions (prevention of blood from reaching all or part of the brain due to atherosclerosis), infections, tumors, sickle-cell anemia, or other causes. Or hemorrhage can result, most commonly from burst aneurysms—weakened regions of blood vessels. The symptoms of stroke vary greatly, depending on the size and location of the damage. Data compiled by the National Center for Health Statistics consistently show stroke to be the third most common cause of death of older people in the United States.

Glucose and Oxygen Fuel the Activity of Neurons

Oxidative metabolism of glucose provides energy (via adenosine triphosphate, or ATP) to fuel the brain's activity and support the synthesis of neurotransmitters. Glucose and oxygen are brought to the brain via the circulatory system, so reduced blood flow or impaired capillary function presumably makes metabolism of these substances more difficult by limiting their supply to neurons. Beyond limitations in the delivery of "raw materials," however, the basic metabolic ability of brain tissue must be considered as well. Even if the blood supply were fully adequate, can the aging brain metabolize glucose and oxygen efficiently enough to fuel its varied activities?

Before addressing this question, it must be noted that blood flow and cerebral metabolism are not independent of one another. If there is an increased demand for glucose and oxygen in a region of the brain, the blood supply to that region normally increases as well. Thus, it is possible that suboptimal metabolic efficiency might be compensated for by increased blood flow, avoiding any dire effects. Of course, if the circulatory system cannot adequately provide the extra blood *and* metabolism has declined with age, the brain would be twice threatened. On the other hand, if decreased demand for oxygen were to accompany the loss or atrophy of neurons with age, the requisite blood supply would be reduced (Meyer et al., 1993). Then a lower level of metabolic activity would be observed, even if metabolic efficiency were normal. Given all of this, it can be difficult to figure out what is going on with respect to aging and cerebral metabolism.

Evidence indicates that declines in the rates of glucose and oxygen use accompany aging, but they typically vary among regions of the brain, individuals, and species. In both humans and other species, the results of various studies are mixed; some studies show a decrease in metabolism, whereas others do not (Duara et al., 1985). The reasons for the discrepancies are unclear, but probable sources of confusion are the failure of some researchers to document their subjects' medical histories (which could affect metabolism) and the state of their sensory systems. When sensory systems are active, the regions of the brain that interact with them increase their metabolic activity; if the sensory systems are not functioning properly, as often occurs during aging (see chapter 7), then those brain regions may display reduced metabolic activity (reduced demand), which could be mistakenly attributed to impaired cerebral metabolism.

Another probable reason for discrepancies is that metabolic activity in various brain regions exhibits different patterns of age-related change. For example, PET studies have found that metabolic activity in the frontal cortex decreased more than that of other brain regions (De Santi et al., 1995; Loessner et al., 1995; Moeller et al., 1996; Salmon et al., 1991). In other cortical regions, variability was found among individuals, irrespective of age. Furthermore, areas such as the basal ganglia, hippocampus, thalamus, and cerebellum may exhibit no consistent age differences (Loessner et al., 1995).

It seems safe to conclude that age-related deficits in the functional capacity or activity levels of certain brain regions are accompanied by reduced metabolic activity. This could simply reflect the reduced demand for oxygen and glucose, secondary to normal or pathological neuronal impairment.It is also likely, however, that indications of reduced metabolic activity (PET, etc.) indicate deficits at the cellular level. As discussed earlier, damage to mitochondria—key organelles in cellular energy metabolism—can accrue with age. Whereas many studies have failed to find age effects in various types of tissue (Masoro, 1985), others have shown changes in mitochondria. One study found changes in mitochondrial function in brain tissue, at least under conditions of high energy demands (Sylvia & Rosenthal, 1979). Other variables that influence glucose metabolism may also become limited with age, possibly including insulin receptors and insulin regulation of glucose metabolism (Hoyer, 1995).

It can be concluded that moderate declines in glucose metabolism at the cellular level may accompany aging in some regions of the brain. However, the various studies on healthy older humans and other species that have shown no deficits in cerebral metabolism (Duara et al., 1985) suggest that fundamental impairment of energy metabolism by surviving neurons is not the rule during healthy aging—at least under resting or baseline conditions. Under stressful conditions, age effects may be more substantial, perhaps indicative of a decline in the "energy pool" available to meet high demands (Hoyer, 1995).

Glial Cells Perform a Number of Important Duties

Glia are small cells that far outnumber neurons. There are several types of glial cells serving various functions. The traditional roles of glia are the production of myelin around axons (Schwann cells in the peripheral nervous system and oligodendrocytes in the CNS), structural and physiological support for neurons (astrocytes), and immunological elimination of nonfunctioning tissue or debris and reactions to infections (microglia).

There is growing evidence that glia play additional roles as well (Sontheimer, 1995; Travis, 1994). For example, oligodendrocytes, in addition to their role in myelination, may produce neurotrophic factors, proteins needed for survival and health of neurons such as nerve growth factor (NGF). Astrocytes produce their own growth factor, glial-derived-growth factor (GDNF), which can influence the health and well-being of neurons. As discussed in chapter 13, neurotrophins may have future importance in allaying neural degeneration. Glia may also help to remove excess neurotransmitter and regulate the external milieu of neurons (e.g., by changing the concentration of important ions such as potassium). Astrocytes appear to play a role in the removal of glutamate, converting it to glutamine, which is returned to the neuron to produce more glutamate (Travis, 1994). Glutamate is an important excitatory neurotransmitter for normal brain function, but it is also an excitatory neurotoxin. That is, too much glutamate can actually damage or destroy neurons. Astrocytes may protect neurons from excitotoxicity by providing a physical buffer and/or regulation of calcium ions that enter the neurons in response to glutamate, causing damage to neurons.

The answer to the question What happens to glia in the aging brain? depends on the type of glia and other variables. Degeneration of dendrites or neurons would likely be associated with the proliferation of the phagocytic microglia, because they are involved with the cleanup of dead material. For example, Vaughan and Peters (1974) evaluated the glial cells of the aging rat cortex and found that microglia increased in density by 65%. The microglia also changed in shape from simple multipolar forms to elongated or spherical forms containing cellular debris. Perry, Matyszak, and Fearn (1993) also found evidence of increased microglia activity in old rodent brains, as did Peters, Josephson, and Vincent (1991) in monkeys.

An enhanced presence of astrocytes (gliosis), including an increase in size (hypertrophy), is a reliable occurrence in older, nonpathological brains, not to mention older brains that have been damaged in some fashion (Beach, Walker, & McGeer, 1989; Finch & Morgan, 1990; Grafton et al., 1991; Shimada, Kuwamura, Awakura, Umemura, & Itakura, 1992; van Swieten et al., 1991). More importantly, immunocytochemical staining of astrocytes shows increased labeling of *glial fibrillary acidic protein* (GFAP) in older brains (Johnson & Finch, 1996; Mann, 1997). GFAP immunolabeling is indicative of the hypertrophy associated with astrocytic responses to tissue insult. Indeed, GFAP has been proposed as a biomarker of aging. Increased GFAP occurs reliably across many species, and age-related GFAP increases can be differentiated from those associated with injury (Johnson & Finch, 1996). Thus, the activity and/or hypertrophy of astrocytes, as indicated by GFAP, may be a more cogent variable than an increase in the number of astrocytes. Indeed, there need not be an increase in the number of astrocytes in older brains in order to have a gliotic response. Although there is a strong relationship between GFAP and aging of the brain, the nature of the relationship is not yet clear. Expression of GFAP and astrocyte hypertrophy can be triggered by a number of factors including neural injury or degeneration, adrenal or gonadal steroids, neural activity, and other variables that affect brain physiology or homeostasis and are likely to accompany aging (Johnson & Finch, 1996).

Compared to microglia and astrocytes, the myelin-producing glia are more likely to be deleteriously affected with age. For example, oligoden-drocytes can suffer damage from a reduction of oxygen or blood supply (Mann, 1997), suggesting their vulnerability to metabolic deficiencies discussed earlier. Anatomical studies have demonstrated age effects in animal models. Peters (1996) evaluated oligodendrocytes in the cerebral cortex of old monkeys and observed a number of changes, such as swellings filled with pigmented inclusions, squashing together of neighboring cells, and degeneration of myelin. Morphological changes were also observed in oligodendrocytes in the cerebellum of aged rats (Monteiro, Conceicao, Roch, & Marini-Abreu, 1995). An electron microscopic study on aging rats found a decrease in mitochondria of Schwann cells, which could affect their ability to function (Choo, Malmgren, & Rosenberg, 1990). As discussed elsewhere, age-related changes in myelin are often observed in the peripheral nervous system and CNS. Thus, in contrast to astrocytes and microglia, these glial cells probably show a downward trend with age.

SUMMARY AND IMPLICATIONS

In this chapter we have seen that many bad things can happen to the nervous system as aging ensues. Neurons die and cannot be replaced, protective mechanisms like the CSF and the blood brain barrier may be compromised, neurons are hounded by various toxins, the supply of blood and metabolism of glucose and oxygen may not be optimal, and it may become more difficult for neurons and glia to carry out the many physiological activities required for proper neural functioning. What is an old person to do? Fortunately, this distressing litany is a qualified one: None of these changes are universal, inevitable, or pervasive throughout the nervous system. Indeed, the reality is that the nervous systems of many thousands of vibrant, active older persons are obviously doing quite well in directing their everyday lives. This attests to the fact that the multifaceted potential for age-related decline is often not realized, even in very old people.

Because the nervous system is a rather mysterious entity, it may help to employ an analogy to think about the way nervous systems might age. Consider a society on an isolated island, where immigration is impossible; furthermore, a potent virus has infected the entire society, rendering everyone infertile, so no new people can be added to the population.

In order to function and survive, the society must accomplish many things. To do so, it is organized into a number of specialized subsets comprised of people devoted to producing food (farmers, food processors), providing fuel (nuclear plant workers, oil drillers) and defense (the military), building and changing the environment (construction workers, engineers), obtaining information (journalists, scientists, scholars, intelligence gatherers), storing and retrieving information (librarians, computer operators, historians), ensuring health (medical and public health personnel), and modulating activity levels (entertainers, weather forecasters, drug manufacturers, bartenders). Subsets of people comprising a central and local governments, in turn, regulate and control much of these other functional subsets. The subsets of this society are specialized, but all are necessary and all must work together and interact.

Now we can sit back and watch this island society "age." In this analogy people are similar to neurons. They are organized into cooperative subsets that communicate with one another and make the whole society and infrastructure work. Our research strategy might be to monitor the age-related changes in the society's "behavior" and, at the same time, determine how the various subsets of people and governments are doing. Like neurogerontologists studying neurons, we would attempt to learn as much as possible about individual people and the way they communicate, and how all this is manifested in the aging society.

Suppose that, as the years pass, many of the societal behaviors decline: Food production has fallen off, the military is slipping, the libraries are in disrepair, and widget production is down. What can be learned about these aspects of aging by looking at the people (a.k.a. neurons)?

Let's focus on the declining widget production: Why are there no longer enough widgets to go around? First, we count the number of widget makers who are still alive and find that 10% of the widget workers have died. Is this the answer to the widget shortage? Not necessarily. If the surviving 90% are now working more skillfully or harder, or if they were overproducing to begin with, a 10% loss of workers would not account for the fewer widgets. We would have to look back at our widget data from when the society was still young to determine what the starting point was, in order to assess the age effect. Simple counting does not tell us much (unless, of course, there was a huge loss of workers).

A different possibility is that the surviving 90% are now older, perhaps ill, and not doing their jobs as efficiently as they once did. We would have to examine individuals and give them a battery of medical and physiological tests. It would be practical to test only a small sample of the large population of workers. Like any group of people, some of these workers will be very healthy, whereas others will show signs of age or fatigue to varying extents. We can't make any general statements about the condition of the workers, other than, on average, they are showing declines. But what are the implications? It may be that, even though they don't feel good, the sick workers are still coming to work and doing their job well, or that the healthier workers are picking up the slack. Unless the general population is really sick, it would be difficult to make conclusions about the impact of the health problems of individual workers.

There are numerous other things to consider. Perhaps the overall environment has changed, due to a buildup of industrial toxins and pollution, and this affects some or all of the workers. Maybe the widget workers themselves are quite healthy, but another subset upon which they depend is sick (e.g., the workers who produce raw materials); the widget workers are not being productive, but it is not their fault. Or, it may be that the general infrastructure is deteriorating, so they cannot do their job well, or that the support and advice of the central governing subset have deteriorated.

From this simple analogy it is evident that understanding the underlying factors that produce age effects are difficult to pin down. By themselves, any of the things that can go awry may have little or no effect on widget production or on the society at large. On the other hand, if problems with a single factor were severe, they could by themselves bring down the whole widget industry, and perhaps the whole society (let's assume widgets are critical to this society). At the other end of the spectrum of possibilities, there could be relatively minor dysfunction of all or most of these factors, and the combined effects could be significant.

Let us expand the analogy somewhat by supposing that there are many isolated island societies such as this one. Depending on the climate, the happenstance of environmental changes, the genetic constitution of the inhabitants, and variations in cultural and educational systems, no two of these societies will age in an identical fashion. Of the various things that can go wrong, one would expect that no two societies will have the same aging profile. They may show similar changes in "behavior" (e.g., most may exhibit a decline in widget production), but there may be many different combinations of factors that are responsible. It would be impossible to make very many generalized statements about the aging of these societies.

There is no question that the first step in understanding aging of either a society or a nervous system is to describe the many changes that occur with age. Great progress has been made in this regard, as is evident from the small sample of research reviewed in this chapter. However, neurogerontology must go beyond the description of lost or ailing neuronal and support systems, and ultimately understand what causes the changes that do occur, why they vary from person to person, and how all of the events interact with one another. The ultimate question is, How do the changes in neuronal physiology affect the ability of the nervous system to function properly? In the next two chapters we begin to examine this question.

APPENDIX: COUNTING NEURONS IN THE BRAIN

It is impossible to count all of the neurons even in a restricted area of the brain. What most researchers have traditionally done is to microscopically examine sample portions of brain tissue and calculate the *packing density* of neurons—the average number of neurons per area of brain tissue section. The volume of the brain structure being sampled is also determined (usually by multiplying the two-dimensional areas of brain sections times the thickness of each brain section times the total number of brain sections containing the structure). The total number of neurons can be estimated by multiplying the density times the volume.

Some studies have reported only the packing density, making it impossible to determine how much the total number has changed. This can be a serious limitation. As shown in Figure 3.6, changes in density do not accurately reflect neuron number unless the volume is taken into account. And estimating the volume of a brain region is difficult if the structure

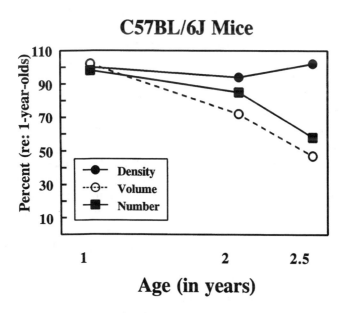

FIGURE 3.6   The relationship between volume, packing density, and cell number. These data are from the octopus cell area of C57 mice. The number of neurons declines in old mice. However, if the packing density alone were examined, there would be no evidence of cell loss. It is only when the volumetric shrinkage is taken into account that the true picture emerges. Data taken from Willott and Bross (1990).

is irregularly shaped or if its appearance changes with age. Furthermore, young brains may shrink more than old ones when prepared for certain types of histologic analysis, giving the illusion that the packing density of neurons is greater in the young brains (Haug, 1984). Obviously, it is important to have good measures of both neuron density and volume to estimate the number of neurons.

Anatomical studies may also be subject to biased sampling of the neurons that are counted. In microscopic sections, smaller neurons are more difficult to find and identify as neurons. If neurons tend to shrink with age, as they often do (e.g., Terry, De Teresa, & Hansen, 1987), older brains would have more small neurons, and the overall packing density could be underestimated. Also, larger neurons are more likely to be split in half by the microtome knife used to cut brain tissue sections for microscopic examination (small cells are more likely to reside completely within the tissue section). In a histological slide, a split cell looks the same as a whole cell, so more half-cells would be counted as whole cells if the neurons were larger. This could result in an overestimation of the packing density in younger brains if they have larger neurons. For these reasons, an apparent loss of neurons in older subjects could be due to smaller size, not to a true loss of neurons.

There has been a trend in recent years to use "unbiased" stereological counting methods, which are designed to overcome these problems (see Morrison & Hof, 1997; Saper, 1996; West, 1993). A caveat is in order with respect to stereological methods, however. Although they certainly have advantages and should be used, it should not be concluded that these methods *necessarily* provide more accurate data than older studies. Many older studies have taken care to determine both volume and packing density, made allowances for split cells and other technical pitfalls, and sampled neurons of all sizes thoroughly (and in some brain regions, neurons are of similar size and do not shrink with age). Thus, many older studies are undoubtedly reliable. By the same token, "unbiased" methods are still subject to sampling errors, poor tissue fixation, poor staining of neurons, improperly delineated boundaries of brain regions, and poor experimenter technique. Furthermore, all histological methods can be subject to the problems with human autopsy material discussed earlier. One gets the impression in reading some recent literature reviews that older studies should be discounted and we should rely exclusively on the findings of stereological studies. This would be a mistake. Stereological methods are a welcome development but not a cure-all.

4

Principles of Neural Communication and Their Neurogerontological Implications

The *raison d'être* of the nervous system is to accomplish the seven basic functions described in chapter 1. To do so, neurons must communicate with one another. We shall now review the basics of how this feat is accomplished and how aging can get in the way. As in earlier chapters, discussions of neurogerontological issues are integrated with a brief review of basic neurobiology. Readers with a background in neuroscience can skip the introductory comments.

ACTION POTENTIALS AND AXONS

By way of analogy, axons can be thought of as the cables by which neurons communicate with one another over distances, much as the outgoing cable of a telegraph. In order for neurons to send messages down their axons, an important question had to be answered by the evolutionary process: How could messages be carried quickly, reliably, and precisely using a form of energy that is readily available and can be installed into animals (using genetic instructions) from available resources? Although electricity might provide an answer (as it does in telegraphs), the type of electricity we are used to (electron-generated) would have required metal wires and generators, things that only existed after humans invented them millions of years after the first animals appeared on the planet. Fortunately, there is another type of electricity that is much easier to produce and harness.

Instead of relying on electrons (like our modern-day electrical devices), ions can also work. An ion is an atom or molecule that has an electrical charge, and ions can be made by simply dissolving chemicals in water. Drop some NaCl (table salt) into water, and it breaks up into sodium (Na^+) and chloride (Cl^-) ions. Na^+ ions have a positive charge, and Cl^- ions, a negative charge. Other important ions include potassium (K^+) and calcium (Ca^{++}). Ions, like electrons, are charged, and they can move into and out of neurons, creating the electrical signals used by the nervous system. Because the world was and is full of the needed ions, early evolution could harness this type of chemically generated electricity for use in neural communication.

For reasons that need not concern us here, entry of Na^+ from the fluid around neurons, through the neuron's cell membrane, generates a sort of electrical chain reaction that arises in the soma and travels to the end of the neuron's axon. Think of a row of dominoes falling or a fuse ignited at one end, burning toward the other end. By producing their own pulselike electrical nerve impulses (action potentials) and conveying them via their axons, neurons can send messages to one another. Information flows to, from, and within the brain in trains of action potentials carried by axons (it should be noted that dendrites of some neurons are also capable of conducting action potentials from one part of the neuron to another, but their functional significance is still a matter of debate; see Johnston, Magee, Colbert, & Christie, 1996).

Ion Channels in the Neuron's Membrane Are Responsible for the Bioelectrical Activity

The full dynamics of action potentials involve the movement not only of sodium ions but of chloride and potassium as well. These ions have a tendency to move into or out of a neuron because of the different concentrations of ions and positive and negative charges on either side of neuronal membranes. Because the ions carry electrical charges, they are key players in the generation of action potentials. The major factor that determines whether the ions actually do enter or leave the neuron is the permeability of the neuron's membrane for each ion—whether or not the membrane will let the ions pass through. The ions have their own special channels—rather complex "pores" that can open and close to varying extents—and this determines the electrical properties of the neurons. Thus, if the channels for sodium open up, Na^+ enters the neurons and an action potential can occur. However, if channels for K^+ or Cl^- open up, these ions can move, thereby being able to exert their influence. Permeability for K^+ or Cl^- makes it more difficult for an action potential to occur. Thus, the relative permeabilities of a neuron's membrane to Na^+, K^+, or Cl^- determine whether an action potential is triggered.

When everything is working properly, the opening and closing of various ion channels work together, generating an action potential, then stopping the process to ensure a discrete impulse and get the membrane back to its resting state and ready to generate another action potential. Any factor that interferes with the proper operation of the appropriate ion channels can create problems for neural communication.

Is aging one of those factors? In general, cell membranes in many types of tissue, including those of neurons, accrue defects with age (Naeim & Walford, 1985). There is some evidence to indicate that ionic mechanisms generating action potentials can be altered, even in healthy older animals. Gyenes, Lustyik, Nagy, Jeney, and Nagy (1984) presented evidence for decreased permeability of neural membranes to K^+ in the cortex of old rats. Scott, Leu, and Cinader (1988) measured electrical properties of mouse neurons (from the dorsal root ganglion) in cell cultures. They found that cells obtained from old mice had decreased electrical excitability and longer duration action potentials; the return of the membrane potential to its resting state was altered as well. (The resting potential of a neuron is the voltage across the membrane in which the inside of the neuron is negative with respect to the outside; a normal resting potential is required for a normal action potential to occur.) They interpreted this as a change in sodium and potassium activity across the membrane. Using an *in vitro* slice preparation from the brain of aged rats, Cepeda, Walsh, Hull, Buchwald, and Levine (1992) found that many neurons had decreased electrical excitability that interfered with optimal generation of action potentials. However, the duration and some other properties of action potentials were normal.

As these examples suggest, there may be alterations in neuronal membrane properties and action potentials, but these are not likely to be the same for all neural tissue.

Calcium

Some age-related changes in membrane potentials appear to involve an augmented role of calcium ions. Like Na^+, Ca^{++} is also found in high concentration outside the neurons, and like Na^+, when given the chance to enter the neuron by the opening of their channels in the membrane, they enter the neuron. Experiments using *in vitro* tissue culture and slice preparations of hippocampus have shown that calcium action potentials and other electrical influences of calcium ions become more prominent with age, and this is associated with an increase in the number of calcium channels in the neuronal membrane (Campbell, Hao, Thibault, Blalock, & Landfield, 1996; Landfield, 1996). Researchers have also observed differences in membrane calcium currents in neurons of the medial septal nucleus and diagonal band (Murchison & Griffith, 1996). Not only would increased calcium influx be expected to alter a neuron's electrical signaling properties, it might be associated with other cellular changes involving calcium. For example, the entry of Ca^{++} is a critical step in the release of neurotransmitters, and this role may be altered with aging (Michaelis, Foster, & Jayawickreme, 1992). Moreover, the risk of cell damage from excessive intracellular calcium (see chapter 3) might be increased.

An Active Ion Pumping System Maintains Ionic Balance Across the Membrane

The maintenance over time of the balance between Na^+ and K^+ inside and outside neurons is accomplished with an active (i.e., using energy from ATP) sodium-potassium "pump." The pump transports Na^+ out of the neurons and K^+ into the neuron to help maintain the proper concentrations and resting potential. Some evidence indicates that ionic pumping may become less efficient with age. Tanaka and Ando (1990) studied membrane potentials in tissue obtained from mouse brains and observed a decline in the resting membrane voltage that was correlated with age. They concluded that decreased activity of the sodium-potassium pump was probably responsible. The same researchers (Tanaka & Ando, 1992) also found that the number of membrane pump sites decreased in very old mice. Calcium pumps exist as well, and evidence has been obtained that their ability to remove calcium from neurons can be diminished with age (see Michaelis et al., 1992). These studies raise the possibility that neuronal physiology could be affected by age-related decreases in ionic pump activity.

Age-Related Changes in Axons and Conduction Speed

Action potentials in axons are the only means by which neurons can communicate rapidly over distance, and it is here that a limitation of ion-generated signals becomes evident. Whereas electron-generated electricity travels extremely fast (practically instantaneously), electricity generated by ionic movement along axons is slow, moving at a speed no faster than 120 meters per second. Therefore, nervous systems cannot act instantaneously. For example, when one is startled by a loud sound, it takes about 10 msec between the noise and the behavioral response; a portion of this time is taken up by the action potentials traveling between the inner ear (where the noise is registered) and the muscles (which contract to produce the startle response). Thus, generation and conduction of action potentials are determinants of the speed at which a nervous system can operate.

Two variables regulate the speed of action potential conduction. First is the diameter of axons. Because of basic electrical properties of cables in general, action potentials travel faster in larger axons. Second is the influence of the insulating lipid substance, myelin, found in sheaths around many axons. Myelination increases the speed and efficiency of the conduction of action potentials, much as plastic insulation is beneficial for the conduction of electricity in wires (although there are gaps or nodes along the myelin sheath that are necessary for neural conduction but would be not be beneficial for electron current). The fastest axons are large and myelinated, and anything that results in thinner or less myelinated axons would interfere with fast conduction.

A number of studies of conduction speed have been performed on axons in the peripheral nervous system, because the peripheral nerves are accessible for measurements. This work has provided much evidence that axonal conduction speed often decreases with age (e.g., Dorfman & Bosley, 1979; MacKenzie & Phillips, 1981). As might be expected, research has also shown a decrease in the average diameter of axons and some loss or alteration in myelin surrounding the axons, as well as the disappearance of some axons (Brody & Vijayashanker, 1977; Spencer & Ochoa, 1981).

Decreases in axon diameter and changes in myelination are also observed in the CNS (Brody & Vijayashankar, 1977; Zhang, Goto, & Zhou, 1995). Some studies have found that changes in myelin accompany aging. For instance, Morell, Greenfield, Constantino-Cellarine, and Wisniewski (1972) and Sun and Samorajski (1972) found that myelin continued to be produced during adulthood in mice, but the composition of the myelin (and perhaps its effects on neural conduction) changed. Peters and colleagues (1996) observed a breakdown of myelin around axons in the brains of old rhesus monkeys, and this was correlated with cognitive changes. Axons can also be afflicted with *neuroaxonal dystrophy,* a condition whose prevalence increases with age in humans and other species (Brody & Vijayashankar, 1977): Axons in various brain regions, but most notably in the gracile nucleus in the brainstem, develop ovoid swellings that presumably affect conduction of action potentials.

As mentioned earlier, it is typically the case that some shrinkage occurs in old brains, and much of this is due to changes in the white matter, the regions occupied primarily by myelinated axons (which provide the whitish appearance). Whereas shrinkage of white matter can be caused by various types of pathology (infarcts, disease, etc.), attrition of myelinated axons probably contributes to varying extents (e.g., Meier-Ruge et al., 1992). The functional consequences of changes in myelin in aging humans are not well understood. However, given that efficient, fast communication among axons is presumably important for optimal brain activity, even relatively subtle changes in myelin could have deleterious effects on the aging brain (e.g., Peters et al., 1996).

Most Communication Between Neurons Occurs at Synapses

When an action potential arrives at the end of an axon branch, its journey ends abruptly because the axon terminal is not connected to the next neuron. (There are exceptions—electrical synapses—but these are not known to be altered with age and will not be discussed here.) The action potential gets short-circuited—it cannot jump the cleft to get to the next neuron's dendrites (this would be like pulling two electric wires apart). Instead of jumping the gap, the action potential causes a small amount of chemical neurotransmitter to be released from the axon terminal, where it quickly diffuses across the synaptic cleft to react with receptors in the postsynaptic dendrite's cell membrane. The reaction between neurotransmitter and receptor causes changes in the postsynaptic neuron.

Fast and slow synapses operate on different principles.   The fastest are *ionotropic synapses.* They act quickly and briefly (milliseconds), as the presynaptically released neurotransmitter molecules cross the synaptic cleft, attach themselves to receptors in the postsynaptic membrane, and quickly open channels for ions (Na^+, K^+, Cl^-). The occurrence of excitation or inhibition is determined by which channels are opened. If, for example, permeability to Na^+ ions is increased by opening Na^+ channels (which facilitates the firing of action potentials), excitation results. If permeability channels for K+ and/or Cl- open, inhibition results, because permeability for these ions tends to prevent the firing of action potentials. Ionotropic receptors can be found for neurotransmitters including acetylcholine (Ach), gamma-aminobutyric acid (GABA), glycine, serotonin, and glutamate.

Some synapses act relatively slowly (e.g., hundreds of milliseconds) and can produce changes in the physiology of the postsynaptic neuron lasting for seconds or much longer. Synapses such as this initiate a sequence of metabolic reactions in the postsynaptic neurons using second messengers, molecules such as cyclic adenosine monophosphate (cAMP) and the gas nitric oxide (NO). *Metabotropic receptors* activate second messengers through the action of *guanosine nucleotide-binding protein*, or G-protein. The family of G-protein-coupled receptors includes α- and β-adrenergic receptors, GABA, glutamate, serotonin, and neuropeptides (note that the same neurotransmitters can have either ionotropic or metabotropic receptors). Other types of receptors that initiate a sequence of "slow" events in the postsynaptic cell are activated by hormones, peptide neuromodulators, and growth factors. The slow synapses can regulate the internal properties of neurons as well as open or close ion channels. The intracellular events that are associated with slow-acting synapses and second messenger systems are numerous, complex, and well beyond the scope of this discussion. Suffice it to say that postsynaptic cellular activity can be altered with age in ways that could affect the efficacy of transmission at slow synapses (e.g., Araki, Kato, Fujiwara, & Itoyama, 1995; Igwe & Filla, 1995; Joseph, Cutler, & Roth, 1993; Sugawa et al., 1996; Young et al., 1991).

The synaptic delay refers to the time it takes to accomplish transmission from one neuron to the next. Obviously, the longer the synaptic delay or the greater the number of synapses in a neural circuit, the longer it takes for the nervous system to accomplish a task. It takes more time to engage complex neural circuits because there are more neurons, which means a greater total length of axons (longer total action potential conduction time) and more synapses (longer aggregate of synaptic delays).

Some Loss of Synapses Can Accompany Aging

A number of research groups have found evidence of reduced densities of synapses in aged brain tissue. Common techniques are to examine the brain tissue with electron microscopy or immunostain the tissue for *synaptophysin*, a protein found in presynaptic terminals. Using these techniques, fewer synapses are evident in various regions of healthy older brains, with the situation being significantly worse in subjects suffering from dementia or cognitive decline (Chen, Masliah, Mallory, & Gage, 1995; Eastwood, Burnet, McDonald, Clinton, & Harrison, 1994; Liu, Erikson, & Brun, 1996; Saito et al., 1994; Scheff, Sparks, & Price, 1996). A large body of research has evaluated synaptic markers for specific neurotransmitters, including measures of presynaptic components (e.g., concentration of the neurotransmitter or enzymes involved with synthesis) and postsynaptic components (e.g., number of receptors for a transmitter, stimulation of second messengers). Substantial variance exists in the research findings, depending on species, brain regions, and other (often unknown) variables. Nevertheless, the majority of studies report some loss of synapses or diminished signs of synaptic activity in various brain regions in healthy aged animals (Morgan & May, 1990; Rogers & Bloom, 1985).

Considering the fact that synapses are the primary site of communication among neurons, one must suspect that a moderate attrition of synapses contributes to age-related changes in brain function observed in healthy older people (discussed in later chapters), let alone those suffering from neurodegenerative disease. However, as the next section indicates, we have a long way to go before we completely understand how synaptic activity is altered with age.

Three Factors That Conspire to Make It Virtually Impossible to Tell the Complete Story About Synapses and Aging

Because the mechanisms and processes associated with synapses are so complex, we may never understand all of the ins and outs of how the brain works, let alone how they change with age. Consideration of three factors provides a sense of the challenge to neurogerontology.

1. A variety of chemical neurotransmitters and postsynaptic receptors are employed at different synapses. The sheer number of chemicals that are believed to act as neurotransmitters in one part of the brain or another is large: dopamine, norepinephrine (noradrenalin), serotonin, histamine, Ach, GABA, glutamate, glycine, taurine, beta endorphin, and many others. This situation is further complicated by the fact that postsynaptic membranes can have a variety of different receptors for the same neurotransmitter. For example, the neurotransmitter serotonin (5-HT) has at least seven "families" of receptors (5-HT$_1$ to 5-HT$_7$), and within these, there are further subtypes (e.g., 5-HT$_{1A}$ through 5-HT$_{1F}$); more 5-HT receptor types are likely to be added to the list. The various receptor subtypes differ with respect to the drugs that affect them. It is certainly the case that the various neurotransmitter systems and receptor types do not all exhibit the same magnitudes, time courses, or directions of age effects (e.g., Morgan & May, 1990; Rogers & Bloom, 1985). Thus, understanding the complete story of aging and the brain will require an understanding of many smaller stories—as many as there are neurotransmitter and receptor systems. What is more, each of these may exhibit a different aging profile when one compares different types of neurons or parts of the brain, even in the same individual.

2. Neurotransmission is a complex, dynamic process. Many interconnected steps are involved in the transfer of information at synapses. The neurotransmitter molecules must first be manufactured or synthesized from precursor substances under the guidance of various enzymes, typically a very complex process that differs greatly from neurotransmitter to neurotransmitter. Then, upon the arrival of an action potential, the neurotransmitter molecules (usually stored in presynaptic vesicles) must be released in the proper amounts, the latter process involving the entry of calcium ions. The released molecules must cross the synaptic cleft and react with the appropriate receptors in the postsynaptic neuron's membrane. The outcomes of this reaction (e.g., change in ionic permeability or modification of intracellular physiology) must unfold in an effective manner. Finally, the effects of the neurotransmitter on the postsynaptic neuron must be stopped or deactivated in order to precisely control the timing of the interneuronal signals and ready the synapse for the arrival of the next action potential. Obviously, if problems in any of these steps were to accompany aging, the older brain could be affected negatively (see Figure 4.1).

The dynamics of synaptic activity make it very difficult for researchers to make solid conclusions about age-related changes. It is not sufficient to simply assay the amount of a particular transmitter in old subjects (not technically difficult) because the balance among the various steps may hold the key to functional changes (e.g., the neurotransmitters, enzymes

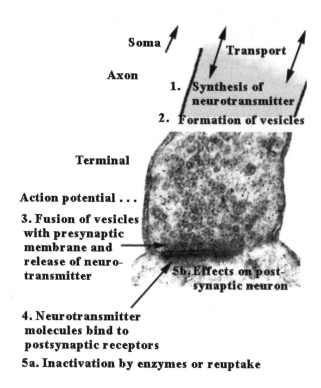

Soma

Transport

Axon

1. Synthesis of neurotransmitter

2. Formation of vesicles

Terminal

Action potential . . .

3. Fusion of vesicles with presynaptic membrane and release of neuro-transmitter

5b. Effects on post-synaptic neuron

4. Neurotransmitter molecules bind to postsynaptic receptors

5a. Inactivation by enzymes or reuptake

FIGURE 4.1 An electron micrograph showing a synapse. Neurotransmitter is synthesized within the neuron, much of this involving transport of substances from the soma to the axon terminal. The axon's terminal is packed with small, round synaptic vesicles, which store neurotransmitter. The arrival of an action potential is associated with the release of neurotransmitter molecules from the vesicles, where they cross the synaptic cleft to the postsynaptic receptors. After this, neurotransmitter activity is terminated by enzymes or reuptake into the terminal. Micrograph courtesy of Jeremy Turner.

that synthesize or break down the neurotransmitters, receptors for the neurotransmitters, processes within the neuron that respond to the transmitter-receptor reaction, etc.). For example, an increase in the levels of a neurotransmitter might indicate an overactive system that is producing extra transmitter, an inability to break down released neurotransmitter molecules, or a system that cannot use its transmitter because its receptors are impaired. Thus, it is often difficult to interpret experimental findings.

Ach, a neurotransmitter in several brain circuits, serves as an example to impart a sense of the types of experiments that are performed and some of the problems in interpreting them in the context of aging (see Rogers & Bloom, 1985, for a detailed review of this literature). Ach is synthesized from choline, which is taken into the neuron by presynaptic terminals, where it combines with coenzyme A, and catalyzed by choline acetyltransferase (ChAT). There is evidence that the uptake of choline is reduced in the aged rat brain, at least under certain conditions. However, there may also be fewer cholinergic neurons in the older brain (i.e., neurons using Ach as their transmitter), and this could confound the measurement of choline uptake for a sample of brain tissue (rather than per capita changes in individual neurons). A reduction in brain ChAT activity has also been reported in aged rodents and humans by some researchers. However, others have reported no age effects for ChAT, and there appear to be individual differences in humans. Thus, it appears that the synthesis of Ach, and therefore the amount available for use by the brain, is reduced in some older individuals, although the cause(s) of this deficit may be difficult to interpret.

If it is established that Ach synthesis becomes diminished with age, can it be assumed that there is less Ach available to neurons? Not necessarily. Reduced synthesis could be counterbalanced by reduced enzymatic breakdown of Ach after it is released. The breakdown of Ach is accomplished by the enzyme acetylcholinesterase (AchE); there appear to be some age-related changes in AchE activity, but they are complex and not yet clear. The actions of Ach can also be affected independently of synthesis or amounts of Ach if some postsynaptic receptors are lost with aging. There is good evidence that the amount of Ach that can react (bind) with receptors is reduced in old age, most probably because of a loss of active receptor sites. This view is supported by experiments using iontophoresis, a technique by which Ach is applied directly to neurons with fine-tipped glass micropipets. The responses normally evoked by Ach can be diminished in the neurons of old animals.

It should be clear that dealing with even one neurotransmitter is a difficult task and that many problems can arise in interpreting experimental findings (see also Morgan & May, 1990). Multiply this by the number of possible brain transmitters, and the challenge of this area of research is evident.

3. Many factors can alter or modulate synaptic activity. The mechanisms that control neurotransmitter activity are, in turn, influenced by a variety of other microenvironmental variables. As discussed in chapter 3, the activity of glia, the blood-brain barrier, the composition and amount of cerebrospinal fluid, the metabolism of glucose, and other variables influence neuronal physiology, and these are all subject to modification during aging. Presumably the effects are often felt at the synapses due to alterations of the biochemical microenvironment and/or physiological processes involved in the various components of synaptic transmission.

A related issue has to do with mechanisms that are designed to dynamically regulate or modulate synaptic activity in the young, healthy brain. Some neurons have widely branched axons designed to influence the activity of many other neurons. For example, the neurotransmitter serotonin is released by neurons whose cell bodies are concentrated in the *raphe nuclei* of the lower brainstem, and these neurons influence many behaviors, such as eating and aggressive behavior. Serotonergic systems have been shown to exhibit some changes with age (Ko, King, Gordon, & Crisp, 1997; Meister, Johnson, & Ulfhake, 1995; Rodriguez-Gomez, de la Roza, Machado, & Cano, 1995; Rogers & Bloom, 1985), and there are indications that these changes might influence the physiology and synaptic activity of other neurons in a variety of ways. For example, Richter-Levin and Segal (1996) presented evidence that treating old rats with a precursor of serotonin (which would increase serotonin levels) reduced spatial learning deficits in old rats. They suggested that this was, in part, due to the modulation of Ach synapses by serotonin, which had declined with age. Another study examined the role of serotonin in modulating daily (circadian) rhythms (Penev, Turek, Wallen, & Zee, 1997). The results suggested that serotonergic modulation in old rats was deficient. Finally, serotonin's modulation of certain neuronal membranes' capacity to incorporate arachidonic acid (involved in second messenger activity) was diminished in old rats (Strosznadjder, Samochocki, & Duran, 1994). It would seem that the fallout from age-related changes in a system such as this would complicate things considerably (see also chapter 10).

Neuromodulators can also complicate the story. Neuromodulators are similar to neurotransmitters in that they are chemicals (often peptides; chains of amino acids) that are released by neurons and affect the activity of neurons. However, neuromodulators can diffuse to other neurons and, rather than having a direct neurotransmitterlike effect on postsynaptic neurons, they facilitate or impede (modulate) the synaptic activity. Neuromodulation is typically slow and long-lasting (as in the slow synapses discussed above). By releasing neuromodulators as well as neurotransmitters, neurons can achieve more subtle and complex modes of communication with their neighbors. Hormones are like neuromodulators in that they can also modify neuronal physiology and synaptic activity in a variety of ways. It follows that age effects in the production, release, membrane receptors, and/or intracellular activity of neuromodulators and hormones could "modulate the modulators." Such effects, perhaps interacting with changes in the neurotransmitter systems per se, could generate extreme mischief at synapses.

Dendrites Are the Key (But Not the Only) Sites of Synapses

In the "traditional" depiction of the synapse, the presynaptic element (releasing neurotransmitter) is the terminal of an axon branch, and the dendrite is the postsynaptic element (possessing the receptors). Such *axodendritic* synapses are very prevalent and thoroughly studied, and we shall focus on this family of synapses. But it should be understood that there are a variety of other arrangements including *dendrodendritic* synapses, where other dendrites actually are presynaptic, *axoaxonic* (axon terminals synapsing on other axons), *axosomatic* (axon terminals upon a neuron's soma), and others.

The primary function of dendrites is, indeed, to receive excitatory and inhibitory synapses and contribute to the integration of these inputs to determine their effects on the postsynaptic neuron. For example, will the excitatory synapses on a dendrite have a greater influence than the inhibitory synapses, thereby triggering an action potential in the postsynaptic neuron? Or will inhibitory synapses prevail, preventing an action potential from firing? The relative effectiveness of the various excitatory and inhibitory synaptic inputs to a postsynaptic neuron is largely determined by their position on the dendritic tree. For example, a synapse located on a portion of the postsynaptic neuron's dendritic tree close to the cell body and initial axon segment (where action potentials are typically initiated) is likely to be more effective than a synapse on a distant, small dendritic branch. Thus, the size, shape, orientation, and complexity of the neuron's dendritic tree (and the location of the synaptic inputs on the tree) are key to the integration process.

There are huge variations in size and shape of dendritic trees and arrangement of synaptic inputs along the dendritic branches. It has been estimated that the human nervous system contains about 10,000 distinct morphological types of neurons based on characteristics of the dendritic trees (Johnston et al., 1996). It is intuitively obvious that, if the number, arrangement, and complexity of dendritic branches and their synaptic inputs determine the information-processing capacity of a neuron, significant damage to dendritic branches with aging could have negative consequences. It is also intuitive that the finely constructed branches of a dendritic tree might be especially fragile when it comes to the various insults associated with aging (much as the smaller branches of a tree might be damaged in a hailstorm, while the tree itself survives). Unfortunately, the latter intuition is supported by a good deal of evidence showing that neurons in older brains often exhibit a decrease in the number of dendritic branches (e.g., Anderson & Rutledge, 1996; Andrews, Li, Halliwell, & Cowen, 1994; Coleman & Flood, 1987; Cruz-Sanchez, Cardozo, & Tolosa, 1995; Duara et al., 1985; Mervis, 1981; Scheibel, Lindsay, Tomiyasu, & Scheibel, 1975; Willott & Bross, 1990). On the positive side, normal-looking dendritic trees are often present in very old brains, and dendritic growth and modification occurs throughout life in some types of neurons (see chapter 13).

Specific examples of altered dendritic trees will be discussed in later chapters, when relevant to a particular topic. At this time, we focus on one particular feature of many dendrites, the spine. Spines are the smallest appendages of dendrites and are particularly vulnerable to age-related damage. For example, Peters and Vaughan (1981) studied cortical pyramidal cells in rats. In young rats, cortical pyramidal cells have a characteristic form, with extensive dendritic trees that are covered with spines. In very old rats obvious changes occur in the dendrites, with reduction in dendritic lengths by up to 50% and a loss of one third of the dendritic spines on the remaining dendrites (not to mention 100% spine loss on dendrites that disappeared). Other studies have also reported significant loss of dendritic spines in various species (Anderson & Rutledge, 1996; Cruz-Sanchez et al., 1995; Jacobs, Driscoll, & Schall, 1997; McGinn, Henry, & Coss, 1984; Mervis, 1981; Ruiz-Marcos, Sanchez-Toscano, & Munoz-Cueto, 1992; Uemura, 1985). Figure 4.2 shows examples of spine loss from cortical neurons of old humans.

The relationship between aging and dendritic spines is an extremely important topic because spines are the sites of many synapses and may serve multiple functions. An understanding of the functions of dendritic spines under normal conditions may provide important insights into certain age effects. That is, can loss or deformity of spines account for certain

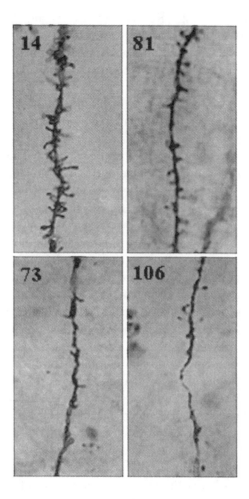

FIGURE 4.2 Dendritic spines in cortical dendrites of young and old humans. The number indicates subject age in years. The 14-year-old's dendrite is covered with spines, whereas those of the older subjects have fewer and less prominent spines. Courtesy of Dr. Bob Jacobs, Colorado College.

changes in brain function? Reviews by Harris and Kater (1994) and
Shepherd (1996) summarize current knowledge about dendritic spines,
and these reviews suggest a number of possible functions of spines and
allow us to speculate about the consequences of spine loss or damage
that accompany aging.

Spines come in a variety of shapes, often with a "head" and narrower
"neck," which is connected to the parent dendrite. It is generally assumed
that dendritic spines play an important role in the processing of information
by neurons. At the most basic level, they provide numerous sites for
synaptic input to dendrites. The relative strength of excitatory and inhibitory synaptic input to a neuron determines whether that neuron will itself
produce action potentials that can signal other neurons (the process of
integration). The majority of excitatory synapses in the CNS probably
occur on spines, usually with only a single synaptic input per spine (with
glutamate being the predominant excitatory neurotransmitter at the spine
synapses). When inhibitory synapses are present, they are on spine stems
or on dendrites per se. This arrangement seems to be ideal for the process
of integration of different inputs to a neuron. Indeed, neurons with dendritic
spines tend to be the principle input/output neurons for a given brain
region—the neurons that integrate input and send action potentials to
other parts of the brain (nonspiny neurons tend to be the local interneurons).
It seems likely that the ability of neurons to process synaptic inputs from
various sources would be impaired if spines were lost to aging.

Spines appear to play an important role in certain types of neural
plasticity associated with learning, such as long-term potentiation (LTP).
As discussed in chapter 8, LTP and other types of neural plasticity are
thought to require the simultaneous synaptic activation of spines to establish an association between events (a requirement of learning that two
events are related to one another). Studies have shown increased numbers
of spines or changes in spine shape (probably representing the growth of
new synapses) after learning and other salient environmental events. If
spines are required for certain types of learning, might a reduced number
of spines limit learning in an aged brain?

The properties of spines are likely to alter the effectiveness of synapses
in various ways, as indicated by the following three examples. (1) Thin
spine necks have a very high electrical resistance (electrical resistance is
inversely related to the diameter of a conducting element). According to
Ohm's law, voltage is increased when the electrical resistance is high
(voltage = current × resistance). The high resistance of spines could

therefore provide a mechanism for amplifying synaptic potentials (voltage). (2) Another electrical property of spines is their very limited capacitance (the ability to store electrical charge). Small capacitance allows neural membranes to respond rapidly to excitatory synaptic inputs (voltage changes are not slowed by the process of storing charge). Therefore, spines could make it easier for neurons to process very rapid inputs. (3) It has been hypothesized that spines could act as a coincidence detector (an AND gate). Suppose that synaptic excitation of one spine was not sufficient to affect a neuron, but the simultaneous activation of two spines was effective because the electrical changes in two nearby spines could summate. A coincidence detector like this could be sensitive to very small differences in the timing of synaptic inputs. These three examples suggest that a loss of dendritic spines could affect the amplitude of synaptic inputs, the speed at which inputs could be processed, and the precision of temporal processing by neurons.

In addition to these sorts of computational functions, neuroscientists have nominated spines for other roles as well. For example, spines may also be sites for modulation of neurons by hormones or drugs. They may function as compartments for biochemical isolation and/or specificity of biochemical action; devices for creating a microenvironment that can be affected by synaptic input and in turn affect the parent dendrite, while being isolated from nearby areas. Spines could also permit increased concentrations of important substances such as second messengers.

One putative function of dendritic spines with especially important neurogerontological implications is their role in preventing damage to neurons from excitotoxicity associated with glutamatergic synapses. It has been hypothesized that the spine might function as a protective compartment, buffering the parent dendrite against the toxic influx of calcium ions at glutamatergic synapses. The compartmentalization of calcium ions could allow high concentrations in the small-volume environment of spines to be more easily lowered by appropriate cellular mechanisms (endoplasmic reticulum and calcium buffers). Thus, spines might help to protect dendrites from changes that would be pathological.

In this regard, spines appear to play an important role in certain brain disorders. For example, spines are absent or distorted in the cerebral cortex and hippocampus of people with mental retardation, epileptic seizures, and neuropathology associated with hypoxia, ischemia, or stroke. It seems feasible then, that age-related loss of spines could exacerbate, mimic, or increase risks associated with disorders such as these. However, it can be difficult to determine where the vicissitudes of spines fit into cause-and-effect scenarios. As might be expected from their front-line position with respect to glutamatergic synapses, spines appear to be vulnerable to damage associated with excitotoxicity. Thus, the loss of spines in neurological disorders or aging might reflect casualties in the battle against excitotoxicity. On the other hand, if other variables (e.g., gene expression, changes in metabolism) had a primary effect on spines (irrespective of excitotoxicity), spine loss could reflect another pathogenic mechanism. In either case, the loss of spines could, in turn, lead to additional problems by disrupting any of the functions just summarized. Spine loss may reflect either cause or effect, or a combination of the two.

SUMMARY AND CONCLUSIONS

The isolated island analogy used in chapter 3, where people played the role of neurons, can be applied here as well. Recall that we were attempting to understand the various possible reasons for the age-related decline in widget production. Variables such as the loss or illness of workers were considered, but another possibility is that many of the workers just don't communicate that well anymore. They might be losing their hearing (input) or voices (output), for example. This would disrupt the efficiency of widget factories, as well as the ability of other population subsets to interact with them, including the central government's widget regulatory board. As gerontological researchers, we would have to test the communication skills (sending and receiving) of a large sample of workers, and also know who is communicating with whom. This is quite a difficult task, particularly because the society is multilingual and multiethnic, with the rules of communications varying from place to place (like synapses in the nervous system, which use different neurotransmitters and receptors). It is possible that if only one ethnic/language group were especially devastated by sickness or death, the whole widget-producing system could be brought down. Alternatively, the loss might not be noticed, depending on the contribution of the ailing group or the ability to switch to speakers of another language to get the job done.

Indeed, the complexity of the problem is even greater than that posed by merely evaluating the mortality and morbidity of the population (refer to chapter 3); now we must understand the consequences with respect to communication among diverse and widely distributed communities of individuals. Trying to do this for the entire population and all of the aspects of each society is beyond herculean and may never be realized. A more reasonable strategy is to cull out small bits of the goings-on and focus on them: We could learn as much as possible about communication in widget making and home in on its various components to see if and how these are affected with aging. A highly focused approach, of course, is the one that neurogerontologists must take in studying the aging nervous system. Ultimately, the pieces will be put together.

Up to this point, we have reviewed the basics of neuroanatomy, neurobiology, and neurophysiology and the various troubles that can arise with aging. Yet to be addressed is the issue of how these features are used by the nervous system to process information, the topic of the next chapter.

5

Information Processing by the Nervous System

The anatomical structures and physiological mechanisms described in chapters 3 and 4 provide the neural infrastructure to support the constant processing of information carried out by the nervous system. Neural information processing comes in many varieties. For example, the raw physical data of the outside world must be transformed or coded (i.e., processed) into trains of action potentials as they enter the nervous system. Here, further processing occurs when the coded data are routed, recoded, and reworked into various formats used for identification, evaluation, streamlining or embellishment, interpretation, integration with other incoming and stored information, storage in memory, and generation of appropriate behavior. Much of the "information" has to do with events that we are not aware of, such as the monitoring of vital functions and automatic reflexes; at the other end of the awareness spectrum, the neurophysiological substrates of "self-generated" thoughts and emotions are also included under the information rubric. The word *information* is employed here to refer to all data being used by the nervous system for whatever purpose. The processing is accomplished by the physiological activity of the nervous system and communication among neurons.

PRINCIPLES OF NERVOUS SYSTEM ORGANIZATION AND THEIR RELATIONSHIP TO INFORMATION PROCESSING

The nervous system is designed to process information. To understand how this is accomplished and, in turn, how it may change with age, some fundamental principles must be considered.

Various parts of the brain are specialized, but there is cooperation among different parts.   As indicated in chapter 1, behavior usually involves elements of various brain functions working in concert. Nevertheless, most brain structures also play a specialized role, and dysfunction of particular parts of the aging brain would be expected to have rather well-defined outcomes. Examples can be drawn for each of the seven neural functions. The chest movements associated with breathing are modulated by certain neurons in the brainstem; specific failure of those neurons will result in death. Sensory systems have their own specialized, primary regions of cerebral cortex; damage to the cortex of a particular modality will produce perceptual deficits specific to that modality. The hippocampus plays an essential role in the storage of information into long-term memory; an impaired hippocampus will result in a deficit in the ability to form new memories. Coordination of serial movements requires neural circuits in the cerebellum; damage to these circuits would result in characteristic motor dysfunction. The amygdala must function properly to experience the emotion of fear; amygdala damage can produce specific changes in this and other emotions. Neurons in the frontal lobes participate in the integration of information needed to plan behaviors; if these neurons are not functioning properly, such integrative processes could falter. Cyclical hormonal activity in women is regulated in part by neurons in specific subdivisions of the hypothalamus; interference with the activity of these neurons would alter the cycle. As these examples suggest, if certain parts of the brain were more or less vulnerable to age-related degeneration in an individual (because of genetic or other factors), some rather specific deficits could accompany aging.

By the same token, because many regions of the brain influence one another to some extent, there could be surprising secondary or tertiary effects of damage in one brain region. One example is *diaschisis*, a phenomenon encountered with brain-damaged patients: An undamaged part of the brain, if it receives synaptic input from the axons of neurons in the damaged part of the brain, is relieved of that input because the source of the input is lost. Diaschisis occurs when the intact brain region no longer functions normally because of the loss of synaptic input from the remote neurons. It is not clear that diaschisis occurs in the context of age-related damage to specific brain regions, but it is a possibility worth considering.

The nervous system has a left and right half.   The nervous system, like the body in general, is bilaterally symmetric: Cutting it down the middle results in two very similar halves (see chapter 3, Figures 3.1 to 3.3). Three aspects of nervous system function stem from this, and each may have neurogerontological implications.

The right and left halves of the brain communicate with each other via bundles of nerve fibers. The most striking of the *commissural* pathways (fiber tracts that connect the two halves of the brain) is the *corpus callosum*, a massive band of axons connecting the left and right cerebral hemispheres. As indicated in chapter 3, there is considerable separation of the two hemispheres, and action potentials conveyed by axons traversing the corpus callosum are required if the hemispheres are to communicate with one another. If aging were accompanied by degenerative changes in the corpus callosum or other commissural pathways, the ability of left and right sides of the brain to interact could be diminished. Several brain-imaging studies have shown that corpus callosum degeneration often accompanies aging in human subjects (Doraiswamy et al., 1991; Janowsky, Kaye, & Carper, 1996; Johnson, Farnworth, Pinkston, Bigler, & Blatter, 1994; Laissy et al., 1993; Weis, Kimbacher, Wenger, & Neuhold, 1993), with the greatest changes typically occurring after age 65, especially in men. When corpus callosum degeneration occurs, it tends to be worst toward the front (anterior) of the brain, suggesting that the connections between frontal and temporal lobes are especially vulnerable. To determine if atrophy of the corpus callosum had behavioral consequences, Jeeves and Moes (1996) performed reaction time experiments that tested the speed of transferring information from one cerebral hemisphere to the other. Older subjects (> 60 years) exhibited significantly slower interhemispheric transfer. In summary, it appears that the corpus callosum of many older individuals undergoes a degree of atrophy and that this could slow the transfer of information between the right and left sides of the brain.

Some functional aspects of the left and right sides of the brain are different. The most well known example of the lateralization of function is the ability of the left cerebral hemisphere to process verbal material versus the right hemisphere's abilities for spatial and quantitative functions. If left and right hemispheres were differentially affected during aging, cognitive abilities could be affected differently as well. There is some evidence, albeit weak, that such changes can occur, and these are discussed in chapter 11.

Some neural pathways in sensory and motor systems cross from left to right.   Several important pathways connecting the cerebral cortex and lower levels of the nervous system cross from one side to the other in the brainstem or spinal cord. For example, sensations of touch or pressure on the left hand, some aspects of auditory sensations from the left ear, and visual sensations from the left portion of a visual scene (the left visual field) are relayed to various regions of the right cerebral cortex for processing into perceptions. Similarly, muscle movements on one side of the body are largely controlled by neural commands (carried by action potentials) originating in the opposite cerebral hemisphere. For everything to work properly, the brain must coordinate these complicated, crossed circuits. If, for example, aging were to affect the precise timing of neural events (see below), it could become more difficult for the older brain to coordinate temporal relationships between bilateral circuits.

NEURAL CIRCUITS

One can conceptualize a nervous system as being organized into mega-conglomerations of large and small neural circuits: neurons and their dendritic trees, which respond to synaptic input from other neurons and, in turn, influence other neurons by sending out action potentials via their axons. The patterns of synaptic "connectivity" (the neurons are not physically connected, of course) and the ways each neuron interacts with those it is connected to characterize the neural circuits that underlie much of what the brain does. It is important to note that neurons influence their neighbors in other, less connectionistic ways as well, such as by producing "local" changes in voltage or by releasing modulating chemicals into the microenvironment. The present discussion, however, will focus on circuits of connectivity, because these have some reasonably well understood properties that might help to account for age effects in information processing by the brain.

Circuits Are Complex

It should come as no surprise by now that the wiring diagrams of neural circuits can be maddeningly hard to unravel, given their sheer complexity. Here is a small excerpt from a literature review (Logothetis & Sheinberg,

1996), describing neural circuits in the brain involved with visual object recognition. The abbreviations need not concern us, but each refers to a region of the brain.

> Area TEO receives feedforward, topographically organized cortical inputs from areas V2, V3, and V4, and has interhemispheric connections mediated mainly via the corpus callosum. Sparser inputs arise from areas V3A, V4t, and MT. Each of these areas receives a feedback connection from TEO. . . . TEO projects feedforwardly to the areas TEm, TEa, and IPa, all of which send feedback projections back to TEO. . . . Cortical projections of area TE include those to TH, TF, STP, frontal eyefields (FEF), and area 46. . . .

And much more. This is only one of thousands of circuits, and probably not a complete description at that. One can imagine that malfunction of neurons in one or a few components of a circuit like this could result in less than optimal processing of information.

Convergence and Divergence Occur in Neural Circuits

An important feature of neural circuits is the ability of neurons to distribute action potentials to many other neurons through diverging branching of axons. Conversely, synaptic inputs from many different sources—thousands in some cases—can converge on the dendrites and soma of individual neurons. Divergence and convergence occur within circum-scribed regions of the brain but also govern the distribution of neural messages through the expanses of the entire nervous system. Both could be affected by loss of neurons, axon terminals, or dendrites (refer to chapters 3 and 4) in obvious ways: fewer postsynaptic sites for convergence of inputs from other axons and fewer axonal branches for divergence of output. The implication is that some neural circuits of older brains may have to get their jobs done with fewer communicating components.

Many Circuit Components Are Topographically Organized

As an organism's brain develops and the axonal circuitry is determined, systematic point-to-point connections are laid down between many of its parts. For example, touch receptors in a particular point of skin on the hand are functionally connected (via a pathway of axons and synapses) to neurons in a particular region of the specialized somatosensory cortex. The adjacent position on the hand is neurally connected to an adjacent region of cortex, and so on. As a result of this topographic projection, a "map" of the hand surface occupies an area of the cortical surface. Topographical organization is also found in other sensory systems, in motor systems, and elsewhere, and is presumably of some functional significance. A growing body of evidence indicates that changes in the representational maps may occur with aging. The possible neurogeronto-logical implications of plasticity of representational maps will be discussed in later chapters.

The Interaction of Excitatory and Inhibitory Synaptic Potentials Influence Neurons' Physiological Output

There is much more to neural circuits than simple "wiring diagrams"; the transfer of information can be modified at each synaptic meeting place between neurons in the circuit. As discussed in chapter 4, the integration of excitatory and inhibitory synapses contacting a postsynaptic neuron often determines whether or not the neuron will fire action potentials (excitation) or be prevented from doing so (inhibition). The outcome of synaptic interactions at the neuronal level can completely change the circuit's behavior. For example, excitatory activity in one part of a circuit can be changed to inhibition, simply by inserting inhibitory *interneurons*. These generate action potentials in response to excitatory synaptic input (i.e., they respond to an excitatory neurotransmitter such as glutamate, released by the axon terminal inputting to them). However, they manufac-ture and release an inhibitory neurotransmitter at their axon terminals that inhibits their target postsynaptic neurons. The greater the excitatory input that drives the interneurons, the stronger their inhibitory output to other neurons. Defective operation of interneurons can greatly disrupt the cir-cuit's behavior.

It is implicit that, under normal operating conditions, some sort of balance between excitation and inhibition exists. This balance undoubtedly differs among neural circuits and components of circuits. In cases where it is best that the circuit remain in the "off" mode, the normal condition is inhibition: The inhibitory inputs predominate. The opposite is true in circuits where it is desirable to have the neurons active or on the verge of being excited easily. Here, excitatory inputs prevail. In many circuits, the relationship between these opposing forces is modified by synaptic input: The balance can swing in one direction or another by activating the appropriate synapses. Presumably, much behavior is generated in this manner. For example, some circuits in the spinal cord produce movement but are normally prevented from doing so by a background of inhibitory synaptic input descending from the brain. The balance can be altered by activating circuit components with excitatory input to this system, thereby overriding the background inhibition. When the excitatory circuit is stopped, the system returns to its inhibited state, providing for precise control (starting and stopping) of movement. If the excitatory components became impaired, nothing would happen, as the constant inhibition would suppress movement. If the inhibitory components were impaired, the balance would be tipped away from inhibition and excessive, uncontrolled movements would occur. This is what happens when a drug like strychnine is administered and causes seizures. Strychnine antagonizes inhibitory synapses that utilize glycine as the neurotransmitter. A less elegant method of removing the descending inhibition from the brain is decapitation—the chicken without a head running around the barnyard.

The gruesome examples of strychnine poisoning and chicken decapitation do serve to make an important point: When the balance between excitation and inhibition is disturbed, some serious consequences can result. Thus, it is of great importance to determine if aging is associated with such imbalances. As we are about to see, this does indeed appear to be the case.

The Decline of Inhibition with Aging

Gerontological research on evoked potentials has suggested that neural inhibition in some circuits may become impaired with age. As reviewed by Prinz, Dustman, and Emmerson (1990): Sensory evoked response amplitudes reflecting cortical activity often increase in amplitude during aging; changes in visual-evoked responses to checkerboard patterns suggest a loss of inhibition; and older people tend to have "augmenting" evoked responses, where increased stimulus intensity produces larger evoked responses.

If inhibition were vulnerable during aging, one would expect to find evidence of changes in inhibitory neurotransmitters. Gamma aminobutyric acid (GABA) is the most important inhibitory neurotransmitter in the CNS. As is typical of the research findings on aging and neurotransmitters, there is no simple pattern of age effects, but many studies have shown a decrease in the synthesis of GABA in various parts of the brain of humans and other species (Rogers & Bloom, 1985). A review of the literature by Morgan and May (1990) concluded that most studies have found about a 20% to 30% reduction in benzodiazepine receptors (associated with the $GABA_A$ receptor complex). Thus, the literature provides strong evidence that some neural circuits using GABA become impaired with age (although enhanced benzodiazepine receptor tone in some brain circuits has also been proposed as a contributor to some age-related changes; see Marczynski, 1995).

The inferior colliculus (IC), a structure in the midbrain predominantly involved in hearing, makes great use of GABA in its neural circuits. Caspary, Milbrandt, and colleagues have provided strong evidence that inhibitory processes involving the neurotransmitter GABA become diminished in the IC of aging Fischer 344 rats (Caspary, Milbrandt, & Helfert, 1995; Caspary, Raza, Lawhorn-Armour, Pippin, & Arneric, 1990; Milbrandt, Albin, & Caspary, 1994; Milbrandt, Albin, Turgeon, & Caspary, 1996; Milbrandt & Caspary, 1995; Milbrandt, Hunter, & Caspary, 1997; Raza, Milbrandt, Arneric, & Caspary, 1994). Older rats are characterized by fewer IC neurons containing GABA (as shown by immunocytochemistry), decreased basal concentrations of GABA, decreased release of GABA by IC neurons, decreased activity of glutamic acid decarboxylase (an enzyme involved in making GABA), changes in GABA receptors at synapses, and a decrease in the number of presynaptic terminals using GABA. Neural responses of IC neurons are altered as well (Palombi & Caspary, 1996a, 1996b). Inhibition also appears to be diminished in the IC of aging mice. For example, an increase in spontaneous neural activity (i.e., action potentials occurring in the absence of appreciable acoustic stimulation) is observed in electrophysiological recordings from individual neurons (Willott, Parham, & Hunter, 1988a, 1988b). The increase in spontaneous activity may very well be caused by lessened inhibition by GABA, which could normally prevent these neurons from firing spontaneously.

Reduction of inhibition in the auditory system is likely to have significant consequences for hearing. Inhibitory processes appear to play important roles in the IC for auditory functions such as sound localization and discrimination of signals in noise. Furthermore, an increase in the level of spontaneous neural activity could decrease the neural signal to noise ratio. That is, sound-evoked responses (the neural signal) would be superimposed on a higher than normal level of background neural activity (the neural noise). On the other hand, neural noise may enhance the performance of sensory systems under certain conditions (Glanz, 1997). In any event, a diminution in inhibition in the central auditory system with aging could help to explain some perceptual problems faced by elderly listeners such as ringing in the ear (tinnitus) and poor hearing in noisy conditions.

Another very important CNS inhibitory neurotransmitter is glycine, but age effects have not been studied nearly as well as they have for GABA. In our laboratory, we evaluated glycinergic neurons in the cochlear nucleus (a part of the auditory system in the brainstem) of young and old C57BL/6J (C57) and CBA/CaJ (CBA) mice by using immunocytochemical staining and a technique (receptor binding) that indicates the number of synaptic receptors for glycine (Willott et al., 1997). As discussed in more detail in chapter 7, adult C57 mice exhibit progressive hearing loss as they age, whereas aging CBA mice retain good hearing (in this respect the two strains are similar to aging humans who do or do not suffer from severe loss of hearing). In old C57 mice (> 18 months) with severe hearing loss, the number of neurons staining for glycine decreased significantly (see Figure 5.1). The number of glycine receptors (as indicated by a measure called B_{max}) decreased significantly as well (refer back to Figure 2.3). Significant effects were not observed in the cochlear nucleus of middle-aged C57 mice (with less severe hearing loss) or in very old CBA mice (which do not exhibit severe hearing loss). The data suggest that old age is associated with deficits in one or more inhibitory glycinergic circuits in the cochlear nucleus, but only when severe hearing loss is also present.

NEURAL CODING

It is axiomatic that the processing of information by the nervous system requires a number of transformations in the way information is represented, or *coded*. For example, neurons in the brain cannot respond directly to the photic or acoustic events of the outside world; rather, the outside world must be transformed into codes that are compatible with the "languages" that the nervous system understands and uses, such as action

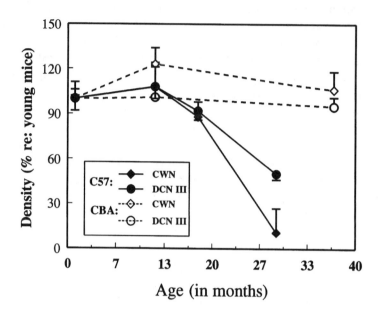

FIGURE 5.1 The packing density (adjusted for volume changes to reflect relative cell number) of glycine-immunoreactive neurons in the DCN of C57 and CBA mice. CWN = cartwheel neurons (a type of interneuron); DCN III = layer III of the DCN. The number of neurons staining for glycine decreases dramatically in old C57 mice but does not change in CBA mice, even at extremely old ages (3 years). Reprinted from Willott, F. F., Milbrandt, J. C., Bross, L. S., & Caspary, D. M. (1997). Glycine immunoreactivity and receptor binding in the cochlear nucleus of C57BL/6J and CBA/CaJ mice: Effects of cochlear impairment and aging. *Journal of Comparative Neurology, 385,* 405–414, with permission from Wiley-Liss.

potentials, metabotropic changes in neurons, and localized electrical activity. Effective operation of the nervous system requires accurate and efficient coding. Thus, when we are looking for reasons why a nervous system is not functioning at its optimal level, as often occurs with aging, neural coding becomes a prime suspect. This section first reviews some basics of neural coding, then evaluates the potential for modifications of coding that might accompany aging.

Uttal (1973) defined a code as *a set of symbols that can be used to represent message concepts and meanings and the set of rules that governs the selection and use of these symbols.* In most cases, we do not yet know with certainty what the neural codes are, and the term *candidate codes* is often used, because it is so difficult to determine if neural events actually are relevant for experience or behaviors. It is relatively easy to identify signs of neural activity associated with behavior or perception: a neural signal that varies as a function of some stimulus variable. However, it may not be responsible for experience or behavior. Rather, the activity may be an epiphenomenon, an event that is correlated with the actual code but does not play a key role in coding. For example, with respect to what makes an automobile move, the sound of the engine is an epiphenomenon; it always accompanies the car's running, but the sound itself does not make the car move. Changes in metabolic activity indicated by PET scans are signs of neural activity, but the variations of metabolic activity per se probably carry little information. Thus, caution is always warranted in making conclusions about neural coding.

Another aspect of neural coding that adds to the confusion is the fact that codes can vary at different parts of the nervous system. For example, information is transmitted over distance via action potential codes but (we presume) is processed locally by synaptic and other local potentials as well. Also, the same information can be represented by completely different codes in different parts of the nervous system.

With these caveats in mind, a number of candidate codes can be identified (cf. Uttal, 1973). When possible, examples of possible age-related changes in these codes are drawn from our own work on the auditory system of mice (Willott, 1984, 1986; Willott et al., 1988a, 1988b). We used microelectrodes to obtain electrophysiological recordings of action potentials emitted by neurons in the IC, a major part of the auditory system discussed earlier. When audible sounds are presented to an animal, they evoke action potential responses in neurons of the IC and other parts of the auditory system. By analyzing the relationship between auditory stimuli and the responses that are evoked, some of the candidate codes can be studied. We compared data from young mice with data obtained from mice that were old but could still hear fairly well (the CBA mouse strain) or from mice that exhibited hearing loss as they aged (the C57 mouse strain).

Labeled Line or Place Codes

The idea of labeled lines goes back to Müller's doctrine of specific nerve energies of the 19th century. It has evolved into the notion that events are coded by which neurons or "lines" of synaptically connected neurons are activated. Another way of putting it is, the activation of certain neurons—a "place" within the nervous system—indicates a specific event or datum; activation of neurons in another place indicates another event or datum. The fact that distinct sensory modalities exist seems to be a general manifestation of this form of coding. The particular neural circuits that are activated determine whether a sensory experience is visual, auditory, tactile, and so on. For example, electrical or chemical stimulation of neurons in the visual system produces visual experiences, as does mechanical activation of the system by pressure against the eye. None of these are visual stimuli, yet they produce visual sensations. The key to getting a visual experience is to activate neurons occupying places within the visual system. If one could cross-wire an auditory pathway to the visual system, an acoustic stimulus would presumably produce a visual experience. At the output side of the nervous system, specific muscles are made to contract by electrically stimulating specific neurons synaptically connected to them in circuits that produce movement. The composite of motor neurons that are activated provide the codes for which muscles contract.

Labeled lines can be reflected by topographic organization and the formation of sensory cortical maps, discussed earlier (although maps probably have additional functional implications). The orderly, albeit distorted, relationship between locations in sensory surfaces and the neural pathways to cortex presumably code the location of the sensory stimulus in space and with respect to other stimuli. Thus, the distortion of topographic maps that may accompany aging (see chapter 7) may perturb labeled-line codes. In the auditory system, the frequency of sound is coded, at least in part, according to a place principle. High-frequency sounds activate the base of the spiral-shaped cochlea of the inner ear, and lower frequency sounds activate parts of the cochlea toward the apex of the cochlea. Thus, the place along the cochlea and central neuronal lines that are activated code the frequency of sounds. In aging C57 mice (as is the case with many aging humans), the high-frequency basal end of the cochlea degenerates with age. The animals can no longer hear high tones because the high-frequency lines (the codes) have been eliminated.

It is important to remember that additional processing of information occurs at various synaptic stations along labeled lines, where the transfer of information can be altered by excitatory-inhibitory interactions and other means. Thus, age-related synaptic changes could affect labeled lines.

With respect to aging C57 mice, it was indicated earlier that inhibitory synapses in the lower part of the central auditory system appear to become impaired (see Figure 5.1; also refer back to Figure 2.3). Behavioral startle responses to closely spaced pairs of brief sounds become exaggerated in these mice (Willott & Carlson, 1995), probably because inhibitory synapses that normally "dampen" the behavioral response to sounds (to prevent overreactions to loud sounds) are diminished. In this case, the relevant "lines" from cochlea to CNS remain intact, but the transfer of coded neural data is altered along the way.

Another aspect of labeled lines should be mentioned. Elements with a given "line" can carry different kinds of information. For example, large and small axons of the somatosensory system, serving the same patch of skin, signal touch and pain, respectively. If aging were particularly hard on one caliber of axon, it would, in theory, be possible to alter the overall informational content of circuit components. The C57 mouse auditory system provides an empirical example. Neural responses in the auditory system are initiated by the activity of two types of hair cells in the inner ear: outer hair cells (OHCs) and inner hair cells (IHCs). IHCs and OHCs have rather different functions in hearing (which we will not go into here). Aging C57 mice lose their hearing because a recessive gene called Ahl results in progressive degeneration of the hair cells (Erway, Willott, Archer, & Harrison, 1993). However, the gene's primary target is the OHCs; these degenerate earlier and more severely than the IHCs. Thus, damage to the high-frequency lines primarily involves OHCs, with the IHCs being less severely affected.

Finally, it should be made clear that the particular neurons (places) that are activated by a stimulus can depend on spatiotemporal patterns of synaptic input, rather than (or in addition to) linear connectivity. An example is the coincidence detector, discussed in the context of dendritic spines in chapter 4. In order to fire an action potential in a particular neuron, simultaneous activation of two excitatory synapses on the same dendrite are required, so that their effects will sum together (neither synapse alone is sufficient to generate a postsynaptic action potential). Because of this design, the firing of an action potential in the postsynaptic neuron would code only the coincidence of the two inputs; if they were slightly out of phase, no response would occur. If the stimulus conditions required for that to happen were fixed and reliable, it would be a type of place or labeled-line code. That is, the occurrence of a response in a neuron signals specific stimulus conditions. Thus, changes in temporal processing could interfere with this type of place code.

Representation of Information in Action-Potential Trains of Individual Neurons

Whereas the individual neurons within neural circuits fire action potentials one at a time, the temporal pattern of firing in a given neuron can vary greatly. A neuron emitting trains of action potentials can be thought of as a *pulse-coded analog device* (Bullock, 1977). The action potentials are discrete, transient events that do not vary in amplitude (like telegraph "dot" signals), but the time intervals between action potentials are graded in an analog fashion. This gives rise to several candidate codes.

Rate of firing.   The number of action potentials per unit of time defines the rate of firing, and this can vary from zero to hundreds of responses per second. The upper limit is determined by the physiological properties of the neuron's membrane and the *refractory period* of the action potentials. The refractory period refers to the time it takes for a neuronal membrane to restore itself to its resting voltage after an action potential has been fired—at least a millisecond or so. Complete or partial restoration of the membrane voltage is necessary before another action potential can fire. There are numerous neurophysiological studies showing that individual neurons increase or decrease their firing rate when put in situations where they seem to be processing information. This is seen in sensory neurons presented with adequate stimuli, motor neurons when movement is occurring, autonomic nervous system neurons when heart or smooth muscle are being modulated, and many, many other examples. The many demonstrations of correlations between firing rate and presumed information processing make it likely that firing rate is often a neural code.

In individual IC neurons of C57 mice, the rate of firing evoked by certain tones changes greatly as the animals age and lose high-frequency hearing (Willott et al., 1988b). Normally, high-frequency tones evoke vigorous firing of action potentials in many neurons located deep within the IC (the high-frequency region of the IC). As cochlear degeneration progresses, high-frequency tones no longer evoke strong firing rates in IC neurons. Although this is to be expected, it is also the case that the response of these neurons to still-audible low-frequency tones improves to the point where abnormally high rates of action potentials are evoked. Presumably, the relationship between sound stimulus and firing rate—the code—has been turned upside down (see chapter 7 for a further discussion of this type of neural plasticity).

Intervals between action potentials. Besides the number of action potentials per unit of time (rate), additional information might be coded by monitoring the time intervals between action potentials. For example many short intervals would indicate rapid firing (mean rate is high), without the necessity of having to count action potentials and divide by time. In addition, the variance of the intervals would indicate how regularly the neurons are firing within a given time period. That is, two neurons could produce the same total number of action potentials in a 1-second time period, but one could fire them at regular intervals, the other in irregular bursts.

In older mice of both the C57 and CBA strains, neurons are more likely to emit action potentials even when no tone is present, and these "spontaneous" action potentials occur at varying intervals. This would appear to add neural noise, making it more difficult to distinguish "meaningful" intervals between action potentials, which might be used as a code.

Macrofluctuations in the action-potential train. The temporal distribution of action potentials following presentation of a stimulus or synaptic input can vary considerably, providing rich opportunities for neural coding. For example, two categories of temporal response patterns evoked by sensory stimuli are "onset" and "sustained." Consider the responses evoked in two auditory neurons by a tone that lasts for 1 second. The neuron with the onset response would discharge one or a few action potentials when the tone came on but would immediately cease firing, even though the tone remained on. The neuron with the sustained response would emit a continuous train of action potentials for as long as the tone remained on. Clearly, these two neurons have different coding capabilities. The onset response signals that a tone has occurred but provides no information about the tone's duration. If the key information to be coded is the occurrence of a sound irrespective of duration (to elicit a startle reflex, for example), the onset response is ideal. The sustained response is linked to the duration and ongoing fluctuations in the tone, so it is well suited to code this type of information. A number of different temporal patterns have been observed in neurons (see Figure 5.2), each of which favors the coding of some type of information.

In C57 mice, about 20% fewer IC neurons of older mice are able to respond to tones with sustained responses (see Figure 5.2C, D), compared to young mice (Willott et al., 1988b). This suggests that coding with sustained responding may be diminished in these mice. On the other hand,

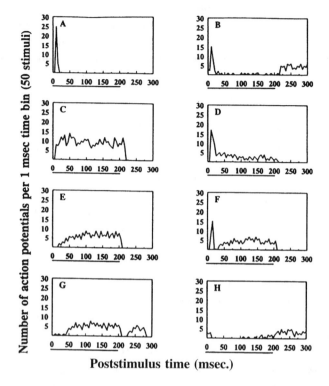

Poststimulus time (msec.)

FIGURE 5.2   Examples of poststimulus time histograms (PSTHs) showing
the temporal pattern of action potential discharges. A 200-msec tone came
on at time 0 (indicated by horizontal line). This was repeated 50 times, and
the action potentials occurring in each 1-msec interval were summed to
produce the PSTHs. All of the examples were obtained from CBA mice older
than 2 years. A. Onset response: A single action potential was evoked only
by the onset of each tone. B. Onset response with inhibition of spontaneous
activity: The neuron fired action potentials spontaneously as in the right
portion of the PSTH, but the tone produced an onset response, followed by
a period of inhibition of spontaneous activity. C. Sustained response: Trains
of action potentials were evoked by the tone for its entire duration. D.
Adapting sustained response: Evoked action potentials decreased between
the beginning and end of the tone. E. Buildup response: The opposite of
adaptation, as more action potentials were evoked later in the tone. F. Pauser:
An onset response is followed by a brief absence of responses, then building
up to a sustained response. G. Long-latency response: Significant action
potentials seen only after 60 to 80 msec into the tone (these neurons do
not response to very brief sounds). H. Inhibition of spontaneous activity:
Spontaneous action potential discharges seen at the right part of the PSTH
were inhibited or "turned off" by the tone. Redrawn from Willott, J. F.,
Parham, K., & Hunter, K. P. (1988). Response properties of inferior colliculus
neurons in young and very old CBA/J mice. *Hearing Research, 37,* 1–14,
with permission from Elsevier Science.

no significant age differences were observed for onset and other responses types, and old CBA mice showed no changes, even in sustained responding (Willott et al., 1988a). The negative findings are perhaps the more remarkable here: Despite old age or hearing loss, the IC neurons retained their ability to generate a rich variety of temporal response patterns. This is evident from Figure 5.2, as all of the examples were obtained from CBA mice older than 2 years.

Coding That Relies on Populations of Neurons

Whereas individual neurons apparently have the capacity to code substantial amounts of information, most varieties of coding probably require neurons acting in concert. Indeed, it is often the case that the code cannot be found in the responses of individual neurons at all. Rather, the information is contained in the behavior of a population, assembly (Hebb, 1949), or ensemble of neurons, particularly in spatiotemporal relationships among responses of many neurons (see Deadwyler & Hampson, 1997; Sakurai, 1996; Uttal, 1973). A population can vary in size from a small assembly of cooperative neurons to huge numbers distributed in networks across the nervous system.

The number of activated neurons. The number of neurons that are activated at any given time provides a relatively simple population code candidate. A few active neurons would indicate one situation; many activated neurons would indicate another. In sensory systems, for example, the magnitude or intensity of a stimulus is often correlated with the number of neurons in which responses are evoked. Usually, increasing stimulus intensity recruits additional neurons into the active pool. This is the case when neurons vary with respect to their thresholds for responding to stimuli. In the auditory system, some neurons have very low thresholds (it takes only a rather faint sound to excite them), whereas others have higher thresholds and respond only to more intense sounds. With low-intensity sounds, only a few, low-threshold auditory neurons are activated. As the acoustic intensity increases, neurons with higher thresholds are recruited to join the low-threshold neurons in responding. That is, the intensity of the acoustic stimulus is directly related to (coded by) the number of neurons that are firing action potentials.

In theory, this candidate code could be constrained by age-related changes in the nervous system that reduce the code's dynamic range (i.e., the difference between few and many activated neurons). First, some reduction in the number and/or physiological status of neurons typically accompanies aging, at least in many brain regions (see chapters 3 and 4). This could limit the maximum number of responding neurons that can be recruited at high-stimulus intensities. In very old CBA mice, for example, an unusually high percentage of IC neurons have "sluggish" responses to sound—the number and reliability of action potentials that are evoked by audible sounds are diminished. The code is affected because "sluggish" neurons cannot contribute normally to the pool of neurons responding to sounds. Second, the sensitivity of sensory systems typically declines with age (see chapter 7) because the peripheral sensory organs can no longer respond to faint stimuli. This would reduce the dynamic range of the code at the lower end of the range, because it would take a relatively intense stimulus to activate any neurons at all. In C57 mice, for example, the percentage of neurons with high thresholds increases greatly with age because of their cochlear pathology. This means that few neurons are being brought into play unless the sound intensity is relatively high.

Spatial and temporal relationships in the activity of neurons. The excitatory and inhibitory activity within a population of neurons can vary as a function of space (which neurons are doing what) and time (when they are doing it with respect to one another). This sets the stage for other candidate codes based on spatial and/or temporal relationships among neurons. In a simple example, all else being equal, if one set of neurons is synaptically excited before another set, this could provide a code that the stimulus activating the first set occurred before the second stimulus. Thus, the temporal relationships among events is a candidate code. Presumably, much more complex information is also contained in the spatio-temporal relationships within populations of neurons.

We can turn again to the auditory system for an example. The ability to determine the direction from which a sound has come relies on the comparison of sounds at the two ears. These *binaural* comparisons can be made on the basis of the time of arrival (a sound arrives at the near ear first) and on the basis of interaural intensity of sounds (the sound is more intense at the near ear; sound to the far ear is partially blocked by the head). Neurons in several parts of the auditory system are quite sensitive to variations in binaural cues. For neurons in the left IC, inhibitory synapses tend to be activated by sounds coming from the left side of the head, whereas excitatory synapses are activated by sounds coming from the right side of the head (the situation is reversed for neurons in the right IC). Because a sound on the left side of the head is more intense in the left ear, it will strongly activate the inhibitory synapses to the left IC neurons while also exciting right IC neurons. As a sound moves toward the right side of the head, the excitatory-inhibitory relationships change accordingly. The net result is spatiotemporal patterns of neural activity that differ considerably between left and right IC, with the patterns varying depending on (hence, potentially coding) the location of the sound.

The ability of IC neurons to reliably code this relationship appears to be diminished in older C57 mice. McFadden and Willott (1994) measured action potentials from neurons in the IC as a sound source was moved to different locations in a 180° arc in front of the mouse's head. In young mice, many IC neurons were excited by tones from the opposite side of the head and inhibited by tones from the same side, the typical mammalian pattern. This pattern was also observed in many IC neurons of older mice, but a number of neurons exhibited an abnormal, reversed pattern, rarely seen in young mice, with sounds from the same side of the head producing excitation (see Figure 5.3). These and other findings suggest that the distribution of excitatory and inhibitory activity (and its putative ability to act as a code) are impaired in these mice. Indeed, a behavioral study showed that middle-aged C57 mice are poor localizers of sounds (Heffner & Donnal, 1993).

Overlapping receptive fields.   The concept of a neuron's *receptive field* is most commonly used in sensory systems to define the portion of the array of sensory receptors that evokes responses in that neuron. Examples of receptive fields are the patch of skin that, when touched, evokes responses in a neuron of the somatosensory system or the area of the retinal surface, which, when stimulated by a photic stimulus, evokes responses in a neuron of the visual system. Theoretically, however, the receptive field concept can be generalized to include the source of effective synaptic inputs to a neuron in any neural circuit. In labeled-line coding, the receptive field of a neuron defines the peripheral end of the line. However, in sensory systems it is often the case that receptive fields are also used in population coding. Populations of neighboring CNS neurons have partially overlapping receptive fields; they respond to some common points on the peripheral receptor array. Information is coded in the overall response of

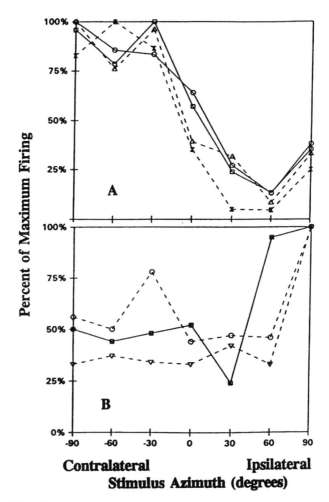

FIGURE 5.3 Azimuth functions from young C57 mice and middle-aged C57 mice with presbycusis. The azimuth functions depict the relative discharge rates for IC neurons as a speaker is moved from one side to the front to the other side of the animal's head. Each curve represents responses of a different neuron to 70dB stimuli. A. Examples of the typical mammalian response seen in young mice; at negative angles (tone on opposite side of the head), the neuron is maximally excited, but at positive angles (tone on same side), the responses decrease greatly. B. Azimuth functions obtained from older mice. The azimuth functions are reversed. Such reversed functions were significantly more prevalent in the older mice. Reprinted from McFadden, S. L., & Willott, J. F. (1994). Responses of inferior colliculus neurons in C57BL/6J mice with and without sensorineural hearing loss: Effects of changing the azimuthal location of an unmasked pure-tone stimulus. *Hearing Research, 78,* 115–131, with permission from Elsevier Science.

the population. An example is the classic Young-Helmholtz theory of color vision, which incorporates three types of color-sensitive visual receptors (cones) in the retina: orange, green, and blue. The combination of receptors that are activated determines the color that is perceived. If one type of color-sensitive retinal cone is missing, a form of color blindness results. The critical feature of this type of population coding is that all components must be able to contribute in order for accurate coding to occur. From a neurogerontological perspective, if one or more components of some neural coding population were especially vulnerable to age-related impairment, the spatiotemporal properties of the population code could be diminished by the loss of this component.

Using the Full Repertoire of Candidate Codes

A variety of candidate codes have been reviewed, but the list can go on well beyond the scope of this chapter. Additional candidate codes may be contained within *microfluctuations in the action-potential train,* transient changes, a missed action potential here or there, or a gap in the train of action potentials. Other candidates may be found in the use of *derived statistical measures,* long-term fluctuations in the pulse pattern, such as the mean or variance, which could contain valuable information (Uttal, 1973). Much important coding is presumed to be carried by processes other than synaptic transmission and action potentials in neural circuits and population activity. Graded voltage changes in local brain regions, the passive (electrotonic) spread and decay of membrane potentials, metabotropic changes in neurons, and many other processes are legitimate candidate codes and are probably used widely by the nervous system.

It is important to emphasize that the nervous system undoubtedly uses many different codes, often in combination. The informational content of most events is multidimensional, and each dimension could be coded in a different manner, and coded information may be used in various ways. For example a person's voice comes from a particular location in space and has intensity, a spectrum of frequencies, timbre, temporal properties, emotional tone, verbal content, and so on, all of which must be coded simultaneously. Somehow, information coded in various fashions is integrated and possibly recoded to produce a unified percept. Obviously, attempting to understand if and how neural coding is modified with age is a daunting endeavor, and we can do little more than speculate at this time.

Aging and Neural Coding

In addressing the possible coding difficulties that may arise with aging, one need first think about the neural substrates necessary for most types of coding. First, each neuron in a circuit must receive input concerning what it is being "asked" to code. Thus, the action-potential coded, presynaptic input must be dependable. Second, the incoming action-potential code must be accurately transmitted and translated (recoded) by pre- and postsynaptic events at the receiving neuron. Third, to reliably recode and send on the information through its own axon, the receiving neuron must be able to generate an appropriate number or temporal pattern of action potentials. In other words, coding in neural circuits requires the processing of input, output, and proper linkage between the two. This is presumably true for coding by individual neurons as well as small groups and large populations (which of course are comprised of many individual neurons). To appreciate the neurogerontological hazards of this multiple input-output arrangement, one need only consider the various factors that have the capacity to disrupt synaptic transmission, reduce a neuron's ability to produce action potentials, and/or otherwise interfere with the optimum physiological status of neurons. This lengthy list, discussed in chapters 3 and 4, suggests that the processing of input and output—and the codes that rely on this processing—are likely to be subject to age effects at practically every turn.

The very first, key variable in an information-processing system—whether a nervous system or a computer—is the condition of the hardware. Missing, broken, or malfunctioning circuit elements, for example, are incapable of participating in the coding process, and the system must get by without them. Presumably, when significant neuropathology accompanies aging, as it often does (see chapter 3), some aspect(s) of neural coding may be compromised. At what point does the loss of neurons become problematic? Essentially, this is the same question posed in chapter 3, and the answer is essentially the same as well. Whether or not a nervous system can continue to function with diminished coding depends on a host of factors, such as the severity and location of the damaged circuitry and the importance of the circuit to survival and/or important behavior. The mechanisms are so complex and varied, it is impossible to make general conclusions.

A heuristic way to delve into this issue is to identify the properties desirable in neural codes and their outcomes, then see if there is evidence that such properties are altered with aging. Consider these three assumptions: (1) Accuracy, speed, and reliability are hallmarks of an ideal neural code. (2) Our working premise is that neural coding is the basis on which the nervous system processes information and operates. Fast, accurate, reliable operation of the nervous system implies the same attributes in coding. (3) The quality of behavior reflects the quality of coding. Thus, by observing age-related changes in behavior, it may be possible to indirectly evaluate the state of neural coding (or, at least, think about gerontological issues from the neural coding perspective). This approach leads to the conclusion that neural codes are often operating at subpar levels in older individuals, whereas in other cases coding remains rather efficient, or is even improved. The evidence for these outcomes is presented in many contexts throughout the remainder of this book.

On the down side, there is ample evidence that speed, accuracy, and/ or reliability of coding almost inevitably decline when it comes to certain activities of the nervous system. For example, the accuracy and speed of operation of sensory and motor systems inevitably decline at some age, cognitive processes tend to slow down, the reliability of memory decreases, the timing of biological rhythms is altered, and so on. The neurogerontological researcher's task, then, would be to determine what aspects of coding have changed in conjunction with the depreciation of behavior. Unfortunately, this itself is a daunting undertaking because of the complex nature of neural coding discussed above. Coding could fail in the peripheral nervous system (inaccurate encoding of physical stimuli into neural events in the sensory organs; unreliable transfer of neural codes from motor neuron action potentials to muscle fiber contractions) or in CNS circuitry. A change in behavior could result because the coding system used by the young nervous system no longer works as well, or because the older nervous system has been forced to abandon an efficient coding strategy and replace it with an alternative that does not work as well, but is still available. There are many possibilities to consider.

On the up side, some neural codes apparently continue to function well, despite advancing age. Well-functioning coding strategies are presumably the rule for those nervous system–supported activities an older person continues to do well. For example, the neural coding that controls vital processes like body temperature or cardiovascular activity *must* be doing an adequate job in every senior citizen who is healthy and robust. This is not to say that coding remains optimal, but that it is fully adequate to accomplish its task of maintaining a good quality of life. Here, the neurogerontological researcher's task is to understand how and why these neural codes persist in good condition, then perhaps use what is learned to ameliorate the more vulnerable coding processes.

Even higher on the up side, some aspects of neural coding continue to improve as people get older, particularly coding in the realm of "mental activity." Behaviors that depend on the accrual of knowledge, the store of past experience, mature social skills or insights, and/or good decision-making are likely to peak in older people. Said differently, even though the hardware may be wearing out, the software is still being revised and improved to produce a better information processor.

SUMMARY

These first five chapters have provided a broad background with respect to neurobiology, neurophysiology, and behavioral neuroscience. Many of the possible ways that the nervous system can be challenged by aging have been reviewed in the general context of neurogerontology. In the following chapters, these challenges are discussed more specifically with respect to the seven basic functions of the nervous system.

6
Regulation of Vital Functions

The first of the seven basic functions of nervous systems is the most fundamental: Keep the body's various physiological systems up and running. Much of this falls under the rubric *homeostasis*—maintaining a relatively constant internal environment. Three key elements cooperate and interact to keep physiological activities within appropriate ranges: the hypothalamus, the endocrine system, and the autonomic nervous system.

THE HYPOTHALAMUS

The hypothalamus is a collection of small clusters of neurons located at the base of the brain. This brain region plays a crucial role in many aspects of behavior, and this is reflected in the array of subnuclei, some of which are shown in Figure 6.1. Neurons in subnuclei of the hypothalamus communicate with structures of the limbic system (e.g., hippocampus, amygdala, limbic cortical structures), reticular formation, thalamus, and cerebral cortex—a necessary arrangement if information of many varieties is to be brought to bear in regulating bodily activity. The hypothalamus is intimately involved with the endocrine system; it both produces hormones (several in cooperation with the pituitary gland) and responds to a variety of hormones that help to regulate behaviors and bodily functions. The hypothalamus also communicates with and influences the autonomic nervous system (see below). Indeed, the hypothalamus plays a role in all of the regulatory functions to be discussed in this chapter, as well as topics dealt with elsewhere, such as emotion and stress (see chapter 10) and sex and reproductive behavior (see chapter 12).

Aging and the Hypothalamus

A feature of the aging nervous system discussed in earlier chapters is the differential vulnerability of brain regions. Given the multifaceted nature

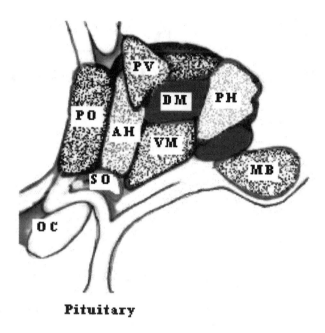

Pituitary

FIGURE 6.1   Some subdivisions of the hypothalamus. This is a midsagittal view of the hypothalamus. Refer to Figure 3.1 for orientation within the brain. PO, preoptic nucleus; PV, paraventribular nucleus; DM, dosomedial nucleus; PH, posterior hypothalamic area; AH, posterior hypothalamic area; AH, anterior hypothalamic area; VM, ventromedial nucleus; SO, supraoptic nucleus; OC, optic chiasm; MB, mammillary body.

of the hypothalamus, it is not surprising that this variability is manifested by hypothalamic nuclei. For example, in an anatomical study of the rat hypothalamus, Sartin and Lamperti (1985) found that only two subnuclei—the ventromedial and arcuate nuclei—exhibited a progressive loss of neurons. The other hypothalamic nuclei examined (dorsomedial, paraventricular, supraoptic, suprachiasmatic, sexually dimorphic, and medial preoptic) did not suffer a loss of neurons with age. In studies on humans (see Hofman, 1997; Mobbs, 1996), a decrease in neurons in the sexually dimorphic and suprachiasmatic nuclei occurred (unlike rats), but no change was observed in supraoptic or paraventricular nuclei (Goudsmit, Hofman, Fliers, & Swaab, 1990). Indeed, hypertrophy and increased activity have been observed in neurons of the paraventricular nucleus, which produce the hormone vasopressin (Goudsmit, Neijmeijer-Leloux, & Swaab, 1992). By and large, then, the number of neurons in most hypothalamic subnuclei is not greatly depleted with age. There are apparent species differences as well.

Despite the apparent stability in the number of neurons in many hypothalamic regions during aging, changes in neurotransmitter and hormone systems are observed, particularly in studies of rodents. For example, decreases in norepinephrine (NE; also called noradrenalin) are observed in the hypothalamus (McIntosh & Westfall, 1987; Rodriguez-Gomez et al., 1995; Rogers & Bloom, 1985; Roubein, Embree, & Jackson, 1986), and such declines could in turn affect the secretion of gonadotropic hormones, growth hormones, and other hormone systems (see below) that can modulate the course of aging (Meites, 1991). The hypothalamus produces peptide *releasing hormones*, which influence the release of hormones by the pituitary gland (see below), and these in turn influence the hypothalamus in a feedback arrangement. At least some of these hormone systems become less responsive with age because of reduced production by hypothalamic neurons, changes in receptor sensitivity for the hormones, and/ or changes in the endocrine glands (Mobbs, 1996; Sadow & Rubin, 1992). Ironically, the loss of sensitivity to hormones might be due to being exposed to these same hormones for a prolonged period of time (Mobbs, 1996).

The fact that relatively small hypothalamic subdivisions control important biological functions has suggested that subtle changes might contribute to aging in a fundamental way (Mobbs, 1996). Bernardis and Davis (1996) noted that experimental lesions of certain subdivisions of the hypothalamus in young animals is associated with changes reminiscent of aging, such as increased body fat, glucose intolerance, and decreased kidney function. This conjures up the notion that hypothalamic "lesions" that might arise with aging could have similar effects, bringing about biological changes observed in older individuals. It is certainly true that, of all the areas of the brain, the hypothalamus has the greatest potential to contribute to age-related changes in physiological systems that are vital to survival.

THE NEUROENDOCRINE SYSTEM

The endocrine system uses a variety of hormones to help regulate and maintain normal physiological functioning (homeostasis). In turn, it is largely under the control of the hypothalamus and other brain regions that communicate with the hypothalamus. Hence, the combined system is termed the *neuroendocrine system*. Neurons in the hypothalamus are able to sense, directly or indirectly, the levels of various hormones circulating in the blood and act like a thermostat, responding to this feedback by increasing or decreasing the hormone levels to maintain the proper average levels.

The major endocrine glands and their hormones include the *pineal gland* (melatonin), *anterior pituitary* (growth hormone [GH], thyroid-stimulating hormone [TSH], adrenocorticotropic hormone [ACTH], follicle-stimulating hormone [FSH], luteinizing hormone [LH], and prolactin), *posterior pituitary* (oxytocin; vasopressin or antidiuretic hormone), *thyroid gland* (thyroxine, triiodothyronine, and calcitonin), *adrenal cortex* (glucocorticoids such as corticosterone, cortisol, and hydrocortisone; mineralocorticoids such as aldosterone; sex hormones such as adrostenedione), *adrenal medulla* (epinephrine and norepinephrine acting as hormones rather than as neurotransmitters), *pancreas* (insulin, glucagon), and *gonads* (estrogens and progesterone in females, androgens such as testosterone in males).

The hypothalamus manufactures various releasing hormones that stimulate hormonal activity by the anterior pituitary gland. These include thyrotropin-releasing hormone, which stimulates TSH; gonadotropin-releasing hormone, which stimulates FSH and LH; and corticotropin-releasing hormone, which stimulates the stress hormone ACTH. The hypothalamus (paraventricular and supraoptic nuclei) also controls the production and release of the posterior pituitary hormones, but this is done with neural connections, rather than releasing hormones.

Aging and the Neuroendocrine System

Pathological alterations in the proper balance of hormones—excesses or deficits—result in a variety of negative medical and psychological outcomes. Thus, it is important to ask, Do alterations in hormone systems occur with aging? And if so, Do they also have negative consequences? The answers are yes and probably. Consider, for example, GH, a hormone that may play a fundamental role in aging. The hypothalamus and pituitary gland regulate the secretion of GH, which affects body fat composition, muscle physiology, various organs (liver, spleen, stomach, pancreas), kidney function, bone growth, and many aspects of the body's metabolic activity. As reviewed by Rudman and Rao (1992), there is a pronounced decline in GH secretion with age ("GH menopause"), and this appears to depend on depletion of neurotransmitters (dopamine and NE) in the hypothalamus, which normally stimulate GH release. The decline in GH is likely to contribute to some of the changes observed in older people such as reallocated body composition (relatively less bone and muscle but more fat) and declines in functional capacity of organ systems. A second example is the hypothalamic-pituitary control of the thyroid gland, which involves TSH. A variety of age effects have been observed in this system in studies of humans and other species (Kunitake, Pekary, & Hershman, 1992). These could lead to various cognitive and emotional conditions commonly associated with changes in thyroid function, as well as general alterations in the body's metabolism.

As mentioned above, the hypothalamus causes the release of stimulating hormones (LH, TSH, ACTH) that activate specific target hormones at an endocrine site (e.g., testosterone, estrogen, thyroid hormone, and glucocorticoids). It appears that peripheral levels of some target hormones can decrease with age, while the stimulating hormone levels remain unchanged. One way to account for this is that aging endocrine glands can no longer produce adequate levels of hormones. These levels are monitored by the brain, so the recognition of diminished glandular performance triggers feedback mechanisms that cause more stimulating hormone to be produced to try to maintain normal function (Mobbs, 1996). Perhaps as a result of this and other mechanisms, it is often the case that neuroendocrine function is maintained quite well during aging.

As the above discussion suggests, age-related changes in neuroendocrine function are likely to stem from a rather complicated series of events involving the condition of glands and their ability to secrete hormones (which tend to decline with age), neuroendocrine sensitivity to circulating hormones (which can potentially increase or decrease), and feedback processes involving the brain. Such processes may be an integral aspect of aging, as suggested by neuroendocrine-based hypotheses of aging involving glucocorticoids (Landfield, 1980; Sapolsky, 1992). Glucocorticoids are hormones produced by the adrenal glands in response to stress. There is evidence showing that glucocorticoids can contribute directly to neural damage during aging. In particular, the hippocampus (where neurons with receptors for glucocorticoids are found) can be damaged by exposure to glucocorticoids. In turn, because hippocampal neurons can inhibit the secretion of glucocorticoids, damage to the hippocampus might reduce that inhibition. Furthermore, hippocampal sensitivity to negative feedback regulation of glucocorticoids may become impaired, resulting in even higher levels of glucocorticoids and more damage. According to this hypothesis, then, glucocorticoid-induced damage has the capacity to contribute to the processes of aging (because this mechanism involves the neuroendocrine response to stress, it is discussed further in chapter 10).

THE AUTONOMIC NERVOUS SYSTEM

Activity of the heart, digestive system, endocrine glands, bladder, blood vessels, and other organs and tissues are modulated by the output of the autonomic nervous system. The autonomic nervous system is influenced by many brain regions such as the cerebral cortex and amygdala. However, the influences of these various regions are generally channeled through and integrated by the hypothalamus, which exerts control over the autonomic system in several ways (see Kandel, Schwartz, & Jessell, 1995). Hypothalamic neurons send axonal projections to the *nucleus of the solitary tract,* a brainstem region that receives sensory information from the viscera and provides output to the parasympathetic system primarily by way of the vagus nerve (which helps to regulate autonomic functions such as temperature and heart rate). Other hypothalamic neurons (e.g., in the lateral hypothalamus) send axons to the *rostral ventral medulla,* which triggers activity in the sympathetic nervous system. Still other hypothalamic projections go directly to autonomic components of the spinal cord. Also, as discussed earlier, the hypothalamus modulates the endocrine system to release hormones that affect the autonomic nervous system.

The pathway between CNS and the autonomic system's target organs involves an intermediate step: Axons leave the CNS to synapse with neurons in the *autonomic ganglia,* and their *postganglionic axons*, in turn, contact the target (see Figure 6.2). The ganglia of the sympathetic division, which marshals responses to dangerous or stressful situations, lie in bilateral chains beside the thoracic and lumbar portions of the spinal cord and in major peripheral sympathetic ganglia (celiac ganglion and hypogastric plexus). The efferents from CNS to ganglion release Ach as the transmitter, and the postganglionic cells respond with nicotinic Ach receptors. Once activated synaptically, their postganglionic axons release (in most cases) the neurotransmitter NE at the synapse with the target tissue. Two types of NE receptors are found on the postsynaptic target tissue—α- and

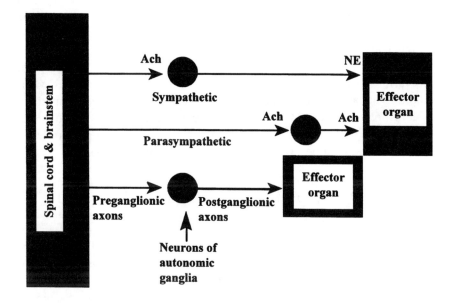

FIGURE 6.2 The autonomic nervous system. The preganglionic fibers exiting the brainstem or spinal cord make cholinergic synapses with neurons of autonomic ganglia, outside the CNS; the sympathetic ganglia are close to the CNS, whereas those of the parasympathetic division are close to the target organs. The postganglionic axons synapse with effector organs (glands, heart, smooth muscle) using NE for the sympathetic division and Ach for the parasympathetic division.

β-adrenergic receptors—based on their pharmacological properties. In general, sympathetic activation is widespread, involving a wide range of target organs.

The ganglia of the parasympathetic division, which counter the sympathetic system by playing a restorative role, are located close to, or in, the target organs. They are activated by preganglionic axons exiting the CNS from cranial nerves or from the lower (sacral) spinal cord. As is the case for the sympathetic system, preganglionic axons utilize Ach as their neurotransmitter and the postganglionic cells possess nicotinic Ach receptors. The neurotransmitter released by postganglionic parasympathetic axon terminals is also Ach, but their targets possess muscarinic Ach receptors (differentiated from nicotinic receptors on the basis of responses to drugs that bind with receptors). In contrast to the sympathetic system, parasympathetic actions can be much more selective with respect to target organs.

When all is working well, the ongoing activity (tone) of both autonomic divisions is properly balanced to maintain an optimal level of activity in the various organs and systems they innervate. Under conditions where emotions are activated or the animal is aroused or stressed, the sympathetic system predominates. This type of sympathetic activity is discussed in chapter 10. For now, discussions of the autonomic system are limited to its role in maintaining homeostasis of vital bodily functions.

Aging and the Autonomic Nervous System

After reviewing the literature on aging and the autonomic nervous system, Cowen (1993) concluded that "few generalizations" can be made, and this certainly seems to be the case. Some anatomical studies have found signs of age-related degeneration in various components of the autonomic nervous system in humans and other species, including loss of neurons, changes in axons, and abnormal synaptic processes. For example, studies on aging mice (Schmidt, Beaudet, Plurad, Snider, & Ruit, 1995) and humans (Schmidt, Chase, Parvin, & Roth, 1990) demonstrated a number of morphological changes in neurons of several sympathetic ganglia. Presynaptic terminal axons and synapses were enlarged and appeared pathological, dendrites exhibited reduced complexity and other changes, and neurons became smaller. Several studies have observed ultrastructural changes in sympathetic ganglia neurons (Vega, Calzada, & Del Valle, 1993). A behavioral study with human subjects measured pupillary reflexes (associated with sympathetic innervation) and found that declines such as diminished reflex amplitude and velocity accompanied aging (Bitsios, Prettyman, & Szabadi, 1996). In the parasympathetic *retrofacial nucleus* (a brainstem structure that contributes fibers to the vagus nerve), Sturrock (1988) observed a loss of neurons and reduced intracellular Nissl substance (which may indicate impaired neuronal health) in old mice.

Other studies have found no signs of aging. For example, research on the superior cervical ganglion (which innervates the iris, submandibular gland, and parotid gland) indicates resistance to age-related anatomical change (Santer, 1993). Thus, aging is probably not uniform across ganglia. Indeed, within the same animals, the absence and presence of age effects (as indicated by the accumulation of lipofuscin) can be found in different autonomic ganglia (Koistinaho, 1986).

There is some evidence that age effects observed in autonomic components may be related to their target organs (Cowen, 1993). For example, Andrews (1996) showed that sympathetic neurons innervating the middle cerebral artery exhibited axonal and dendritic atrophy with age, whereas this was not the case for neurons innervating the iris. One interpretation of these and other similar findings is that changes in the availability of neurotrophic factors provided by the targets are responsible for the differential vulnerability of autonomic ganglia.

Gerontological research has tended to focus on physiological and neurochemical aspects of the autonomic nervous system, particularly the sympathetic division (e.g., see Docherty, 1993). One fairly consistent finding is that NE levels of older people are generally higher, increase more in response to sympathetic stimulation (e.g., exercise, standing upright, mental stress), and remain high longer when compared to young adults (Borst, 1996; Finch & Landfield, 1985; Kuchel & Kuchel, 1993). Circulating levels of NE reflect the activity of sympathetic postganglionic nerve terminals and, to a lesser extent, the adrenal medulla. The increased NE levels may represent a reduced ability to clear out excess NE or, more probably, increased release by the sympathetic neurons. A possible explanation for the increased NE release is that the sensitivity of the target organs to NE tends to decline with age (e.g., fewer receptors), so more NE must be released to compensate. Another factor might be decreased sensitivity of the baroreceptors that monitor blood pressure (see below). Impairment of the reflex results in greater sympathetic activity and therefore higher levels of NE. Another possible contributor to increased NE levels is the loss of α_2-adrenergic (NE) receptors which are found presynaptically and negatively regulate NE release (Marin, 1995).

The complexity of autonomic regulatory functions and the relatively small amount of neurogerontological research limit our understanding of aging and autonomic regulation of various organ systems. Mitigating this shortcoming somewhat, it seems that most age-related autonomic dysfunctions are not severe enough to be clinically significant (but see discussions below), unless combined with coexisting disease processes or the use of drugs that interfere with autonomic function (Supiano & Halter, 1992).

THE REGULATION OF SPECIFIC FUNCTIONS

Now that we have a general background with respect to how the hypothalamus, endocrine system, and autonomic nervous system are organized and interact, we can focus on the specific functions that are regulated to maintain homeostasis and how each fares with age.

Cardiovascular Function

The heart's rate and pumping properties are modulated by the relative activity of sympathetic and parasympathetic divisions of the autonomic nervous system. Sympathetic neural activity increases heart rate and predominates under stressful conditions, whereas parasympathetic activity slows it and predominates when the body is at rest.

As Lakatta (1990) noted, gerontological studies of these systems are complicated by the high prevalence of cardiovascular disease in the senior population. It is difficult to find cardiologically healthy subjects, since about 60% of men who live into their 50s have substantial narrowing of at least one major coronary artery. Furthermore, coronary disease is often occult, so researchers may be unaware of its presence in some of their "healthy" subjects. Also, cardiovascular function is affected if healthy subjects have ceased exercising regularly, as is often the case with senior citizens. And, even in the absence of disease, older people usually exhibit changes in the structure and function of arteries and other tissue that can affect cardiovascular function (e.g., Marin, 1995). Despite these potential hazards, overall cardiac performance is generally not greatly altered in older, healthy, active people *under resting conditions* (Lakatta, 1990).

In contrast to the resting condition, however, exercise stress often poses problems for seniors. Declines in the heart's maximum functional capacity under exercise stress are often observed, and autonomic control of the heart can become less precise (Goldberg, Kreider, & Roberts, 1984; Lakatta, 1985, 1990; Marin, 1995). The factors that contribute to this are complex, involving heart structure, morphological and compliance changes in heart tissue, and vasculature, autonomic innervation, and dynamic adjustments to acute stress.

During high levels of exercise, sympathetic control of the heart dominates. Lakatta (1985) points out that changes in sympathetic function alone could, in principle, account for a number of common age-related changes in cardiac function: a decrease in the maximum heart rate and the degree to which the heart contracts, increased impedance of the aorta to blood flow, and changes in the regulation of blood flow to the muscles. Evidence for this comes largely from pharmacological studies. For example, isoproterenol (a drug that mimics NE) has a reduced effect on the heart, and the effects of β-adrenergic receptor blockers (beta blockers) are diminished in older subjects. Although these drugs might have other effects on cardiovascular function besides altering sympathetic regulation (Lakatta, 1990), there is good evidence that diminished responsiveness of the heart to β-adrenergic stimulation can alter the heart's response to exercise stress. This does not appear to be due to a decrease in the secretion of NE or epinephrine during exercise. Rather, the capacity of heart muscle to respond to these neurotransmitters probably diminishes with aging. Evidence suggests that the change may lie in various steps in the β-adrenergic pathway within cells after the receptor has been activated (Scarpace, 1986).

The arterial baroreflex (*baro* = blood pressure) acts as a buffer against changes in arterial pressure and regulates minute-to-minute blood pressure. The receptors for this reflex are located in arteries of the upper body. When blood pressure increases, the vessels expand, and the baroreceptors are activated. This triggers reflexive inhibition of sympathetic activity to reduce heart rate and the resistance of peripheral blood vessels, thereby lowering blood pressure. The reflex inhibition of sympathetic activity is often impaired in older people. One contributor to this problem is likely to be reduced sensitivity of the baroreceptors themselves; the arteries become more rigid with age and are less capable of signaling an increase in blood pressure (Borst, 1996; Roberts, Snyder, Johnson, & Horwitz, 1993). However, faults in the central components of the reflex may be implicated as well. Hajduczok, Chapleau, and Abboud (1991) found that the ability to maintain inhibitory neural activity is diminished in central pathways that mediate baroreflex inhibition of sympathetic activity. Johnson and Felder (1993) studied physiological properties of neurons in the *medial nucleus of the solitary tract* (mNTS), which receives major input from the arterial baroreceptors. Whereas age effects were not pronounced, some changes in mNTS neurons were observed (e.g., more neurons with high electrical resistance), and these might affect the baroreflex. Other researchers have also provided evidence of age-related changes in the central components of the baroreflex (Barringer & Bunag, 1991; Eriksson, Kerecsen, & Bunag, 1991; Roberts et al., 1993). Whatever the exact mechanisms, the result is reduced ability to adjust blood pressure to changing conditions, as well as a general increase in blood pressure because of increased sympathetic activity.

Sympathetic stimulation of β-adrenergic receptors also mediates the postural hemodynamic response, which responds to the drop in upper body blood pressure when one stands up rapidly. Reduced β-adrenergic responsiveness (from altered receptor-coupled responses) affects this type of blood pressure adjustment, as well as the response to exercise stress (Borst, 1996). Declines in α-adrenergic receptors in heart and veins may contribute to problems with the postural adjustments as well.

Parasympathetic innervation of the heart is provided by the vagus nerve. There is evidence that the vagal tone declines with age in some cases. This is associated with a decrease in the intrinsic resting heart rate with a concomitant reduction in the need of the parasympathetic system to slow the heart rate (Borst, 1996; Low, Opfer-Gehrking, Proper, & Zimmerman, 1990).

Respiration

The function of breathing is to bring in sufficient oxygen (O_2) to support life, and to expel carbon dioxide (CO_2) after the oxygen has been extracted from air and transferred to the blood. Breathing is controlled by respiratory centers in the brain, primarily the medulla and pons. As in any function the brain performs, certain information must be acquired, in this case the amounts of O_2 and CO_2 available. Specialized sensors (receptors) in the brainstem are designed to monitor the blood for concentrations of these blood gases. This information is then used to control the respiratory neurons of the medulla and pons, which modulate output to the muscles of the chest and abdomen, causing them to constrict or relax in a manner that controls expiration and inspiration of the lungs. All of this is done automatically and involuntarily, although we obviously have some control of our breathing. The nervous system also coordinates activity of muscles of the larynx and pharynx to keep the airway clear (e.g., coughing). Because breathing and heartbeat go hand in hand, the two functions are coordinated by the nervous system.

The most serious threats to respiration in older people have to do with changes in the structure and capacity of the lungs and breathing muscles and exchange of oxygen and carbon dioxide. This is most often associated with tumors, smoking, and disease. The literature does not provide strong evidence that neural control of respiratory adjustments to changing demands for oxygen becomes consistently altered with age. However, when age effects are observed, central deficiencies are likely to be involved (Cherniack & Altose, 1996). One source of difficulty is the diminished ability of respiratory control neurons in the brain to monitor the requirements for oxygen and status of lung and respiratory muscle tissue, particularly if the tissue elasticity has been altered or affected by respiratory illness. The coordination of heart rate and respiration can be diminished with age as well (Davies, 1975).

Changes in the autonomic nervous system might also affect respiration. For example, bronchial smooth muscle is innervated by the parasympathetic vagus nerve and cholinergic stimulation constricts the airway. This response can be exaggerated with age, apparently because of a decrease in acetylcholinesterase available to terminate the synaptic action of Ach (see chapter 4). Also, β-adrenergic receptors in the submucosal glands and bronchial arteries in the lungs are involved with counteracting parasympathetic constriction of the bronchial smooth muscles that modify the airway. Age-related declines in these β-adrenergic receptors have been observed in animals and could result in breathing problems (Borst, 1996).

Gastrointestinal Control

The movements of smooth muscles in various parts of the digestive system are coordinated by the CNS, the autonomic nervous system, and the *enteric nervous system.* The latter is found in the wall of the gut in the *myenteric* and *submucosal* plexuses and is primarily controlled by hormones. Because digestion is inhibited by the sympathetic nervous system and facilitated by the parasympathetic system, autonomic dysfunction may contribute to gastrointestinal difficulties many older people experience. The problems can include difficulty swallowing, slower gastric emptying and intestinal transit time, constipation, and reduced absorption of calcium and fat (Borst, 1996). One factor that might contribute is a loss of myenteric neurons and other age effects, which have been observed in a number of studies on humans and rodents (de Souza, Moratelli, Borges, & Liberti, 1993; Gomes, de Souza, & Liberti, 1997; Santer & Baker, 1993). Impaired autonomic control could be significant for older individuals with digestive problems.

Regulation of Body Temperature

The body must function within a rather narrow range of its core set point of 37°C. The brain dictates behavioral strategies that facilitate temperature regulation, such as staying in an indoor climate-controlled environment or annually migrating between New England and Florida. Of course, these measures are not sufficient to maintain thermal homeostasis by themselves, and physiological thermoregulatory mechanisms are constantly being engaged. The two major mechanisms to conserve heat and increase body temperature are *vasoconstriction*, which reduces the heat transfer from the body to the outside by reducing peripheral blood flow, and *thermogenesis*, the production of heat from metabolic activity. The latter is associated with shivering. Increasing physical activity also increases heat production, but this also increases blood flow to muscles, which counteracts the vasoconstriction mechanism. To lower body temperature, mechanisms such as sweating (which cools by evaporation) and vasodilation (which allows heat to dissipate from blood to the outside) are engaged. Morphological features of the body are also important, including the amount of subcutaneous fat (which retains heat) and body size (a large body loses less heat because of the smaller surface-to-volume ratio).

The components of the "thermostat" that maintains temperature around 37°C are found primarily in the hypothalamus, with the *preoptic area* and *anterior hypothalamus* being particularly important. Neurons here receive information about body temperature from thermoreceptors distributed throughout the skin, viscera, and spinal cord, and they have their own thermoreceptors to monitor the core temperature as well. The latter are believed to modulate the firing of certain neurons in the hypothalamus to regulate temperature. In response to an increase in body temperature, neurons in the preoptic area come into play and, with the cooperation of the autonomic nervous system, cause dilation of blood vessels and suppression of shivering. Decreased body temperature triggers responses of hypothalamic neurons, which cause constriction of blood vessels and shivering (also with autonomic participation). The hypothalamus also influences body temperature by regulating the release of thyroxine, which increases tissue metabolism to create more body heat. In addition, animal experiments have shown that hypothalamic regions facilitate the learning of behaviors that affect body temperature, such as gaining access to cool air.

Various lesion-behavior experiments have shown that damage to the hypothalamus in young animals impairs thermoregulation. Thus, if aging were associated with dysfunction of the thermoregulatory regions of the hypothalamus and other participating brain regions, problems would be expected in maintaining the temperature set point. Is there evidence that such problems tend to occur in older people? The ability to tolerate heat and engage appropriate cooling responses (e.g., sweating) are typically not greatly compromised in older people who are healthy and physically fit, although the literature is not in complete agreement on this issue (Pandolf, 1997). Cold tolerance, on the other hand, can be more problematic for older people, although here too there is a good deal of inconsistency in the literature (Young & Lee, 1997). One generally supported finding is that the ability to reduce peripheral blood flow by constriction of blood vessels during mild or brief cold exposures tends to occur more slowly in older people. Some research also indicates that increased metabolic heat production from shivering becomes muted as people age, and this may be more problematic for men than women. These factors may contribute to the higher prevalence of hypothermia (core body temperature less than 35°C) and risk of deaths from hypothermia observed in the older population (Young & Lee, 1997). However, even though the hypothermic risk increases with age, it is still a rare primary cause of death (Young & Lee, 1997).

In summary, the brain mechanisms and other physiological responses required for temperature regulation appear to fare reasonably well in healthy older people, as indicated by their generally adequate ability to tolerate heat and cold stress.

Eating and Weight Regulation

A person's eating behaviors and weight are influenced by a number of familiar variables such as metabolic activity and demands, physical exercise, general health, drug therapies, psychological factors such as depression, what and how much one eats (appetite), and even ill-fitting dentures—all of which can be altered with aging. Most of the research in this area falls within the disciplines of nutrition, endocrinology, exercise physiology, sociology, and other areas of gerontology, which are beyond the scope of this book (see Ausman & Russell, 1990; Blumberg, 1996; Goldberg, Dengel, & Hagberg, 1996; Goldberg & Hagberg, 1990; Mobbs, 1996; Morley & Korenman, 1992; Rolls & Drewnowski, 1996). For our purposes, we focus on the neural mechanisms that underlie eating and the cessation of eating, hunger and satiety, and the regulation of body weight.

People tend to eat less as they age (Morley, 1996). The intake of energy-producing foods and certain nutrients tends to decline, and many older people are at increased risk of malnutrition. Paradoxically, however, the prevalence of being overweight and having more body fat increases with age. This suggests that the ability to properly regulate food intake in response to nutritional requirements may be upset in older individuals, and there is evidence that this is the case in both humans and other species (see Rolls & Drewnowski, 1996). This leads us again to the hypothalamus, hormones, and autonomic nervous system.

Experimental or pathological damage to various areas of the brain can alter eating and weight regulation. It follows that, if age-related changes were to occur in these regions, similar effects might occur. Although key aspects of the damage and the mechanisms involved can be difficult to pin down, many experiments have shown that lesions in the region of the lateral hypothalamus result in undereating and weight loss; damage in the regions of the ventromedial hypothalamus and paraventricular nucleus of the hypothalamus result in increased eating and weight gain. It is important to note, however, that none of these is a "center" for eating or satiety; rather, they are components of complicated neural circuitry that controls eating and weight regulation.

The neural circuits that underlie the experience of hunger or satiety and the initiation or cessation of eating are influenced by several variables, including the palatability and taste of food, the distention of the stomach and intestines, the secretion of the hormone cholecystokinin (CCK) and other peptides in the intestine, and blood levels of glucose and other nutrients. The availability of nutrients is also modulated by the release of the pancreatic hormones insulin (which promotes entry of glucose into cells) and glucagon (which stimulates the liver to convert stored glycogen to glucose), and this is tied into the neural circuitry as well. Other hormones and neurotransmitters also play important roles, including neuropeptide Y, NE, galanin, dopamine, serotonin, and estradiol (Kalat, 1998). In addition, psychological factors such as the time of day and daily eating routines come into play.

Age-related changes in the aforementioned variables could lead to anorexia (Rolls & Drewnowski, 1996). For example, the senses of taste and smell often become blunted with age, as discussed in chapter 7. For those who enjoy a good meal, this probably makes the eating of good-tasting foods less enjoyable and compelling and could contribute to reduced food intake. Indeed, amplifying the flavor of food can be an effective treatment for anorexia in older people (Schiffman & Warwick, 1988).

Gastrointestinal changes also occur with age, and these could alter neural messages signaling stomach or intestine distension. If the system erred toward signaling premature distension, satiety could be reached earlier. Also, reduced gut motility could influence meal patterns. Studies of aging rodents have also shown that CCK can have a greater appetite-suppressing effect (Morley & Silver, 1988).

Neuropeptide Y is synthesized in the *arcuate nucleus* of the hypothalamus and secreted into the paraventricular nucleus. When this occurs, eating behavior is stimulated. Thus, the initiation of eating appears to rely, at least in part, on the synthesis, secretion, and response to neuropeptide Y. It is of interest, then, that the neuropeptide Y system and its ability to respond to increased nutritional needs after fasting are diminished in old animals (see Mobbs, 1996). Other relevant neurotransmitter and hormonal systems can also change with age, including serotonin, NE, dopamine, and estradiol (discussed elsewhere).

Given all of this, it is clear that the potential exists for the regulation of eating and weight to be thrown out of kilter by many, if not all, of the interacting mechanisms and variables involved. We can add age-related changes in the autonomic nervous system, since these influence the digestive system and other aspects of eating behavior, as well as psychological conditions like depression. It is not surprising that many older people are faced with a constant struggle to maintain an optimum level of nutrition and body weight.

Drinking and Hydration

To maintain the proper amount of fluids in the body, there must be a balance between the water and salt that is lost (from breathing, evaporation, urination, sweating) and what is taken in through drinking and eating. The need for water is accompanied by the psychological experience of thirst; the need for salt is experienced as salt appetite. *Osmotic thirst*, which occurs when cells become dehydrated, is monitored by osmoreceptors in the viscera, vasculature, and brain. Osmotic information is available to the supraoptic and paraventricular nuclei of the hypothalamus, which control the excretion of vasopressin (antidiuretic hormone) by the posterior pituitary gland. Vasopressin enables the kidneys to reabsorb water. A reduction in blood volume also triggers thirst (*hypovolemic thirst*). Changes in blood volume are detected by vascular baroreceptors, as well as by hormonal mechanisms. The kidneys respond to blood loss by releasing the hormone *renin*, which ultimately leads to the production of another hormone, *angiotensin II*, which constricts blood vessels to compensate for the loss in blood pressure. Information from the baroreceptors reaches the brain via the nucleus of the solitary tract, whereas angiotensin II in the blood stimulates neurons in the *sensory circumventricular organs* of the brain (e.g., the *subfornical organ* and others). These organs lie outside the blood-brain barrier, where they can monitor the blood more effectively. From here, information is relayed to the complex circuits in the brain that include the preoptic area of the hypothalamus. The activity of these circuits motivates drinking and salt intake. Water and sodium homeostasis is also influenced by the hormone *aldosterone,* which is produced by the adrenal cortex when the body's reserves of sodium are low; the result is increased intake and conservation of sodium, reduced urine production, and conservation of water. In addition to vasopressin, renin, angiotensin, and aldosterone, a number of other neurotransmitters and hormones influence the regulatory system (e.g., endogenous opioids, serotonin, and NE).

Serious dehydration is a significant geriatric condition, but it is usually associated with illness, disease, or drugs (Wilson & Morley, 1996). Nevertheless, even in the absence of such factors, aging is typically associated with reduced fluid intake.

Several variables that may interact with one another are likely to contribute to hypodipsia in older people (Mooradian, 1992; Wilson & Morley, 1996). First, the ability of the aging nervous system to employ at least some of the neurotransmitters and hormones implicated in drinking and thirst can decline. For example, there is evidence that the production, metabolism, and/or activity of renin, angiotensin, and aldosterone can be compromised with aging (Mooradian, 1992). In the CNS, impairments in adrenergic circuits that modulate vasopressin activity might contribute to age effects. Also, reduced efficacy of opioid circuits (lower neurotransmitter production and/or loss of receptors) in older subjects has been linked to hypodipsia and reduced thirst (Wilson & Morley, 1996).

Second, monitoring the hydration status and water needs of the body may become impaired with age. Age-related changes in the baroreceptor system (see above) could interfere with the hypovolemic thirst mechanism, and reduced sensitivity of osmoreceptors could interfere with osmotic thirst. Also, a cardiac hormone, atrial natriuretic hormone, responds to blood volume changes, and this system may be altered in older people in a manner that affects thirst and drinking (Mooradian, 1992).

Third, diminution of kidney functions typically accompany aging. This can impair the ability to filter and concentrate urine or respond to vasopressin and may disrupt the renin-angiotensin system (Phillips, Johnston, & Gray, 1993).

Fourth, older people may drink less because of secondary factors. Thirst perception may be impaired in older people, leading to reduced water intake despite an existing need. Reduced drinking also accompanies anorexia: As food intake drops, so does the amount of water taken in.

Finally, various socioeconomic variables may contribute to the type and amount of fluid consumed.

SUMMARY AND CONCLUSIONS

Most serious problems with homeostasis and the efficacy of vital functions that occur in older people are likely to be associated with illness, chronic disease, nonneural aspects of aging, or the use of medications. In most cases, the nervous system's role in the dysfunction is probably secondary or minimal, as the target organs or systems are the site of primary damage or pathology. Indeed, maladies of the heart, lungs, gastrointestinal tract, and other organ systems are common in older people, and changes in body composition and general health problems are often independent of neural regulation per se. In short, one does not "need" to have faulty neural control in order for a system to fail.

When we speak of healthy older people, we are implying that none of the vital neural control systems has deteriorated too much. On the other hand, it is apparent from the literature that homeostatic mechanisms in older people are not likely to perform as effectively as they once did, even in the healthy. This is particularly the case when the system is challenged by some sort of stressor or extreme condition.

The take-home message is that relatively minor functional defects tend to accrue in the hypothalamus, neuroendocrine system, and autonomic nervous system in a variety of regulatory contexts. Whereas individually these changes may not be life-threatening or even problematic in most situations, their composite effects will be felt. They are part and parcel of what constitutes "normal aging." A neurogerontological perspective would seem to be rather important in dealing effectively with most geriatric issues involving these systems, if the quality of life is to be optimized in older people.

7
Obtaining Information with the Sensory Systems

The second basic function of nervous systems is to obtain information about the environment, a task assigned to the various sensory systems. The neural means by which sensory stimuli are experienced involve multistage processes requiring high-quality representation of stimuli by the peripheral sensory apparatus, undistorted neural messages carried by action potentials into the brain, and accurate processing of the information by the central sensory systems (CSSs). Disruption of any of these processes with age would have the potential to cause problems in the sensory domain. Thus, an understanding of the relationships among aging and the sensory systems must take into account factors that might degrade the neural messages sent to the brain, as well as factors that affect the brain and its ability to process those messages.

A note on terminology: In referring to the experiences and behavioral consequences of sensory system activity, we shall use the terms *sensory* and *sensations* when emphasizing the role of these systems. However, the terms *perception* and *perceptual*, which imply further neural elaboration of sensations, are often appropriate as well. It is often the case that either terminology seems applicable; sensory experiences are also perceptual ones and vice versa. However, perception often encompasses a good deal more, such as assigning cognitive understanding or learned meaning to the sensory information (largely involving parts of the brain outside the sensory systems per se). Indeed, another person's attitudes and intentions can be "perceived" mentally even in the absence of current sensory information. On the other hand, sensory phenomena need not be perceived. For example, sensory input from stretch receptors in the muscles are constantly engaging postural reflexes that are not directly experienced.

AGING AND SENSORY ABILITIES

The sad truth is, our sensory abilities almost inevitably decline with age. The rate and severity of the decline may vary considerably among individuals and across sensory modalities within individuals, but few if any octogenarians possess the same sensory capacities they started out with. This conclusion is evident in the numerous books, chapters, reviews, and articles addressing this topic (e.g., Abramson & Lovas, 1988; Birren, 1996; Corso, 1981; Ordy & Brizzee, 1979; Verrillo & Verrillo, 1985; and many others cited below).

Audition

The term *presbycusis* or *presbyacusis* is typically used to describe the changes in hearing associated with aging. Hearing disorders are among the most common health problems of the senior citizenry; depending on the clinical criteria, testing methods, and so on, 25% to more than 50% of septuagenarians have clinically significant degrees of hearing loss that can be detected by routine hearing tests (audiograms). Whereas the most commonly mentioned manifestation of presbycusis is a loss of sensitivity for high-frequency sounds, the types of hearing problems confronting older listeners extend to suprathreshold stimuli, including speech perception, hearing in noisy backgrounds, hearing in suboptimal conditions, distorted loudness of sounds, and tinnitus (ringing in the ears) (Gordon-Salant, 1996; Willott, 1991). Age-related changes in a variety of auditory abilities must be implicit in the term *presbycusis*. Thus, a formal definition (Willott, 1991) is *hearing impairment associated with various types of auditory system dysfunction, peripheral or central, that accompany aging and cannot be accounted for by extraordinary ototraumatic, genetic, or pathological conditions. The term* hearing impairment *implies deficits in absolute thresholds and/or suprathreshold perception.*

Vision

A host of visual deficits may accompany aging (Corso, 1981; Kline & Scialfa, 1996; Morgan, 1986; Rubin, Roche, Prasada-Rao, & Fried, 1994; Spear, 1993; Verrillo & Verrillo, 1985). Thresholds for detection of low light levels become elevated; susceptibility to glare increases; the critical flicker frequency (the rate at which a flickering light appears to become a continuous light) decreases (i.e., poorer temporal resolution); visual acuity, the ability to discriminate fine details, decreases, especially at lower light levels, for both static and moving stimuli; the ability to see close objects declines; contrast sensitivity is reduced; depth perception may diminish slightly. Changes in color vision tend to be minimal until relatively late in life, at which point shorter wavelengths (blues and greens) may be affected.

Somatosensation

The somatosensory system encompasses a number of submodalities, including the senses of touch, pressure, vibration, heat, cold, pain, joint position, and musculoskeletal movement (kinesthesia). Aging is usually accompanied by some losses in somatosensory sensitivity (Corso, 1981; Kenshalo, 1979; McBride, 1988; Stevens & Cruz, 1996; Verrillo & Verrillo, 1985; Weisenberger, 1996). The ability to detect a light touch or discriminate two points on the skin tends to decrease with age. Age-related losses are well documented for the vibration sense. The loss of sensitivity is great for higher frequency tactile vibrations (40 to 500 Hz) and minimal for lower frequencies (10 to 40 Hz)—a pattern analogous to the loss of sensitivity for high-frequency tones in presbycusis (although the mechanisms responsible are different for the two systems). The research on temperature sensation is somewhat inconsistent, but older people may be less good at discriminating different temperatures and perhaps less sensitive to heat stimuli. It is important to note that somatosensory age effects can vary in different regions of the body. For example, loss of vibration sensitivity tends to be greater in the lower extremities, and loss of tactile acuity is greater in the finger than in the forearm and lip.

It is difficult to study pain for ethical reasons and the fact that the experience of pain is influenced by various psychological factors such as anxiety, which might be different in older people (see chapter 10). Not surprisingly, then, there is some disagreement with respect to whether sensitivity to pain becomes altered with age (Harkins & Scott, 1996). Reports of increased, decreased, or no effect on pain sensitivity or tolerance for pain in older subjects have all been published.

Some discrepancies in findings on aging and somatosensation are likely to be the result of methodological differences. For example, Stevens and

Cruz (1996) noted that gerontological studies of tactile sensitivity typically use single brief threshold tests that produce considerable "scatter" in thresholds; thus, some individual thresholds of older subjects can be lower (more sensitive) than some thresholds of younger subjects. However, when these researchers used more thorough, repeated testing, all of the older subjects tested worse than the worst of the young subjects for tactile detection of gaps between points, orientation of lines, and length of line. The more thorough testing approach suggests that a loss of acuity for touch is likely to have declined in nearly every elderly person.

Balance and Postural Control: Proprioception, the Vestibular Senses, and Vision

The combined input from the visual system, the vestibular system, and the proprioceptive systems (the somatosensory submodalities for body position and movement) are used to control posture and center of gravity, maintain balance, and orient oneself in space. Age-related changes in proprioception include diminished awareness of foot position (Robbins, Waked, & McClaran, 1995), reduced ability to detect movements of the joints (in particular the lower joints and especially when the movement is slow), vibration sensitivity in the ankles, visual difficulties (described above), and less effective vestibular capacities (experiencing acceleration or rotation). These can combine to cause vertigo, increased sway, trouble regaining balance after stumbling, falling down, and alterations in locomotion (Cohen, Heaton, Congdon, & Jenkins, 1996; Horak, Shupert, & Mirka, 1989; Katsarkas, 1994; Woollacott, 1996; see also chapter 9). The interaction between visual and vestibular systems (e.g., vestibulo-ocular reflex, control of eye movements, and visual pursuits) can also show declines with age (Paige, 1994).

Olfaction

The ability to identify odors and enjoy the flavor of food and drink rely heavily on the sense of smell. Olfactory thresholds of people over 65 are often substantially higher than those of young adults; in addition, the perceived strength of odors declines, and older people may have difficulty in naming specific odors (Bartoshuk & Weiffenbach, 1990; Murphy, 1993;

Schiffman, 1996; Stevens & Dadarwala, 1993). Even over a 3-year period, longitudinal testing can detect declines in smell identification in healthy subjects (Ship, Pearson, Cruise, Brant, & Metter, 1996). Olfactory sensitivity is strongly affected by exposure to chemicals and other environmental events, and these can interact with changes that are associated with aging per se (Corwin, Loury, & Gilbert, 1995). The negative implications of diminished olfaction are not restricted to pleasures of the palate. Reduced ability to detect household gas or other toxic molecules can have dangerous consequences.

Gustation

The sensations of sweet, sour, salty, and bitter combine with olfactory sensations to produce the flavor or "taste" of foods and other substances. A number of studies have shown that many older people exhibit some declines in taste sensitivity (Bartoshuk & Weiffenbach, 1990; Schiffman, 1996; Stevens, Cruz, Hoffman, & Patterson, 1995). There is some disagreement with respect to the prevalence of diminished taste sensitivity, however. Stevens and colleagues (1995) noted that, in studies where many subjects are tested (but each in a single test session), there is a great deal of scatter in thresholds as a function of age, suggesting that many older people have excellent taste sensitivity. When subjects are repeatedly tested, however, clearer age differences are observed. Whereas the data of Stevens and colleagues (1995) suggest that many older people have some loss of taste sensitivity, there is still substantial variability among individuals. It is also important to note that when taste is greatly altered in older people, medications and medical disorders are likely to have contributed significantly.

AGING AND THE SENSORY PERIPHERY

The peripheral interface between information processing by the brain and stimuli on "the outside." If information about the physical world is to be used by the brain and/or experienced, it must be translated into neural signals and sent to the brain for further processing. The information finds its way into the brain via the spinal and cranial nerves and is carried by action potentials, the signals that transmit neural information over distances in the nervous system. *Transduction* refers to the operations by which various forms of external energy or entities are changed into neural events (graded potentials leading to action potentials) for further processing by the brain. Transduction is initiated by *sensory receptors,* specialized cells designed to be affected by certain physical stimuli in a manner that produces a neural event (usually a change in the voltage across the receptor cell's membrane). Examples of receptors and the stimuli that affect them (called *adequate stimuli*) are the rods and cones in the eye's retina that are chemically altered by light, taste buds that react to certain types of molecules (e.g. salt, sugar), and free nerve endings that respond to physical perturbations of the skin (e.g., pressure, temperature change, pinpricks). The primary reaction between stimulus and receptor (mechanical or chemical) is an essential step in the processing of sensory information.

Generating action potentials to carry the information from sensory receptor cells to the brain.   In some cases (e.g., olfactory receptor cells, free nerve endings), the receptor cells are modified neurons with their own axons, capable of generating action potentials that are sent directly into the CSSs. For these receptors, the adequate stimuli produce graded depolarizations of the receptor cell membrane, which, if sufficiently strong, trigger action potentials. In other cases (e.g., rods and cones, auditory and vestibular hair cells, taste buds) the receptor cells do not have axons. Their membrane voltages are altered by their intercourse with adequate stimuli, and this causes the release of a neurotransmitter at a synapse with another neuron. If these synaptic potentials are sufficiently strong, action potentials are generated in the sensory neurons and sent to the CSS.

Prereceptor modification of stimuli.   Before the physical stimuli "out there" ever reach the sensory receptors, they may be modified by specialized structures. The structures can filter out irrelevant or unimportant information, as well as amplify or enhance particularly important stimuli. The prereceptor modification can have profound effects on sensory stimuli. The most familiar example is the eye. Before light reaches the rod and cone receptors in the back of the eye, it is refracted and focused by the cornea and lens. In addition, the size of the pupil is adjusted to regulate the amount of light entering the eye, and motor systems controlling the position of the eyes and head determine which part of the visual field enters the eye to reach the retina. A breakdown in any of these events will disrupt the system's efficiency.

With the exception of the auditory system (see below), the other sensory systems do not require the same extent of prereceptor stimulus modification, and in a number of cases there is little modification of stimuli before they encounter the receptors. An example is the olfactory system, where odor-producing molecules are simply drawn into the nasal cavities to contact olfactory receptors. There is some nonneural modification even here, however, as the flow, concentration, and temperature of the odor molecules can be modified by the sniffing process.

To summarize, it is obvious that problems would be created in the sensory domain by factors that reduce the number or efficiency of receptors, impair their ability to transduce stimuli into neural events, or interfere with the prereceptor modification of stimuli. Not surprisingly, these peripheral stages of sensory processing are often negatively affected by aging, as seen below.

The Peripheral Auditory System

Of all the sensory systems, the process by which acoustic stimuli are converted to action potentials is the most convoluted—a seeming Rube Goldberg arrangement involving various prereceptor processes. The auditory system's task is to detect and analyze movements and rapid vibrations of objects in the environment (between 20 and 20,000 Hz for human hearing). When an object vibrates rapidly, it displaces molecules of air (or water or solids), which in turn displace other molecules. Repeated back-and-forth movements result in a wave of displacements outward from the sound source. When the air molecules are pushed together within the wave, the air pressure increases slightly; when they are pulled apart, air pressure decreases.

These minute pressure changes are what the auditory system has got to work with, and this is problematic. The sensory receptors (hair cells) are located in a fluid-filled duct; the cochlea, embedded in the temporal bone of the skull. Even if air pressure changes could reach the cochlea, they would have little effect because fluid is much heavier (has a higher impedance) than air and is hard to move using air pressure changes.

Some mechanical amplification is required, and evolution has provided an answer. The mammalian auditory system features an air-filled middle ear whose opening to the outer ear canal is covered by an elastic eardrum. When the air pressure of a sound wave is greater in the ear canal than the air pressure inside the middle ear, the eardrum is pushed in; when the low pressure part of the wave arrives, the eardrum is pulled out. Because the middle ear is air filled (low impedance), this works well. The next step is to transfer these movements to the fluid-filled cochlea, and this is done using a chain of three bones, the middle ear ossicles. One end of the ossicular chain is attached to the eardrum and moves with it; the other end of the chain is attached to an elastic membrane (the oval window) that opens into the cochlea. Because of leverage and a focusing of force from the relatively large eardrum to the small oval window, the movement of the ossicular chain is able to move the fluid column in the cochlea. At this point, outside air pressure changes have been transduced into mechanical movements.

Inside the cochlea is another elastic structure, the basilar membrane. The basilar membrane is moved (displaced) by movements of the fluid column, which had been moved by the ossicular chain. It is on the basilar membrane that the auditory receptors are found, a row of inner hair cells (IHCs) and three rows of outer hair cells (OHCs). The hair cells (mostly the IHCs) make synaptic contact with auditory nerve fibers. When the basilar membrane moves, the hair cells are moved, and this causes the release of excitatory neurotransmitter molecules, generating action potentials in the auditory nerve fibers, which are transmitted to the brain. The transduction process is complete.

Whereas it might be expected that aging would have a significant effect on the complicated mechanical transduction process, this is typically not the case. Some older people have hearing loss caused by changes in the elastic properties of the eardrum or altered movements of the ossicular chain, but the primary cause of presbycusis involves damage to the cochlea. Six varieties of cochlear pathology and corresponding "types" of presbycusis can be recognized (this classification was proposed by Willott [1991] to incorporate observations by H. Schuknecht, J. Hawkins, and others): (1) sensory presbycusis (primary damage is to the OHCs); (2) neural presbycusis (primary damage is to the spiral ganglion cells, whose axons form the auditory nerve); (3) sensorineural presbycusis (a combination of IHC, OHC, and spiral ganglion cell damage—probably the most common age-related cochlear pathology); (4) metabolic or strial presbycusis (dysfunction of the *stria vascularis*, the tissue that provides the primary metabolic and microenvironmental support to the cochlea); (5) mechanical presbycusis (changes in the mechanical properties of the basilar membrane, which in turn affects the responses of the hair cells); and (6) vascular presbycusis (impaired cochlear physiology caused by a reduced blood supply from altered capillaries and/or blood vessels). "Pure" cases are relatively rare, as most aging cochleas probably exhibit some degree of each type of change. In all cases, however, the result is diminished and/ or distorted transduction of acoustic stimuli into neural events.

Because the link between the cochlea and the central auditory system is provided by the axons of spiral ganglion cells (which form the auditory nerve), attrition of these neurons in sensorineural presbycusis diminishes the amount and quality of auditory input to the brain. The loss of spiral ganglion cells is often severe, as shown in Figure 7.1; although this example is from mice, a similar picture is often the case with elderly humans as well. Thus, both the quality of auditory information processed by the cochlea and its central transmission are reduced.

Schmiedt, Mills, and Boettcher (1996) showed that even when sensori-neural degeneration is not severe, changes in the fibers of the auditory nerve may occur in old gerbils. Auditory nerve fibers come in two varieties: high- and low-spontaneous activity (i.e., the rate of action potential firing in the absence of acoustic stimulation). The researchers found that, in old gerbils, the number of low-activity fibers decreased. The low-spontaneous-activity fibers are thought to code wide ranges of acoustic intensities, preserve information about the timing of sounds, and convey information in the presence of noise. Schmiedt and colleagues (1996) suggested that a loss of low spontaneously active axons could account for the difficulty older listeners have hearing rapidly changing sounds or hearing in noisy conditions.

The Peripheral Visual System

Reflected or transmitted patterns of light (electromagnetic waves within a restricted band of wavelengths) provide a great deal of information about the world, which is exploited by the visual system. Patterns of light are focused on the retina after entering the eye via the cornea and lens. The retina is, embryologically, an extension of the brain and contains a complex network of neurons, in addition to the sensory cells that transduce light into neural responses, the rods and cones. Action potentials in the optic nerves carry the information from the retina to the brain, where further information processing occurs.

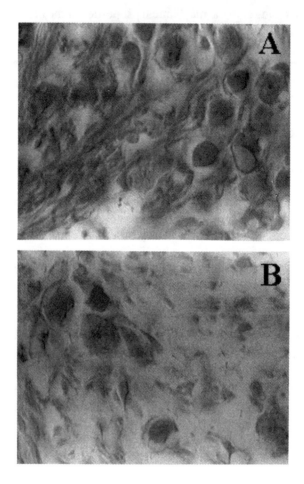

FIGURE 7.1   Loss of spiral ganglion cells with age. A. Numerous spiral ganglion cell somata and axons are seen in the basal end of the young cochlea of a C57 mouse. This is typical of normal-hearing individuals. B. Only a few spiral ganglion cells remain in this cochlea of a 2-year-old mouse. Obviously, little information can now be transferred from cochlea to CNS.

The initial, preretinal processing of visual information is optical rather than neural. In order to be projected onto the retina, visual stimuli must first pass through the cornea at the eye's surface; through the anterior chamber, which contains clear liquid (aqueous humor); through the focusable lens, and then the gelatinous vitreous humor, which fills the interior of the eye, ultimately reaching the retina. The amount of light entering the eye through the pupil is regulated by the iris.

The eye's optical system is subject to age-related change at each of these prereceptor stages, degrading the quality of the image projected upon the retina (Kline & Scialfa, 1996; Ordy & Brizzee, 1979; Pierscionek & Weale, 1996; Verrillo & Verrillo, 1985). The cornea is prone to yellowing, particularly around its periphery, a condition known as arcus senilis. The aqueous fluid in the eye's anterior chamber must circulate between the chamber and bloodstream, and glaucoma occurs when this flow is obstructed and the intraocular pressure increases with the potential to damage the optic nerve where it enters the eye. Glaucoma can cause serious visual impairment and becomes increasingly common with age. The lens can become yellowish with age, but more importantly, it typically becomes stiffer and thicker, making it impossible to focus on near objects (accommodation). This condition is called *presbyopia* and is usually quite evident by age 45.

Another lens-related problem is the occurrence of cataracts, an opaque region of the lens that blocks the passage of light. A decrease in the size of the pupil (senile miosis) makes it difficult to obtain adequate light under low levels of illumination. The gelatinous vitreous humor can become thinner with age, facilitating the appearance of "floaters," bits of fibrous components of the vitreous fluid.

Fortunately, the most serious of these age effects can be treated. Glaucoma usually can be controlled with drugs, cataracts can be corrected with surgery, and presbyopia is readily corrected with reading glasses or bifocals.

The condition of the retina's sensory receptors, cones (for high-illumination, daytime, and color vision), and rods (low-illumination, nighttime vision) tends to decline with age in various species, with some loss and/or changes in receptor cells (Curcio, Millican, Allen, & Kalina, 1993; Gao & Hollyfield, 1992; O'Steen & Landfield, 1991; Spear, 1993). The rods appear to be more susceptible to damage, although they may increase in size to compensate for lost cells (Curcio et al., 1993). By and large, however, age-related loss of retinal receptor cells tends not to be severe, although factors such as smoking, atherosclerosis (Pierscionek & Weale, 1996), and chronic stress (O'Steen, Sweatt, Eldridge, & Brodish, 1987) may exacerbate the damage. A pathological condition, *macular degeneration,* affects the portion of the retina (the macula and fovea) that is most sensitive to fine details. Some forms of this disease are more prevalent in older individuals (senile macular degeneration). Recently, a gene has been discovered that can cause this disorder in humans (Pennisi, 1997).

The Peripheral Somatosensory System

The receptors for the various adequate stimuli of the somatosensory system are distributed as needed throughout the surface and interior of body. The adequate stimuli define the type of receptors, which include mechanoreceptors for touch, pressure, and vibration, thermoreceptors for heat and cold, nocioceptors for pain, and proprioceptors for position and movement of body parts. The somatosensory receptors are associated with free nerve endings as well as specialized structures, including Pacinian and Meissner's corpuscles, Merkel disks, and Ruffini cylinders. The precise relationships between receptor type and adequate stimuli are not completely worked out, but all types exhibit age-related changes in form (Weisenberger, 1996). In addition to morphological changes, which probably alter their functional properties, there is typically a decrease in the number of Pacinian and Meissner's corpuscles. In contrast, Merkel disks and free nerve endings appear to be relatively stable in form and number. There is also evidence for loss of spinal root fibers and diminished circulation interfering with peripheral neural function, all of which could attenuate or distort sensory input to the central nervous system.

Prereceptor modification of stimuli occurs in various ways in the somatosensory system. The very fact that stimuli are typically applied to the body surface and the receptors are located beneath the surface produces some modification. For example, heat may be dispersed or absorbed by the skin surface, and the skin may be warm or cold to begin with (indeed, lower skin temperature in older people can modify somatosensation). A number of changes typically occur in the skin (Klingman, Grove, & Balin, 1985), such as changes in elasticity, wrinkling, loss of capillaries and small vessels, changes in hirsuteness (e.g., loss of hair on the head or gain of hair in the nose and ears), and reduced sweating, any of which might have subtle effects on somatosensation in some instances.

The Pacinian corpuscles are examples of specialized structures that provide nonneural processing of stimuli. They are onionlike, layered structures that surround nerve endings sensitive to vibration. Pacinian corpuscles are well suited to transmit high-frequency (but not low-frequency) vibrations from the skin to nerve ending within the capsule. Age-related changes in the Pacinian corpuscles and/or the central circuits to which they are connected are a likely candidate for the loss of high-frequency vibrotactile sensitivity that accompanies aging (Van Doren, Gescheider, & Verrillo, 1990).

Painful stimuli activate both myelinated axons (A-delta fibers) and very thin, unmyelinated axons (C fibers). These mediate two different pain experiences: fast-occurring, pricking pain (A-delta fibers) and slower-occurring, tonic pain sensations (C fibers). There is some evidence that A-delta fibers are more vulnerable to degeneration during aging than C fibers (Harkins, Davis, Bush, & Kasberger, 1996). Thus, the experience of pain in older people may tend to rely primarily on C fiber activation, whereas both types of fibers contribute more equally prior to old age (Chakour, Gibson, Bradbeer, & Helme, 1996). Whereas such findings suggest that pain experience might be altered by deficits at the peripheral level, there is little consistent evidence that pain threshold or pain tolerance is altered with age (Harkins & Scott, 1996).

One condition that strikes older people is trigeminal neuralgia (*tic douloureux*). Pain sensations for the face are mediated by the cranial trigeminal nerve system, and abnormal activity in this system (probably peripherally) results in excruciating paroxysms of pain.

The Peripheral Vestibular System

Embedded in the temporal bone, next to the cochlea, are the receptor organs for the vestibular system. The semicircular canals and the otolith organs (utricle and saccule) signal dynamic changes in position of the head and the static position with respect to gravity. There are age-related losses in the receptors found within these structures (Corso, 1988; Kenshalo, 1979). The hair cells in the semicircular canals exhibit losses after 50 years of age, and especially after age 70 (Rosenhall, 1973; Rosenhall & Rubin, 1975).

The Peripheral Olfactory System

The olfactory receptors are modified neurons in the nasal mucosa or epithelium, with extensions (cilia) that extend into the nasal passages and respond to odorous molecules. The olfactory receptors detect many qualities of odor, and their axons communicate directly with the brain via small openings in the intervening bone. Thinning of the olfactory epithelium, loss of olfactory receptors, and reduction in capillaries have been reported to occur with age (Bartoshuk & Weiffenbach, 1990; Naessen, 1971). There is evidence of increased degeneration in the receptor cell axons and the sites (glomeruli) where they synapse with olfactory bulb neurons in the CNS (C. G. Smith, 1942); in some older people, the degree of degeneration can be quite pronounced. A complicating factor for gerontological studies is the ability of these cells, unlike most CNS neurons, to be continually replaced throughout life, with an average turnover time of 30 days. Thus, the important variable may be the efficacy of regeneration as aging ensues, rather than the virulence of degeneration per se.

The Peripheral Gustatory System

The receptors for gustation are organized as aggregates (taste buds), which are found in specialized structures on the tongue (papillae). The receptors are designed to detect four basic taste qualities: salty, sweet, sour, and bitter. As is the case for the olfactory system, the receptor cells are also replaced throughout life. The oral environment provides some prereceptor effects on the substances to be tasted. Changes in salivary glands (with consequent dryness of the mouth) and other modifications of the oral environment may contribute to changes in taste sensations of older people (Verrillo & Verrillo, 1985). Smoking may also reduce taste sensitivity and may be responsible for some age-related declines, particularly for bitter substances.

As is the case for the psychophysical literature, there is some disagreement as to the magnitude of age-related losses of gustatory papillae and taste buds, but various studies have indicated minimal losses in humans and other species (Bartoshuk & Weiffenbach, 1990; Misretta, 1984). It would seem that, in contrast to some of the other sensory systems, many elderly individuals maintain a strong complement of gustatory receptors.

Other Factors Affecting Sensory Receptors

In addition to straightforward damage to receptors, we need also consider other processes that could be altered with age. These include receptor adaptation and central control of receptor sensitivity.

Receptor adaptation.   It is a normal occurrence that, if a sensory stimulus is presented for a period of time, the response of receptors may decrease or even cease. Such receptor adaptation reduces or eliminates the stream of sensory information from receptor to brain. Thus, for example, shortly after we encounter a vile odor, we may no longer notice it because olfactory receptors have undergone adaptation. The speed of adaptation in different types of receptors ranges from phasic, where responding decreases rapidly, to tonic, where receptors continue to report input for long periods of time. Phasic receptors are well suited to signal abrupt changes in stimuli, whereas tonic receptors can monitor ongoing stimuli that may vary more subtly. In this respect, it is probably important that receptors adapt the way "they are supposed to" to ensure that proper sensations arise.

In the somatosensory system, adaptation occurs when a stimulus is maintained for some period of time and the receptor responses decline. In a study of rats, Reinke and Dinse (1996) measured action potentials from nerve fibers innervating cutaneous receptors that were either fast adapting or slow adapting. Fast-adapting fibers respond well to the onset of a tactile stimulus but cannot sustain a response, whereas slow-adapting fibers continue to respond to maintained stimulus. In young adults, 49% were of the slow-adapting type, but only 29% were of this type in 2-year-olds. This could mean that slowly adapting receptors tended to die off with age or that they became fast adapting. In either case, the data suggest that receptor adaptation was altered in the old rats.

In the auditory system adaptation refers to the effects of fairly intense auditory stimuli that reduce the sensitivity to subsequent sounds for a period of time. If the adapting sound is very intense, the reduced sensitivity can be substantial (temporary threshold shift) or even permanent. It is really not clear if the old ear is more or less susceptible to adaptation of this kind, and there is considerable variability among individuals (Mills, Lee, Dubno, & Boettcher, 1996). It appears from animal studies that when the adapting stimulus is moderately intense and the threshold shift is temporary, there may be no age difference (McFadden et al., 1998; Sun, Bohne, & Harding, 1994). However, when very high levels of noise are involved, age may be associated with greater vulnerability (McFadden et al., 1998). Studies on mice indicate that genetic influences may play a role as well (Erway & Willott, 1996; Li & Borg, 1993; Shone, Altschuler, Miller, & Nuttall, 1991).

If the adapting auditory stimuli are not very intense, sensitivity to subsequent, less intense sounds lasts for only a brief period (this is also called forward masking). Walton, Frisina, and Meierhans (1995) presented data on forward masking in C57 mice with presbycusis and found little change in the auditory nerve response compared to young, well-hearing mice. However, when they evaluated forward masking in the auditory midbrain, they found it to be significantly greater in the mice with presby-cusis. Their findings suggest that central mechanisms can contribute to the magnitude of auditory adaptation in presbycusic mice.

In dark adaptation of the visual system, the term *adaptation* actually involves enhanced sensitivity. Dark adaptation improves the ability to see in dim light. In going from bright sunlight to a dark room, it may take more than a half hour to gain maximum sensitivity (a process involving the retinal rods). Whereas this time course remains fairly constant in older people, the maximum sensitivity to light tends to be reduced (Morgan, 1986; Scialfa & Kline, 1996). Thus, some older people may encounter greater difficulty seeing at night.

Receptor adaptation has not been well studied in the context of gerontol-ogy, yet this is a potentially important topic. Age-related changes in adaptation—were they to occur in various sensory systems—could have pluses and minuses. As mentioned in the example above, olfactory adapta-tion can rescue us from unpleasant odors. On the other hand, it blunts the flavor of food and drink, which is generally a bad thing (assuming the food tastes good to begin with). Thus, a change in olfactory adaptation might cut both ways. An example of somatosensory adaptation is "getting used to" very hot or cold water (the heat or cold receptors cease re-sponding). Being able to tolerate a hot bath or cool swimming pool are good outcomes, and facilitation of adaptation with aging might be generally desirable. On the other hand, one may need to detect stimulus changes after adaptation has occurred, and if adaptation were facilitated by aging, this could be a bad thing (e.g., not being able to detect a slow increase in the temperature of a hot tub).

Central control of receptor sensitivity. CSSs do not simply receive incoming (afferent) action potentials from the receptors; they also send (efferent) action potentials back out. One function of the sensory efferents is to adjust the sensitivity of receptors, making them more or less sensitive as warranted by the situation. This can be accomplished by modifying the prereceptor processes, as, for example, when the iris causes the pupil to change the amount of light entering the eye. Efferent control can occur closer to the receptors as well. For example, efferent fibers to the OHCs in the cochlea are able to alter the mechanical properties of the cochlea, and this changes the sensitivity of the IHCs. The fate of sensory efferent systems during aging has not been well studied, but they can certainly contribute to age effects. The two forms of efferent control just mentioned provide examples. The size of the pupils may decrease with age (miosis), and the degeneration of OHCs in older ears is likely to alter cochlear mechanics.

AGING AND THE CENTRAL SENSORY SYSTEMS

The Central Components of Sensory Systems

The CSSs must process the action-potential-coded sensory information originating in the sensory receptors. Before discussing the processing of sensory information by CSSs, it is important to point out that the central components of sensory systems are threatened by two adverse correlates of aging. First, changes in the structure or function of the brain's neurons occur in the context of biological aging (see chapters 3 through 5). This can presumably cause difficulties in the neural processing of sensory material (this, of course, holds for the other basic functions of the nervous system as well). Second, otherwise "healthy" central components of sensory systems may be secondarily affected by the elimination of portions of the peripheral input from damaged receptors. The removal or attenuation of sensory input might affect the CSS because reduction of synaptic input, physiological or anatomical, can alter the physiological properties of postsynaptic neurons. Because the altered neurons provide input to other neurons, the effects could spread throughout the CSS. Also, central neural circuitry would be disrupted or altered because various circuit components (neurons) have become abnormal or nonfunctional to a greater or lesser extent.

Because the CSSs of aging individuals might be affected in two rather different ways, it is useful to differentiate two types of age-related central changes (Willott, 1991). The term *central effects of biological aging* (CEBA) refers to sensory changes stemming from age-related changes in neurons, metabolism, support systems, and other elements of the CNS discussed in chapters 3 through 5. The term *central effects of peripheral pathology* (CEPP) also refers to sensory changes associated with modifications of neurons and neural circuits in the brain. However, these are secondary to the removal or alteration of input by sensory receptor damage.

A note on terminology: The phrase *effects of* implies causation, thereby flirting with the semantic and logical conundrum that "aging causes aging," as discussed in chapter 1. However, CEBA refers to centrally mediated sensory experiences or codes that are the outcome of neural activity; biological changes in neurons do indeed have effects on such information-processing phenomena. Similarly, changes in the periphery associated with CEPP may be part and parcel of aging, but they in turn have effects on the CSSs.

It would be expected that CEBA and CEPP often occur in combination, since many older people have some loss of receptor function as well as various CNS deficits. Indeed, it is often difficult to distinguish between the two. To determine the presence of CEBA, it should be shown that the age-related CSS changes can occur in the absence of significant peripheral pathology or pathophysiology. To do so, one obviously needs to study some old individuals with minimal peripheral damage. The most conclusive way to demonstrate CEPP is to show that an age-related CSS change *only* occurs in individuals or genetic strains that exhibit peripheral pathology. To do this, one needs access to subjects with a range of severity of peripheral impairment.

Even if the appropriate subject pool is accessible, the manifestations of CEPP can be tricky, even paradoxical. As discussed later, our laboratory has studied CEPP using mouse strains that have peripheral damage with onset prior to old age. Generalizing from this work suggests that anatomical or histological degeneration associated with CEPP is likely to be most severe in (or even restricted to) those CSS structures that receive primary synaptic input from the impaired peripheral structures. This is presumably due to the heavy loss of trophic support and/or reduced postsynaptic activity resulting from the diminished peripheral input. By contrast, physiological changes in neural responses may not conform to this scenario, as changes in higher level neural circuits, synaptically well removed from the primary inputs, may be even more pronounced than those interfacing with the periphery. This presumably occurs because the lower level CSS structures contribute to excitatory and inhibitory circuits ascending to higher anatomical levels. Thus, for example, if lower level damage removed inhibitory input to a higher level circuit (see chapter 5), it could become hyperexcitable; this hyperexcitability could, in turn, affect still higher levels, an so on. It is clear that the manifestations of CEPP can be both complex and difficult to predict.

Principles of Central Sensory Coding

Sensory systems are composed of numerous nuclei and subnuclei containing a variety of different types of neurons. Sensory stimuli have a number of attributes. These include magnitude (e.g., loudness, brightness), quality (e.g., timbre, hue), duration, temporal order or rate of repetition of brief stimuli, and spatial properties (e.g., location, spatial relationships among two or more stimuli). Two or more of these dimensions are typically coded simultaneously, but they usually involve different neural codes and central neural circuits. For example, the frequency of a sound is coded by the location of activated IHCs on the basilar membrane and the central neurons that are synaptically connected to those cochlear regions; the sound's intensity is in part coded by the firing rate of certain central neurons, and the direction of the sound source is coded by comparison of central neural activity evoked by the left and right ears. Different types of neurons, anatomical structures, and neural circuits within the central auditory system contribute differently to each of these dimensions.

The "parallel" processing of sensory qualities is a well-documented example of the principle of multiple neural structures and circuits. For example, two divisions of the central visual system, the parvocellular and magnocellular systems, have different capabilities and reside in different anatomical neighborhoods in the thalamus and the cortex (Livingstone & Hubel, 1988; Merigan & Maunsell, 1993). Neurons in the parvocellular system have good acuity, are sensitive to color, and respond best to slowly moving or slowly changing visual stimuli. Neurons in the magnocellular system are "color blind" but can respond to rapidly moving stimuli. Although they are largely specialized (with some overlap), these parallel systems together provide information about the whole range of spatial detail, colors, speeds of movement, and so on.

A second example is found in the auditory system. The auditory nerve fibers are the axons of spiral ganglion cells in the cochlea, and they provide the input from inner ear to brain. As these nerve fibers enter the auditory brainstem, they branch into each of the three main subdivisions of the *cochlear nucleus*: the anteroventral, posteroventral, and dorsal divisions. In the dorsal division, most of the terminals of auditory nerve branches synapse in the deeper parts, with few fibers terminating in the more superficial portions. This pattern of afferent innervation has important consequences for CEPP because neurons in these regions are directly affected by diminution of synaptic input due to age-related cochlear dysfunction. In C57 mice, which exhibit presbycusis by middle age, a loss of neurons and general loss of tissue volume are only observed in the regions that are directly innervated by the auditory nerve. In the superficial dorsal cochlear nucleus and in higher level structures, such as the inferior colliculus (IC), that do not receive direct cochlear innervation, these changes are not observed (Willott, 1996a; Willott & Bross, 1990; Willott et al., 1987; Willott, Jackson, & Hunter, 1987). These findings suggest that anatomical changes resulting from cochlear damage (i.e., a manifestation of CEPP) differ significantly depending on the degree of innervation arising from the sensory receptors.

The multiple, parallel principle has potential relevance for both CEPP and CEBA. The manner in which central processing is affected could be complicated by differential vulnerability of two or more parallel pathways that include certain sensory receptors (CEPP) or components of central circuits (CEBA). For example, the ability of the parvocellular visual system to appreciate color relies on color sensitivity of cone (not rod) receptors, and would be affected by changes in one or more types of color-sensitive cones. By the same token, if the cones continued to function well, but age effects occurred in the central parvocellular system (irrespective of the magnocellular system), color vision would also be affected (thus far there is little evidence that this occurs, however; see below). Similarly, the three divisions of the cochlear nucleus participate in different neural circuits and functions.

To summarize, the coding of different sensory functions or qualities by different neurons, structures, and circuits in the brain implies that, if aging were to affect some of these differently, certain sensory functions would be affected more than others. As discussed in chapter 3, variability of age effects within the nervous system is well documented and is likely to be manifested in sensory systems. It should also be noted, however, that the different sensory dimensions are only quasi-independent, and they often interact. For example, the experience of loudness is influenced by both frequency and intensity of acoustic stimuli. Age-related changes in the neural coding of either frequency or intensity might affect loudness.

Topographic organization and plasticity of sensory maps.   The principle of topographic organization was discussed in chapter 5. It refers to the orderly organization of connections between one part of the nervous system and another. Topography in the sensory systems involves the organization of anatomical connections from points on the receptor array to the CSS and within the CSS as well. Topography can affect age-related changes, because the loss of sensory receptors is often not uniform. For example, in the auditory system the loss of hair cells tends to be greater for the high-frequency end of the cochlea, and in the somatosensory system, the feet tend to lose tactile receptors to a greater extent than some other areas. What this means is, the regions of the CSS that are normally innervated by these vulnerable portions of the receptor array will be relieved of their input to a greater extent than other areas (an example of CEPP). Thus, the topographical dimensions of aging sensory systems must be considered in order to understand how the systems age. Furthermore, the loss of input from peripheral receptors induces modifications in the central maps of the receptor surface. This sort of neural response change or *plasticity*—reorganization of central maps after partial deafferentation—is probably a general reaction of the brain to the peripheral receptor damage (Kaas, 1991). Thus, the way stimuli from still-normal portions of the receptor surface are processed can be altered.

The Central Auditory System

The axons of the cochlear spiral ganglion cells form the auditory nerve. The axons branch and their terminals synapse with neurons in the three subdivisions of the cochlear nucleus in the lower brainstem. From here, the central auditory pathways are rather complicated, involving various subdivisions of the *superior olivary complex, nuclei of the lateral lemniscus*, and IC (all of which are in the brainstem), the *medial geniculate body* in the thalamus, and several auditory cortical areas (see Figure 7.2).

Quantitative studies of the aging human central auditory system were performed by Konigsmark and Murphy (1970, 1972), who evaluated the size (volume) and number of neurons in the ventral division of the cochlear nucleus of postmortem patients ranging in age from infancy through 90 years. They found no evidence of age-related change in the number of neurons but did find a loss of three-dimensional volume (32% decrease between ages 50 and 90), which probably reflects some loss of dendritic branches. Ferraro and Minckler (1977) saw a significant loss in fibers of the lateral lemniscus, a major fiber tract in the auditory system, but age-related changes were not striking. In studies of other species, Feldman and Vaughan (1979) found no evidence of cell loss in the cochlear nucleus of old rats whose hearing loss was not severe, although electron microscopy showed some neurons with "watery-appearing" cytoplasm and a

Central Auditory System

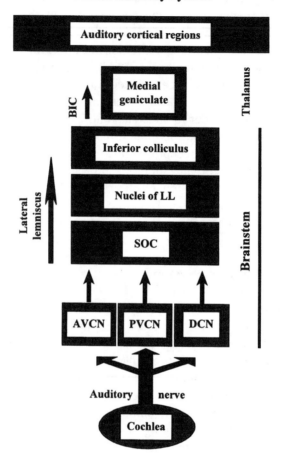

FIGURE 7.2   Schematic of the central auditory system. **Auditory nerve fibers leave the cochlea and branch to innervate the anterior ventral cochlear nucleus (AVCN), posterior ventral cochlear nucleus (PVCN), and dorsal cochlear nucleus (DCN). The axons leaving these structures follow different pathways to the upper brainstem, involving the superior olivary complex (SOC), nuclei of the lateral lemniscus (LL), and inferior colliculus (IC). Major fibers tracts are the LL in the brainstem and brachium of the IC (BIC), which provides input to the medial geniculate nucleus of the thalamus. From here, axons project to several auditory cortical regions, which are interconnected.**

reduction of organelles. Like the study by Konigsmark and Murphy (1972), volume of the ventral cochlear nucleus of the oldest animals was reduced. Similar findings were observed in old mice of the CBA/J strain (Lambert & Schwartz, 1982; Willott et al., 1987). In a study of the human auditory cortex, Scheibel and colleagues (1975) used Golgi stains to demonstrate swelling and "lumpiness" of cell bodies, loss of dendritic spines, progressive loss of dendrites, and cell death in older subjects.

From these and other anatomical studies (see Willott, 1991) certain commonalities emerge in comparing the histopathological material obtained from humans and other species, and several conclusions can be drawn. First, whereas very old individuals are likely to have a reduced number of central auditory neurons, the losses are typically modest. Second, the volume of central auditory structures tends to be smaller in old individuals, with loss of dendrites probably contributing significantly. Third, there is considerable variability among individuals in the number of neurons surviving to old age. Material from rodents suggests that genetics plays a strong role in this regard, since significant strain differences have been observed.

Neurophysiological studies on rats and CBA mice that do not suffer from severe presbycusis have generally shown some age-related changes, particularly with respect to neural inhibition, increased spontaneous activity, and the appearance of "sluggish" neurons (see chapter 5). However, the changes in response properties of auditory neurons are generally not dramatic (Finlayson, 1995; Palombi & Caspary, 1996a, 1996b; Willott, 1986; Willott et al., 1988a). Similarly, auditory evoked potential studies on older human subjects whose hearing was not greatly deteriorated have not provided consistent evidence of significant central changes (Willott, 1991).

CEBA/CEPP. Because aging rats and CBA mice do not exhibit severe cochlear pathology, the modest neurophysiological changes just described probably reflect CEBA and may not accurately reflect what happens in individuals suffering from severe cochlear degeneration (CEPP). Because many people are so afflicted, our laboratory has investigated the central auditory system in C57BL/6J (C57), a strain that exhibits genetically determined cochlear pathology during middle age.

Topographic organization in the auditory system is *tonotopic*: Neurons in a particular location respond to tones within a limited band of frequencies, and there exists an orderly relationship between the effective frequencies and the location of neurons within that region of the auditory system. For example, neurons in the dorsal portion of the IC respond to low frequencies; neurons at progressively more ventral locations respond to progressively higher frequencies. This tonotopic organization is one principle by which frequency is thought to be coded in the central auditory system (e.g., there are neural maps of frequency in various regions of the brain).

Tonotopic organization depends on the existence of anatomical connections from the cochlea to the appropriate tonotopic region. For example, high-frequency regions of the basal cochlea must connect via some anatomical pathway(s) to high-frequency tonotopic regions of the central auditory system. Young adult C57 mice exhibit sensorineural pathology in the basal region of the cochlea with concomitant threshold elevations for high-frequency sounds (Henry & Chole, 1980; Li & Borg, 1991; Mikaelian, 1979; Willott, 1986)—the pattern of hearing loss typical of people with presbycusis (Willott, 1991). The result is the removal or attenuation of neural input to the tonotopically organized regions of the central auditory system that normally respond well to high-frequency sounds only (e.g., the more ventral regions of the IC). The loss of high-frequency sensitivity in C57 mice results in changes in frequency coding in the central auditory system.

After the high-frequency regions of the IC and auditory cortex have been relieved of their ability to respond to the absent high frequencies, they become increasingly responsive to lower frequencies (Willott, 1984, 1986; Willott, Aitkin, & McFadden, 1993; Willott et al., 1988b): Lower frequency sounds now evoke vigorous responses in these neurons, whereas such stimuli are normally ineffective in high frequency tonotopic regions. In addition, the "best frequency" (the frequency for which a neuron's sensitivity is best) shifts downward for many neurons. Indeed, virtually the entire IC and auditory cortex of middle-aged C57 mice come to respond well to those middle and low frequencies that remain audible (see Figure 7.3). Because this central change is induced by age-related peripheral pathology, it is an example of CEPP.

The degree of hearing loss–induced plasticity differs at different levels of the central auditory system (Willott, Parham, & Hunter, 1991; Willott et al., 1993). Plasticity is greatest in the auditory cortex, followed by the IC, and then by the ventral cochlear nucleus (an example of more pronounced physiological CEPP at higher CSS levels). The differential plasticity across anatomical levels has interesting implications, because these central audi-

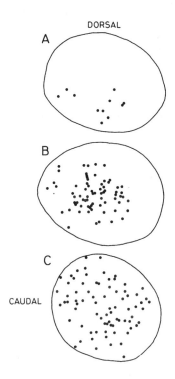

FIGURE 7.3 **Plasticity of frequency maps in the central auditory system.** These drawings were made by the superposition of cortical maps for frequency representation in C57 mice. Each point represents the location in the map, where the neurons responded best to the middle frequencies of 10 to 13 kHz. A. Maps from young, well-hearing mice show that the bottom half of the auditory field contains neurons responding best to the middle frequencies, but other regions do not (these regions respond best to higher or lower frequencies). B. As the mice begin to lose high-frequency hearing, more regions of the map now respond best to middle frequencies. C. As hearing loss gets worse in older mice, the entire auditory cortical field contains neurons that respond best to the middle frequencies. The tonotopic maps are drastically altered. Reprinted from Willott, J. F., Aitkin, L. M., & McFadden, S. M. (1993). Plasticity of auditory cortex associated with sensorineural hearing loss in adult C57BL/6J mice. *Journal of Comparative Neurology, 329,* 402–411, with permission of Wiley-Liss, Inc.

tory system structures undoubtedly play different roles in various auditory perceptual capacities. The functions that depend on them should likewise be affected to different extents by neural plasticity. For example, auditory functions mediated primarily at subcortical levels (e.g., auditory reflexes) might be less plastic than those mediated cortically (e.g., many perceptual processes). Certain aspects of auditory perception may be affected by neural plasticity, but the extent could depend on which central auditory system pathways are involved.

The Central Visual System

The neural processing of visual information begins in the retina and involves several types of neurons, including *horizontal, bipolar, amacrine,* and *retinal ganglion cells.* These cells are distributed differentially in retinal layers. Although degenerative changes have been observed in all retinal layers (Weisse, 1995), most neurogerontological research has focused on the retinal ganglion cells and/or their axons, which form the optic nerve. Action potentials in optic nerve axons transmit coded information to the *dorsal lateral geniculate nucleus* (LGN) of the thalamus and the *superior colliculus* in the midbrain. The LGN relays information to the visual cortex, which has several iterations of varying information-processing complexity (see Figure 7.4).

The literature on aging and retinal ganglion cells/optic nerve fibers is inconsistent, with reports of no change (see Kim, Tom, & Spear, 1996) but mostly reports of decreases with age (e.g., Celsia, Kaufman, & Cone, 1987; Curcio & Drucker, 1993; Gao & Hollyfield, 1992; Jonas, Schmidt, Muller-Bergh, Schlotzer-Schrehardt, & Naumann, 1992; Porciatti, Burr, Morrone, & Fiorentini, 1992; Trick, Trick, & Haywood, 1986). As Spear (1993) pointed out, however, many studies showing age-related decrease in optic nerve fiber counts of humans did not obtain statistically significant findings, the magnitudes of age effects were typically small, and the between-subject variability was typically high. Furthermore, the extent to which losses of ganglion cells in human studies were influenced by the factors that often plague studies of human autopsy material (refer to chapter 3) is always difficult to determine. Thus, it is of interest that Kim and colleagues (1996), using an unbiased counting method, observed no loss of retinal ganglion cells of old rhesus monkeys who were in good health when euthanized. Similarly, Morrison, Cork, Dunkelberger, Brown,

Central Visual System

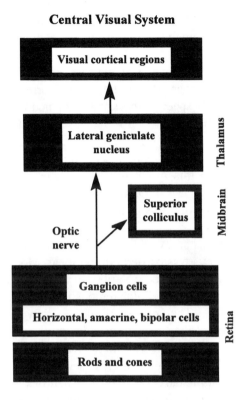

FIGURE 7.4 **Schematic of the central visual system. The retina contains various types of cells, including the rod and cone receptors, which react chemically to light; horizontal, amacrine, and bipolar cells, which begin to modify neural information; and retinal ganglion cells, whose axons leave the retina as the optic nerve. The information is sent to the superior colliculus of the midbrain and lateral geniculate nucleus (LGN) of the thalamus. LGN neurons project to various visual areas of the cortex for further neural processing.**

and Quigley (1990) found only a nonsignificant trend toward a loss of axons in old rhesus monkeys. All in all, it would seem that retinal ganglion cell loss is usually not terribly severe in older humans and rhesus monkeys.

The electrical activity of the retina evoked by flashes or patterned light stimuli (the electroretinogram, or ERG) can become altered in older people, although again, the findings vary from study to study (Birch & Anderson,

1992; Elsner, Berk, Burns, & Rosenberg, 1988; Spear, 1993; Wright, Williams, Drasdo, & Harding, 1985). Unfortunately, interpretation of changes in ERGs is somewhat limited because they are influenced by optics and other variables.

Morphometric studies have been performed on the LGN of rhesus monkeys (Ahmad & Spear, 1993) and rats (Satorre, Cano, & Reinoso-Suarez, 1985). In both species, the number of neurons remained stable with age, although the LGN volume increased, presumably because of growth of dendrites, blood vessels, and/or glial cells. LGN neuronal soma size also increased in old rhesus monkeys and Wistar rats (Villena et al., 1997), suggesting that this might represent some sort of compensatory neuronal growth (Spear, 1993). On the other hand, there is some evidence that metabolic activity of LGN neurons decreases in old rats (Diaz et al., 1996).

A neurophysiological study on the responses of LGN neurons in young and old rhesus monkeys was carried out by Spear, Moore, Kim, Xue, and Tumosa (1994). They measured a variety of response properties in both the parvocellular and magnocellular regions of the LGN but found little if any age differences. The sorts of properties they measured included color coding, latency of responses to visual stimuli, receptive fields (how the neurons respond with respect to the location of stimuli on the retinal surface), spatial resolution, and contrast sensitivity. There were some tentative findings that the parvocellular LGN neurons of old monkeys did not process low contrasts or changes in contrast as well as neurons of young monkeys. There was also a small increase in spontaneous firing of action potentials (i.e., irrespective of visual stimuli) in older neurons. By and large, however, aging was not associated with much of a change in LGN responses.

LGN neurons send their axons to the primary visual cortex. Some studies have reported a loss of visual cortical neurons in older individuals (Brody, 1955). As indicated elsewhere, however, early studies of various cortical areas of human subjects may have overestimated neuronal loss, and this may be true of the visual cortex as well. Some more recent studies have failed to find evidence of age differences in the density of visual cortical neurons in humans (Haug, 1984; Leuba & Garey, 1987) or monkeys (Vincent, Peters, & Tigges, 1989). On the other hand, signs of dendritic degeneration have been well documented in the visual cortex of old rodents (see Spear, 1993), and some changes have been seen in humans (Scheibel et al., 1975) and monkeys (Vincent et al., 1989).

Evoked potential studies have provided evidence for age effects in the physiological responses of the visual cortex (reviewed by Spear, 1993). These include reduced evoked potential amplitude and prolonged response latencies (i.e., slowing of neural processing). When patterned or moving visual stimuli are employed, the age changes are greatest for high-spatial frequencies (fine detail requiring acuity) and slowly changing light patterns (Bobak, Bodis-Wollner, Guillory, & Anderson, 1989; Porciatti et al., 1992). Furthermore, comparisons between the cortical potentials and the ERG responses from the retina suggest that the age changes are occurring at the LGN and/or cortical levels, not in the retina. These findings would be expected if the central parvocellular pathway were especially affected (Crassini, Brown, & Bowman, 1988; Porciatti et al., 1992). On the other hand, some psychophysical studies have suggested that the magnocellular pathway is also vulnerable to age effects (Spear, 1993).

In summary, anatomical and neurophysiological studies have yet to reveal evidence of prominent age-related changes in the visual pathway from retina to cortex. Does this mean that such changes do not occur, or that they have not yet been found? There is reason to believe the latter, in light of psychophysical studies showing visual perceptual deficits that are likely to depend on central processing of information (Kline & Scialfa, 1996; Spear, 1993). Age differences have been demonstrated for binocular summation (improved performance when two eyes are used together), acuity for moving targets, depth perception, temporal resolution (the ability to see rapidly changing stimuli such as flickering lights), motion perception, and the ability to search visually. Declines such as these cannot be attributed to optical or retinal changes alone and are presumably due to changes in the central visual pathways, in both the parvocellular and magnocellular systems.

Various regions of the cerebral cortex other than the primary visual cortex participate in complex visual perception. Grady and colleagues (1994) performed a PET study (regional changes in cerebral blood flow) on human subjects to evaluate age effects in these cortical regions. Their findings suggested faster processing and more efficient use of some visual areas in the young subjects. The older subjects exhibited different overall distributions of neural activity across cortical regions, perhaps indicating a reliance on different cortical circuits. The age differences applied more to cortical regions coding spatial vision than those coding object vision.

CEBA/CEPP. Because the retinal rods and cones are generally not greatly damaged during aging, one can assume that significant CEPP does not arise from receptor damage. Whether or not the optical changes in the aging eye may trigger central changes is unknown. However, it is of interest to note that the central visual system readily makes adjustments to optical distortions (e.g., inversion or lateral shifting of the visual field caused by the donning of prism eyeglasses). Thus, optical changes might have the capacity to induce CEPP. It is doubtful, however, that optical changes have significant effects on the neural organization of the central visual system. It seems most likely that the neural substrates of age-related changes in visual perception are associated with CEBA. However, as the literature review suggests, little is known about those neural changes at present.

The Central Somatosensory System

Axons from the periphery link somatosensory receptors with central neurons in the spinal cord or brainstem. The ascending somatosensory pathways include synaptic stations in the medulla (*gracile* and *cuneate nuclei*), thalamus, and somatosensory cortical areas. However, submodalities such as tactile sensation and pain follow different pathways in the CNS; in some respects, these pathways are parallel.

Very little work has been done on aging and the central somatosensory systems, and what literature there is on neuronal loss in somatosensory cortex is not consistent across species. Brizzee (1973) observed neuron loss in somatosensory cortex of old rhesus monkeys, but losses were not found in old mice (Curcio & Coleman, 1982) or rats (Peinado et al., 1997). The latter group did, however, observe an increase in glial density, some decrease in soma and nucleus size, and changes in neuron shape, all of which suggest some age effects. Bigham and Lidow (1995) evaluated the distribution and density of synaptic receptors in the somatosensory cortex of young and old (> 20 years) monkeys. Age-related decreases in receptor density occurred for adrenergic $\alpha 1$ receptors in the superficial cortical layers, $\alpha 2$ receptors in most cortical layers, adrenergic β receptors in the deep cortical layers, and serotonergic 5-HT_1 receptors in most cortical layers. In a study of synapses in human brain tissue, however, I. Adams (1987) observed no age effects for the number or appearance of synapses in somatosensory (postcentral) cortex, although changes were observed in the motor cortex.

Most of the neurophysiological research on the central somatosensory system has utilized evoked potentials, and most of these studies have found that it takes longer for information to be transmitted from the peripheral receptors to the somatosensory cortex (Ferri et al., 1996; Hume, Cant, Shaw, & Cowan, 1982; MacKenzie & Phillips, 1981; Shaw, 1992). What happens to conduction of information within the cortex is more complicated. For example, Kakigi (1987) obtained evoked potentials throughout the somatosensory system in human subjects following stimulation of the posterior tibial nerve. The time course (latencies after stimulation) of evoked potentials indicated that in older subjects, conduction time was slower up through the spinal cord, through the brainstem (from the medial lemniscus to the thalamus), and from the thalamus to the somatosensory cortex. However, conduction within the cortex was not slowed. Although this suggests smaller age effects in cortical circuits, other evoked potential studies have not found this to be the case (Desmedt & Cheron, 1980; Luders, 1970). Simpson and Erwin (1983) measured the latency of somatosensory evoked potentials from two different cortical locations and found that one peak increased in latency but the other did not. The evoked potential story is not a simple one.

Besides the response latency, the other basic parameter of evoked potentials is the amplitude of the various waves of neural activity. Evoked potential amplitudes can be difficult to interpret because they are influenced by the placement of recording electrodes and other mundane variables. Furthermore, the size of an evoked potential presumably depends on both the number of neurons responding and the synchrony of action potentials or synaptic potentials from many neurons. Therefore, an age-related change in evoked potential amplitude might be due to any number of factors. Not surprisingly, then, gerontological studies of somatic evoked potentials have produced varying findings—decreases in amplitudes as well as increases (Desmedt & Cheron, 1980; Ferri et al., 1996; Hume et al., 1982; Kakigi, 1987; MacKenzie & Phillips, 1981). In general, the literature suggests that amplitudes tend to become smaller in the subcortical pathways, whereas in cortex findings are variable but often include an enlargement of amplitudes. It is not clear what would cause evoked potential amplitudes to increase in size in an older cortex, but one possibility is a reduction in inhibition (see Prinz et al., 1990). If this were the case, increased amplitudes could signal abnormal information processing in the somatosensory cortex. Weaker inhibition could result from a decline in GABA neurotransmission, as discussed in chapter 5.

The hypothesis that neural processing is perturbed in the aging somatosensory cortex is bolstered by animal research on tactile receptive fields—

the area of skin surface that, when touched, causes action potentials to fire in a particular cortical neuron. Spengler, Godde, and Dinse (1995) measured the receptive fields within cortical somatosensory maps (hind-paw representation) in old rats and observed that the receptive fields became much larger and overlapped greatly with one another. That is, there was a diminished, less precise point-to-point relationship between an area of skin stimulated and the cortical neurons that responded to this small area. Presumably, this would alter the coding of tactile sensations.

CEBA/CEPP. Because peripheral somatosensory receptors often exhibit declines with age, it is feasible that CEPP could be significant in some cases. What, if any, manifestations of CEPP might occur are unknown at present, however. Furthermore, it is difficult to distinguish CEPP and CEBA from the available data. For example, Reinke and Dinse (1996) found that responses of peripheral somatosensory fibers of old rats were not deleteriously affected to the same extent as cortical neurons. This suggests that alterations in the central circuitry had become exacerbated compared with peripheral changes. It is not clear if the central changes were instigated by loss of peripheral sensitivity (i.e., physiological CEPP exhibited at a higher CSS level), if they involved cortical changes that were independent of the peripheral changes (CEBA), or whether they reflected some combination of both. In any event, central changes did not simply mirror but added to those that occurred peripherally.

The Central Vestibular System and Proprioception

Peripheral vestibular afferents synapse in several central *vestibular nuclei* in the brainstem. Information is then distributed to the cerebellum, spinal cord, structures involved with multisensory control of posture and movement, and elsewhere. The aging central vestibular system has received little attention from neuroanatomists. Recently, however, Lopez, Honrubia, and Baloh (1997) performed a quantitative morphometric study of the human vestibular nuclei, using subjects as old as 93 years. They estimated that there was a 3% neuronal loss per decade from ages 40 to 90. However, viewed differently, there were only about 8% fewer neurons in 75- to 85-year-olds (about 230,000) than in 35- to 45-year olds (about 250,000). Subjects ages 85 to 95 years had about a 16% loss. This suggests an accelerating loss of vestibular neurons that remains rather minor until a rather old age. The percentage of neuronal loss was greatest in the superior vestibular nucleus and least in the medial nucleus. Significant accumulation of lipofuscin was observed as well. Lopez and colleagues concluded that the overall rate of neuronal loss was comparable to that observed at lower levels of the vestibular system.

Other than this article, there is not much literature on aging and the vestibular nuclei. Sturrock (1996) found a decrease in the number of large neurons of the lateral vestibular nucleus of mice (ASH/TO strain). In studies of rats, some dendritic swelling and a shift in the type of axon terminals with respect to the shape of the vesicles that contain neurotransmitter were observed (Johnson & Miguel, 1974). A study by Cransac and colleagues (1996) reported that the amount of NE decreased in old rats, whereas serotonin levels increased and dopamine levels were unchanged with age. There also appeared to be changes in the synthesis and/or metabolism of NE that might represent a compensatory response. Although these findings are difficult to interpret, they suggest some age-related change in central vestibular processing.

The Central Olfactory System

The axons of the olfactory receptor cells form the olfactory nerve as they enter the olfactory bulbs of the brain, synapsing with dendrites of *mitral cells* and *tufted cells*. From here, important pathways communicate with structures in the limbic system, such as the amygdala and piriform cortex, involved in emotional and motivated behaviors (see chapter 10).

Bhatnagar, Kennedy, Baron, and Greenberg (1987) described the morphology of the human olfactory bulb in some detail, using subjects as old as 102 years. Their main findings were a decrease with age in the thickness of the olfactory bulb's several layers, shrinkage of mitral cells (especially during middle age), and a loss of mitral cells from about 50,000 in young adults to 14,500 in subjects over age 90. Although the loss of cells is striking, the large age difference must be viewed with caution. The olfactory receptor neurons interface directly with the outside air and various toxins and are vulnerable to environmental damage. However, the subjects' premortem health status or history of exposure to toxic agents was not available in the study by Bhatnagar and colleagues. Furthermore, both Alzheimer's disease (see chapter 11) and Parkinsons's disease (Hawkes, Shephard, & Daniel, 1997) are associated with pronounced changes in the olfactory system, so the possible presence of these diseases could have affected the results as well.

Thus, while it is clear from this study that significant degeneration occurs in some older people, it is not clear if these are typical of healthy aging. Indeed, studies of rodents suggest that olfactory bulb changes may not be so severe or universal. The number of mitral cells in the olfactory bulb has been shown to decrease in old Sprague-Dawley rats (Hinds & McNelly, 1977) but not in Fischer 344 rats (Forbes, 1984) or Charles River rats (Hinds & McNelly, 1981). On the other hand, a study on dogs found substantial atrophy of the olfactory bulb (Hirai et al., 1996) more similar to what was found in humans than in rats. Of course, dogs live much longer than rats and, as pets, are exposed to many of the same environmental insults as their human companions. The variability of the research findings suggest that species/genetic differences and environmental variables may be potent modulators of aging in the olfactory system.

Beyond cell counts, subtle age effects may occur in the rodent olfactory bulb. Alterations in the dendrites of mitral cells have been observed in old mice (Machado-Salas & Scheibel, 1979), and a moderate decrease in immunolabeling for GAP-43 (a protein associated with neuronal plasticity) has been observed in the olfactory bulb of rats (Casoli, Spagna, Fattoretti, Gesvita, & Bertoni-Freddari, 1996). A sometimes confusing variety of age differences in neurotransmitters (e.g., dopamine, NE) and their metabolites has been reported in olfactory bulbs (Baker, Franzen, Stone, Cho, & Margolis, 1995; Dluzen, 1996). Concentrations or activity of these substances appear to exhibit age-related changes in various directions, with considerable degree of variability and strain differences. Although the data suggest the presence of age effects of some sort, it is impossible to conclude much more at this time.

The regenerative properties of the olfactory system are evident in the olfactory bulb, where new synapses are continually formed. Hinds and McNelly (1979) found that, in aging Sprague-Dawley rats, mitral cells of the olfactory bulb exhibited large gains in synapses (270%) between 3 and 27 months of age. It was only between 27 and 30 months that a loss (26%) of synapses occurred. The overall decrease in synapses appeared to be due to a dying off of mitral cells (Hinds & McNelly, 1977) rather than a loss in the density of synaptic contacts per neuron. Increases in synapses, as well as the volume of olfactory bulb layers and size of mitral cells, was also observed in Charles River rats through 27 months before declining in very old rats (Hinds & McNelly, 1981). Morrison and Costanzo (1995) assessed the ability of previously transected olfactory nerve axons to transport horseradish peroxidase, a tract-tracing method, as an indication of regeneration. The capacity for regeneration persisted in 2-year-old hamsters (the average life span age). Baker and colleagues (1995) found no evidence for changes in the size of the olfactory bulb or in the expression of a protein found in olfactory receptor neurons in several strains of rats and mice as the animals aged. Granule cells, another type of olfactory bulb neuron, also have the ability to regenerate, and this appears to be maintained well into old age in rats (Kaplan, McNelly, & Hinds, 1985), although fewer regenerated cells survived in older animals. These findings suggest that the olfactory bulb, its afferent inputs, and presumably the replacement of receptor neurons can fare relatively well in at least some genetic strains of aging rodents.

A study of olfactory evoked potentials in humans revealed changes associated with age (Evans, Cui, & Starr, 1995). Using amyl acetate as an odorant stimulus, a significant correlation was observed between the latency of the second positive evoked potential wave (P2) and declines in performance on an odor identification test. Smaller amplitudes of the N1 and P2 waves evoked by amyl acetate were also observed in older subjects (Murphy, Nordin, deWijk, Cain, & Polich, 1994). These evoked potential studies indicate that changes occur at the early stages of olfactory stimulus processing (i.e., the waves with short latencies).

CEPP/CEBA. Based on correlations between changes in receptor cells versus olfactory bulb, Smith (1942) attributed changes in the human olfactory bulb to a loss of receptor cells. Hinds and McNelly (1981) made similar conclusions regarding rats. This being the case, the age-related changes in the olfactory bulb probably represent CEPP. This conclusion is further indicated by the finding that anatomical changes in the piriform cortex, which receives synaptic inputs from the olfactory bulb, were minimal in old Sprague-Dawley rats compared to declines in the olfactory epithelium and bulb (Curcio, McNelly, & Hinds, 1985). The less-severe degeneration at higher anatomical levels is reminiscent of that discussed earlier for the auditory system of C57 mice. Again, the notion is that more centrally located neurons are relatively less dependent on peripheral input for trophic support because they receive more synaptic input from other central neurons which are not diminished with age.

The Central Gustatory System

The gustatory receptors in the taste buds are connected to the brain via three different cranial nerves, each innervating a different part of the tongue and mouth. The *nucleus of the solitary tract* in the medulla receives action potentials from the peripheral nerves and in turn sends information on up the brainstem (to the *parabrachial nucleus* in particular). Further processing occurs in the thalamus, the hypothalamus, and the cerebral cortex. The "painful" properties of spicy foods are transmitted by the *trigeminal nerve system*. Little research has addressed aging and the central taste pathways, and it is not known if changes in central processing contribute to the reduced perceived intensity of taste stimuli that often occurs in older people (Schiffman, 1996).

SUMMARY AND IMPLICATIONS

We began this chapter by briefly reviewing psychophysical and behavioral literature, showing that sensitivity and other capacities tend to decline with age in all of the sensory systems. Can the neurobiological findings explain the psychophysical findings? The answer is yes, up to a point, when it comes to the sensitivity of the systems. The "yes" part of the answer stems from the fact that the ability to detect stimuli is closely tied to the condition of the sensory receptor cells and nonneural modifying processes, both of which exhibit negative changes in older individuals. The "up to a point" part of the answer reflects our lack of understanding of possible changes in the CSSs that might further modulate the peripheral declines, in the context of either CEBA or CEPP. In other words, degeneration of the peripheral receptors sets limits in sensitivity but does not tell the whole story about how information is processed centrally.

With respect to suprathreshold perception, which involves considerable central processing, we have a long way to go. Little is known about aging and the sensory systems when it comes to the complex or dynamic aspects of sensory stimuli such as modulation of intensity or frequency, movement, multiple stimuli, location, stimuli embedded in noise, distorted stimuli, or otherwise difficult stimuli. The appropriate neurophysiological studies have simply not been done, in large part because of the sheer difficulty of studying the neural coding of complex sensory stimuli in young adults, let alone older subjects.

Indeed, when central changes that affect the processing of stimuli are observed, it is difficult to determine the implications for perception and behavior. For example, plasticity of frequency representation in the central auditory system has potentially positive and negative consequences for hearing. After the reorganization of frequency maps in hearing-impaired individuals, more central neurons respond to sounds that are still audible. This could provide a sort of central amplification of sounds that are heard, as suggested by behavioral work (Willott, Carlson, & Chen, 1994). Whereas this could be a potential benefit, it is well known to audiologists that amplification of sounds is often deleterious to hearing in listeners with sensorineural hearing loss, particularly if the amplified sound is interfering noise. Therefore, plasticity could have negative consequences. Another potential negative exists because, with disruption of normal tonotopic organization, the "rules" have been changed with regard to frequency coding. A basic central place-coding theory of hearing implies that spectral components of sounds (at least higher frequencies) are coded according to the specific sets of tonotopically organized neurons that are responding: If neurons in high-frequency tonotopic regions are responding, the sound is perceived as containing high frequencies. After central reorganization, however, these same "high-frequency" neurons are responding when middle frequencies are present. Thus, there is the potential for the brain to make errors in frequency coding leading to altered perception. In summary, if frequency map plasticity were to occur in people with chronic high-frequency hearing loss, as is typical with aging, this could both help and hinder auditory perception.

The occurrence of CEBA and CEPP have clinical implications for gerontology and geriatrics, because dealing with the clinical aspects of CEBA and CEPP requires somewhat different strategies (Willott, 1996b). Understanding CEBA and devising clinical interventions must take neurogerontological approaches for studying the aging brain and apply them to the CSSs. For example, it must be determined if certain CSS regions, nuclei, subnuclei, or types of neurons are more or less vulnerable to age effects, if age-related changes in the functioning of particular neurotransmitter systems are altered in a way that could affect CSSs, whether normal neuronal metabolism is maintained throughout the CSS in older people, and the extent to which central sensory changes interfere with cognitive processes that affect perception. With respect to CEPP, two general strategies can be used: intervening at the periphery or within the CSSs. The first approach attempts to counteract the peripheral pathology causing

CEPP. Examples are using hearing aids to make the cochlea provide input to the brain that is more normal, engaging prophylactic measures to reduce cochlear damage (e.g., controlling exposure to noise), or using cochlear prostheses to restore lost neural input. To the extent that such measures work, CEPP is ameliorated because the quality of neural input to the brain is enhanced. The second approach is to counteract changes within the CSS that are caused by the existence of peripheral pathology. This tactic demands that we know what types of anatomical and physiological changes are induced in the brain by sensory receptor dysfunction (Willott, 1996b).

As a final note, it must be kept in mind that various nonsensory processes also influence sensation and perception. These include learning, cognition, social or sexual contexts, arousal, attention, emotional state, and neurode-generative disease. All of these processes vary during aging, as discussed in the chapters that follow.

8
The Storage of Information: Learning and Memory

The ability of animals to use information obtained by their sensory systems to modify their behaviors advantageously (learning) and store what was learned for future retrieval (memory) has obvious adaptive benefits. Thus, these capacities appear, with varying degrees of sophistication, in most animal species. Whereas learning and memory are intimately interwoven, we will view learning primarily as the acquisition of new information, behaviors, or behavioral modifications, focusing on the neural mechanisms and circuits that underlie this process. We will view memory with respect to how material is stored and retained for varying periods of time and retrieved when needed. Of course, when knowledge and skills are summoned up, acquisition, retention, and retrieval must each have functioned adequately.

Older people can learn many things as well as ever and certainly continue to remember vast amounts of information. However, numerous studies, as well as everyday observations, make it clear that age-related declines occur for some aspects of learning and memory, such as the ability to recall recently learned names. At this point, we cannot answer the question What neurobiological processes are responsible for deficits in learning and memory? In part, this is because the neurobiological mechanisms of learning and memory are not completely understood, irrespective of aging. Thus, it is difficult to determine what age effects are truly relevant or what parameters of neural change are most important. The best we can do within the scope of this chapter and the current state of the neurogerontological art is to outline the behavioral findings, identify the brain structures and circuits that have been implicated in learning and memory, review the literature to determine the extent to which age-related changes have occurred in these structures and circuits, and evaluate the correlations between behavioral and neurobiological changes.

LEARNING

The behavioral literature on aging and learning has been reviewed in a thorough and comprehensive book by Kausler (1994), as well as in recent chapters and review articles (Freund, 1996; Kausler, 1991; Powell, Buchanan, & Hernandez, 1991; Woodruff-Pak, 1990; Woodruff-Pak & Port, 1996). Some basic conclusions are drawn from these sources in the following brief review of the behavioral literature. Any discussion of this sort must recognize that learning comes in many forms. These undoubtedly make use of different but often overlapping constellations of neural circuits and structures. To a large extent, neurogerontological investigations will probably have to address them one by one.

Classical Conditioning

In classical or Pavlovian conditioning, a neutral *conditioned stimulus* (CS) is paired with a biologically meaningful event, the *unconditioned stimulus* (UCS), which naturally evokes an *unconditioned response* (UCR); after a sufficient number of pairings the CS, when presented by itself, becomes capable of eliciting a response similar to that originally produced by the UCS. The response that is now evoked by the CS is called the *conditioned response* (CR). Both somatomotor and visceral-autonomic responses can be modified by classical conditioning.

Eyeblink conditioning and other types of classical conditioning have been used in a number of gerontological studies of humans and other species. Consistent findings indicate that the rate of conditioning (number of CS-UCS pairings to reach a criterion for learning) typically slows with age. Older subjects have also performed more poorly in the more difficult *trace conditioning* paradigm, where there is an interval between CS offset and UCS onset. Furthermore, once conditioning has occurred, *extinction* (the persistence of the learned behavior in the absence of additional presentation of the UCS) tends to be slower.

Operant and Instrumental Conditioning

In operant conditioning, the subject behaves freely, encounters the consequences of that behavior, and subsequently modifies the behavior to maximize beneficial consequences or minimize negative ones. For example, for rats placed in a Skinner box, pressing a bar sometimes causes food to be released into a hopper; by repeatedly pressing the bar and frequently receiving food, the rat learns to press the bar to get food when it is hungry. Instrumental conditioning is similar (indeed, some psychologists do not distinguish it from operant conditioning), but the responses are typically structured in discrete trials, and the responses can be more complex (e.g., learning a sequence of responses). For example, each time a rat runs through a maze (a trial), it is either rewarded or not, depending on the (sequential) choices it makes; after a sufficient number of trials, it learns to make the turns that bring the reward.

Older subjects tend to make more errors and acquire instrumental responses more slowly, particularly when the task is more difficult. *Avoidance conditioning* is a commonly employed type of operant or instrumental conditioning in gerontological experiments with animals. The subject learns to engage in behaviors that prevent exposure to some negative event (a *negative reinforcer*, such as painful stimulus). A number of behavioral experiments have demonstrated poorer avoidance conditioning in old rats. The greater the complexity of the task, the greater the age-related deficit. Human studies have been less common due to ethical concerns of exposing subjects (particularly older ones) to negative events.

Experiments using *positive reinforcers* (e.g. food, money), where the conditioned behavior increases access to the consequential events, have not provided consistent evidence of age effects in rodents or humans. Although acquisition of learning is likely to be slower, some studies have shown that, with an appropriate reinforcement regimen, the rate of responses can be effectively augmented in old subjects.

Spatial Learning

Learning often involves spatial behaviors—where to go in an open space or a maze. A commonly used spatial task for rodents is the Morris water maze. A rat is placed in a large tub filled with milky water and must swim until it locates a platform just below the surface but not visible. The rat's ability to learn the location of the safe platform and find it at some later time serves as a measure of spatial learning and performance. Radial arm mazes, where the rat must choose one food-baited runway arm from many possible runway arms that radiate out from the start box, are also used in spatial learning experiments.

Old rodents learn Morris and radial arm mazes more slowly than young ones, although it is usually the case that a sample of old animals contains both good and poor learners. Many older humans also have difficulty with spatial relationships. For example, in everyday life, older people tend to acquire less knowledge about novel environments, such as learning to navigate a new travel route (Wilkniss, Jones, Korol, Gold, & Manning, 1997). The task difficulty can have a significant impact, however, and for simple spatial learning, age differences may be negligible. This might be due in part to factors other than learning ability per se; poorer maze learning might be due to increased distraction from the relevant stimuli or reduced motivation to engage in a more difficult task. In any event, older subjects, both rodent and human, often seem poorer at constructing a cognitive map of space, which is often assumed to be required for spatial memory.

Skill or Motor Learning

Many learning tasks in everyday life require a person to acquire one or more motor responses (perceptual-motor learning). Because new situations and behavioral demands continue to arise during one's later years, such learning is of great practical importance. Learning of tasks such as keyboard manipulation or moving the hand a specified distance tend to take more time and be subpar for older learners. Deficits usually occur whether the motor tasks involve discrete responses such as typing or continuous responses such as tracing figures in a mirror. The slowing of skilled behaviors need not be inevitable, however, as well-practiced, proficient skills are usually less seriously affected. For example, older expert typists can type as fast as younger ones. Thus, skills that are used regularly are usually maintained well throughout life, albeit at slower rates in some cases. Difficulties encountered by older people are most serious when it comes to the acquisition of new skills.

Perceptual Learning

The ability to improve the processing of sensory stimuli constitutes perceptual learning. Older subjects are fully capable of perceptual learning, but they tend not to do as well as younger people. For example, practice improves detection of target stimuli (e.g., a visual feature in a complex pattern) in older subjects, but they still may perform below the level of young subjects because they started out at a lower performance level before learning. Thus, the relative degree of improvement in older subjects may be comparable to that of younger subjects.

This illustrates another important principle: If an older person has a diminished capacity to perform but learns to improve just as well as younger subjects, he or she will still end up performing more poorly than the younger subjects. This is not by virtue of a learning deficit, but because of a lower baseline level of performance. The learning curves are parallel but shifted.

Verbal Learning

A special type of learning that is relevant only for humans is verbal learning, where the material to be learned is comprised of words or syllables. For example, in *paired associate* learning, the subject must learn that certain words or syllables are linked together (e.g., two parallel lists are presented). A number of studies have shown that older subjects are generally less proficient at paired associate learning; they do not perform at a high level and take longer (more practice trials) to reach a certain performance criterion. Elderly subjects are also likely to exhibit poorer *serial* learning, where a single list must be learned; age differences are most pronounced when the words are presented at a fast rate.

MEMORY

One need only listen in on a group of 40-somethings talking about movies to realize that memory for names and other facts begins to decline during middle age: "That movie starred what's-his-name; you know, the one that was married to the blond actress who was in that other movie." Whereas difficulty in retrieving stored memories such as these may constitute a mere inconvenience, more serious degrees of memory impairment associated with Alzheimer's disease can be debilitating. The ubiquity of minor memory loss in healthy older people and the devastation of memory associated with Alzheimer's disease have spawned a great deal of gerontological research on memory. Most of the research has been done using human subjects and is best characterized as cognitive psychology rather than neurogerontology. Many reviews are available (e.g., Craik & Jennings, 1992; Hultsch & Dixon, 1990; Kausler, 1991, 1994; A. D. Smith, 1996), from which the following gerontological highlights have been gleaned.

As is the case for learning, different types of memory can be identified. However, these typologies are organized along several dimensions. For example, memory can be defined by the nature of what is stored, usually with the assumption of different, interacting memory systems. *Declarative memory* refers to the knowledge, facts, or information one has learned; material that can be consciously remembered and stated (also called *explicit memory*). Two subtypes of declarative memory are *episodic memory*, which applies to personally experienced events (episodes), and *semantic* or *generic memory*, our store of permanent knowledge about the universe (without necessary reference to where, when, or how it was acquired by us). *Nondeclarative, implicit,* or *procedural memory* refers to the skills and behaviors one uses, knowing how to do things without necessarily being able to explain them or even be conscious of learning them. Episodic memory typically becomes substantially poorer as people age, whereas declines in semantic memory tend to be minimal. Most forms of nondeclarative memory are generally not impaired much if at all with age, and in those studies that have found age differences, the magnitude of the deficits is usually small (there is no universal agreement on this issue, however).

Types of memory can also be distinguished with respect to their time course and duration. Although there is no general consensus, many psychologists recognize three or four different types of memory along the temporal dimension. The shortest, transient memories are called *sensory memories* and are essentially the briefly lingering neural traces of sensations (mostly visual and auditory). Sensory memory can be viewed as the initial stage of processing, making information available for further processing. *Short-term* or *primary memories* last for a number of seconds, then disappear unless "rehearsed" by reiterating the information verbally or mentally (e.g., reading an unfamiliar phone number and remembering it only long enough to make the call). The term *intermediate-term memory* is used by some psychologists to refer to those memories that may last for days or weeks (e.g., what you ate for dinner a few days ago) but are not long-lasting or permanent. Persistent memories are referred to as *long-term memories* and constitute the sum of our stored knowledge and life experiences (e.g., where you were born, the name of your kindergarten teacher). Sensory memory lasts for about 1 second (visual) to 2 seconds (auditory) in young adults, and there do not appear to be significant age-related changes in duration. Therefore, the availability of information for short-term memory remains intact (assuming the sensory system is functioning adequately). Only minimal to moderate age effects are typically observed in studies of short-term memory. However, a conceptual cousin of short-term memory, *working memory*, suffers some limitations, as older people tend to have a limited capacity to perform simultaneous cognitive tasks. The most significant memory deficits are evident for intermediate- and long-term memories, the ability to remember specific events or facts.

Memory can also be conceptualized according to the processes required for long-term storage. Three processes are usually identified: *encoding* (the information is processed in short-term or working memory to be made available for long-term storage), *consolidation* (the process by which the memory is permanently stored), and *retrieval* (finding the stored information and bringing it out). Memory can potentially fail at any of these stages, and there is evidence that each (particularly retrieval) usually exhibits deficits in older people. However, various situations and variables can mitigate or exacerbate the age differences, and the cognitive literature is complicated and challenging (see reviews cited above).

VARIABLES THAT MODULATE LEARNING AND MEMORY

Learning entails neural coding processes that establish associations among stimuli, consequences, and responses; memory requires enduring neural changes to store what has been learned and mechanisms to find and retrieve stored information. Whereas the neural substrates that underlie these processes are fundamental to the efficacy of learning and memory, other aspects of neural function are also highly relevant.

Sensory Processes

Although it may be true that people can learn from internal, "mental" processes using information already stored in memory (e.g., gain insights or understanding), learning typically requires sensory input. The CS, UCS, verbal stimuli, reinforcers, and other components of learning are all delivered by the sensory systems. Clearly then, age-related deficits in the sensory systems, as discussed in chapter 7, can affect learning. Whereas this may seem obvious, experiments on aging and learning have occasionally failed to appreciate this obvious point. This is particularly true when it comes to rodent models. Three of the inbred mouse strains most widely used in biomedical and behavioral research, C57BL/6, BALB/c, and DBA/2, exhibit severe loss of hearing by 1 year of age (Erway et al., 1993; Willott, 1996c). Other widely used mouse strains, C3H and CBA/J, can hear well as they age but have retinal degeneration genes that render them blind. Nevertheless, studies have appeared showing deficits in learning in these strains using auditory or visual CSs and attributed the deficits to impaired learning ability.

The potential occurrence of sensory declines should always be controlled for in gerontological experiments. Furthermore, it should be appreciated that, even if an older subject can detect stimuli required for learning (i.e., the stimuli are above threshold), the quality, perceived magnitude, speed of processing, or salience of the stimuli may be altered. Similarly, if the stimuli contain rapidly fluctuating or repetitive components or are embedded in "noisy" or distracting backgrounds, sensory processing deficits could become relevant.

Whereas age-related changes in sensory systems usually make it more difficult to learn, this need not always be the case. As discussed in chapter 7, partial impairment of peripheral sensory receptors can induce neural plasticity in the central sensory systems that can make some stimuli more salient. Experiments from our laboratory suggest that such enhanced salience can actually facilitate learning. Recall that C57 mice exhibit early presbycusis, losing the ability to hear high-frequency sounds. However, the still-audible middle frequencies (e.g., 12 kHz, a middle frequency for mice) become overrepresented in the central auditory system. We have found that the overrepresented frequencies become more effective CSs in a learning paradigm called *fear-potentiated startle*: If a subject learns to associate a CS (e.g., a tone) with a negative UCS (e.g., a mild foot shock), presentation of the CS alone comes to elicit fear; the learned fear is manifested by a potentiated startle response when the subject is startled in the presence of the CS. In C57 mice (see Figure 8.1), learning with a 12-kHz tone CS resulted in a much greater magnitude of fear-potentiated startle in mice with presbycusis (high-frequency hearing loss) than in

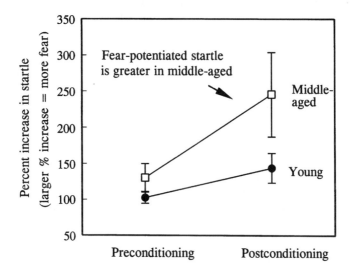

FIGURE 8.1   **Fear-potentiated startle in young and middle-aged mice. Fear-potentiated startle is a type of learning in which the subject associates a CS (in this case a 12-kHz tone) with a negative UCS. After fear has been conditioned, if the subject is startled when the CS is present, the startle amplitude increases. The subject has learned the significance of the CS. This figure shows the effect of a 12-kHz tone (CS) on startle before and after conditioning. The startle amplitude increased by about 30% in the young mice after conditioning, and this was statistically significant. In the middle-aged mice with high-frequency presbycusis, the CS was much more salient, and startle amplitude more than doubled. This is presumably a result of central neural plasticity, which made the middle frequency 12-kHz CS more effective in the hearing-impaired mice. From Willott et al. (1996).**

young adults with normal hearing (the age difference did not occur with a light CS). Paradoxically then, presbycusis can actually make a still-audible sound more salient as a CS.

Motor and Autonomic Output

In order to demonstrate that learning has occurred, behavior must be exhibited. In other words, learning must be *inferred* from performance.

This is a concern because learning and performance can vary independently of one another. For example, even though a behavior was not learned, it might be emitted by chance (a lucky guess on a test). On the other hand, a behavior might have been learned, but the subject does not exhibit the learned behavior for some reason (e.g., fatigue, lack of motivation, inability to execute a motor or autonomic response). In the latter case, if an experimenter were to infer that an older subject had not learned, it would be a mistake. This type of error (a false negative) can be especially problematic in gerontological research because of the potential for age-related changes in various factors that could interfere with performance irrespective of learning, as discussed throughout this book.

As is the case for sensory processes, gerontological studies of learning and memory must be sensitive to limitations in the production of behavior that may be exhibited by older subjects. From an applied, practical standpoint, the task older individuals are asked to learn should be appropriate to their performance ability.

Emotion and Arousal

Most forms of learning and the concomitant memories have a requisite emotional component. For example, in appetitive conditioning the reinforcer of the learned behavior has a positive (e.g., pleasurable) emotional tone. In avoidance conditioning, negative emotion (e.g., fear) may be necessary to learn the appropriate behavior that prevents exposure to an aversive stimulus. In other words, without positive or negative emotional components, many forms of learning would not occur. Furthermore, the intensity of emotion modulates learning and memory, as emotionally charged material is more readily learned and remembered.

Arousal also plays an important role in learning and modulates the formation of long-term memories, with a moderate level usually optimal. The experimental setting itself can produce arousal, being both novel and associated with aversive or positive reinforcers. If older subjects were more or less reactive to the arousing stimuli, their behavior or performance might be altered in ways that could be mistaken for age differences in learning ability.

Emotion and arousal are discussed in detail in chapter 10, but suffice it to say that aging is associated with altered arousal and emotions. These age effects could in turn influence learning and memory.

NEURAL MECHANISMS OF LEARNING AND MEMORY

Behavioral neuroscientists have made considerable progress in understanding the neural bases of learning and memory, although there is still a long way to go. The advances that have been made provide an excellent framework from which neurogerontological research can gain insights into the neural changes that may underlie the age-related deficits in learning and memory.

Synaptic Plasticity

It is generally assumed that learning and memory involve modifications (plasticity) of synapses in neural circuits. In the simplest of conceptualizations, repeated simultaneous activation of circuits mediating the CS and UCS-UCR strengthens synapses that link the CS to the unconditioned behavioral circuitry; ultimately, the CS becomes capable of producing this or a similar behavior, the CR. Presumably, most learning entails synaptic changes (strengthening and/or weakening) in rather complex circuitry, but the notion of alterations in synaptic communication is still the key. The synaptic changes might be presynaptic (e.g., the amount of neurotransmitter released; modulation of neurotransmitter release by axoaxonic synapses near the presynaptic terminals), postsynaptic (e.g., the number of receptors), a change in the number of synapses (synaptogenesis), a change in the size of synapses, and/or growth of dendrites or dendritic spines. Other types of postsynaptic mechanisms might include changes in the neurons involving second messenger activity, intracellular calcium regulation, changes in protein properties (e.g., phosphorylation), gene expression, and synthesis of proteins (Rosenzweig, Leiman, & Breedlove, 1996). As seen in chapters 3 through 5, virtually all of these variables are subject to age effects. Clearly, there are many potential avenues by which learning and memory could be affected as organisms age.

Neural Speed

At the neural level, age-related changes in axonal conduction speed, synaptic transmission, and other physiological processes (as discussed in chapters 4 and 5) presumably make it more difficult to acquire rapidly occurring information or quickly retrieve data from storage. Indeed, a large amount of evidence has been assembled by cognitive psychologists showing that various mental and perceptual abilities become slower as people age (refer to chapter 11). The processes of encoding and retrieval are among those that occur more slowly, presumably contributing to poorer memory in older people. There is a good deal of evidence that the slowing of neural processing is a major impediment to efficient learning, memory, and other aspects of cognition (see chapter 11).

Long-Term Potentiation

In the hippocampus and other parts of the brain, appropriate parameters of electrical stimulation of axons providing synaptic input results in a long-lasting increase in the magnitude of neural responses (e.g., higher rate of action potentials firing, augmented excitatory postsynaptic potentials) called long-term potentiation (LTP). LTP can be demonstrated *in vivo*, as well as *in vitro*, using brain slice preparations. The extent to which LTP occurs naturally (i.e., without electrical stimulation) is debatable, but it is nevertheless an attractive model with which to study learning and memory at the neuronal level: It can be induced rapidly, lasts for days or weeks, and demonstrates other similarities to learning/memory (Geinisman, deToledo-Morrell, Morrell, & Heller, 1995; Hawkins, Kandel, & Siegelbaum, 1993; Rosenzweig et al., 1996).

Neurogerontological studies are beginning to reveal relationships among aging, learning, and LTP in the hippocampus. Fairly consistent findings are: LTP tends to be acquired more slowly in old rats or rabbits; however, once acquired, potentiation is often as strong in old animals as in young; on the other hand, once acquired, LTP declines more rapidly in old animals compared to young ones (Geinisman et al., 1995; Landfield, McGaugh, & Lynch, 1978). The declines in LTP appear to correlate with behaviorally measured age differences as well. For example, Barnes and McNaughton (1985) induced LTP in rats and found that both the rate of forgetting of spatial information and the waning of LTP were accelerated in older rats.

A variable that appears to be important in the demonstration of age differences in potentiation is the duration of the electrical pulse trains used to induce potentiation. Long trains have generally resulted in the absence of age differences in the acquired magnitude of LTP in hippocampal preparations just alluded to. However, when short pulse trains are used, greater age differences in the strength of potentiation have been revealed (e.g., Deupree, Turner, & Watters, 1991; Diana, Scotti de Carolis, Frank, Domenici, & Sagratella, 1994; Landfield et al., 1978; Moore, Browning, & Rose, 1993; Norris, Korol, & Foster, 1996). *Post-tetanic potentiation* (PTP) is a term often used to describe potentiation of shorter duration. Diana and colleagues (1994), using hippocampal slices, observed no differences in LTP between young rats and old rats that varied in their ability to perform spatial learning. They did, however, find that shorter lasting PTP in the dentate gyrus was diminished in the old rats that performed poorly on the spatial task. Landfield and colleagues (1978) also reported a delayed rise in PTP in old rats. Perhaps the clearer age effects with shorter potentiation have something to do with the observations that LTP does not develop as rapidly in old animals (Geinisman et al., 1995).

Synaptic activation of glutamatergic receptors allows Ca^{++} influx into the cells, which initiates various changes in proteins and other intracellular processes; LTP is dependent upon these events (Hawkins et al., 1993; Rosenzweig et al., 1996). Thus, one might look here to explain the age-related changes in LTP that have been observed. Lynch and Voss (1994) stimulated the *perforant path* (input fibers from the entorhinal cortex to the hippocampus; see Figure 8.2) in young and old rats *in vivo* and observed an increase in neural responses (excitatory postsynaptic potentials). In the young rats, the potentiation lasted for the entire 45-min experimental period, but the activity had returned to baseline in half of the old rats. The age differences in LTP were correlated with glutamate release at synapses. A loss of NMDA glutamate receptors associated with *Shaffer collateral* axons (input from the CA3 to CA1 region of the hippocampus; see Figure 8.2) appears to play a role in reduced LTP (Barnes, Rao, & Shen, 1997). Diminished ability of synapses to be adequately depolarized (allowing repetitive synaptic excitation to summate) may be another contributor to LTP deficits (Rosenzweig, Rao, McNaughton, & Barnes, 1997). Another study used a drug treatment that enhances glutamate receptors, and this increased hippocampal neural activity and improved spatial learning and memory in middle-aged rats (Granger et al., 1996). Lanahan, Lyford, Stevenson, Worley, and Barnes (1997) found that the ability to sustain LTP was reduced in old rats, and their evidence implicated altered calcium regulation. A role of calcium mechanisms was suggested by the findings of Diana, Domenici, Scotti de Carolis, Loizzo, and Sagratella

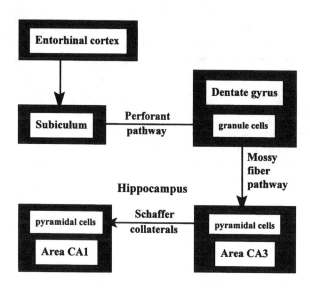

FIGURE 8.2   Some connections in the hippocampal formation. Neurons in the entorhinal cortex project to the dentate gyrus by way of the subiculum, via the perforant pathway. Neurons in the dentate gyrus project to the hippocampus proper by way of the mossy fiber pathway. Neurons in hippocampal area CA3 project to area CA1 via axons called Schaffer collaterals.

(1995). Increasing the extracellular Ca^{++} concentration in hippocampal slices produces LTP when input fibers are electrically stimulated. Old rats that had performed poorly in spatial learning exhibited less calcium-induced LTP than either young rats or old rats that did well on the spatial task. Moreover, as discussed in chapter 13, the calcium-blocking drug nimodipine affects both learning deficits and hippocampal neuronal responses in old subjects.

A structural element that might be involved in age-related changes of LTP in certain areas of the brain is the dendritic spine. Spines may play an important role in LTP (Harris & Kater, 1994); they receive glutamatergic synapses and regulate calcium entry into postsynaptic neurons, both of which are aspects of LTP. As discussed in chapter 4, loss of spines is frequently observed in older neurons. Thus, for example, spine loss was observed in hippocampal neurons of senescence-accelerated mice that displayed learning deficits (Kawaguchi, Kishikawa, Sakae, & Nakane, 1995).

Other stimulation-induced synaptic changes. Electrical stimulation of hippocampal inputs induces still other changes in neural excitability that may be related to the modulation of LTP. Landfield and colleagues (1978) measured *frequency potentiation*, the growth of neural activity during repetitive stimulation. Frequency potentiation was reduced in old rats, and this correlated with behavioral declines.

Another stimulation-induced form of neural plasticity is *long-term depression* (LTD), a phenomenon in which low-frequency electrical stimulation depresses synapses that have undergone LTP. Norris and colleagues (1996) suggested that the decrease in LTP might result from the augmentation of mechanism(s) that depress potentiated synapses, namely LTD. Using a hippocampal slice preparation, they tested the potency of LTD as a function of age. Old rats were indeed more susceptible to LTD and consequent reversal of LTP. LTD is also mediated by calcium, and the researchers speculated that alterations of Ca^{++} mechanisms might contribute to the enhanced LTD.

Summary. The story on synaptic changes associated with stimulation of inputs to the hippocampus, and what they might tell us about aging and learning, is a promising one with an element of confusion. This approach has promise because far more is known about synaptic potentiation than any other neural model of learning in mammals. Many sophisticated neurobiological techniques can be applied. Furthermore, old rats that differ in performance on learning tasks can be identified, and these can be used to establish neurobehavioral relationships within the same aged groups. Thus, much has been learned about the physiological modifications that can accompany aging in general, and deficits of learning and memory in particular. The confusion, which will undoubtedly be sorted out, stems from the various types of synaptic changes that can be observed, each of which can be differentially affected in older subjects. There are also differences in the properties and mechanisms of LTP in different regions of the hippocampus that we have not delved into here (e.g., Barnes, Suster, Shen, & McNaughton, 1997), not to mention other regions of the brain. Thus, like everything else in neurobiology, this story is an unfolding, complex one.

Protein Synthesis and the Formation of Long-Term Memories

It has been known for some time that the synthesis of proteins is important for the formation of long-term memories and for the occurrence of relevant phenomena such as LTP (Rosenzweig et al., 1996). For example, treatments that prevent protein synthesis (e.g., the antibiotic anisomycin) prevent the consolidation of long-term memory without affecting short-term memory. The synthesis of intracellular proteins that affect cellular physiology and/or the formation of new synapses, dendrites, and spines are likely to be required for the formation of memories.

A large body of research has demonstrated age effects with respect to protein modification and protein synthesis in neural tissue (Danner & Holbrook, 1990; Johnson & Finch, 1996). If these effects encompass the protein-related mechanisms of long-term memory, the implications with respect to declines in memory associated with aging could be extremely important.

CIRCUITS AND STRUCTURES INVOLVED IN LEARNING AND MEMORY

A number of neural circuits and structures have been implicated in learning and memory. A potentially fruitful approach to understanding the neural processes that underlie age-related deficits in learning and memory is to expand these lines of research in neurogerontological directions. In some cases, this has already begun, as correlations between neural and behavioral age effects have been demonstrated.

In reviewing the literature, we focus on one brain structure at a time, knowing full well that most of these are functionally interconnected with one another—a principle that should always be kept in mind. Trying to deal with the variety of specific circuit models that have been proposed would be prohibitively baffling, and we shall not attempt to do so.

The Hippocampus

The hippocampal formation (the hippocampus proper, along with the neighboring *dentate gyrus* and *subiculum*; see Figure 8.2, as well as Figure 3.3) plays a critical role in various aspects of learning and memory

(Geinisman et al., 1995; Powell et al., 1991; Rosenzweig et al., 1996; Zola-Morgan & Squire, 1993). The hippocampal formation and neighboring regions of the medial temporal lobe (*perirhinal, parahippocampal,* and *entorhinal* cortices) are essential for consolidating information into long-term declarative memory. The hippocampus seems to act like a memory buffer in the computerese sense of the word, holding and shepherding information into long-term storage, primarily involving neocortical locales. The hippocampus plays an especially critical role in spatial learning and memory and in learning where some delay is involved, such as delayed matching tasks (e.g., a time period passes between the acquisition trials and the response to be performed). The hippocampus is involved in trace conditioning and discrimination-reversal learning (the subject must learn that the meaning of the CS has changed).

Hippocampal lesions in young subjects produce learning and memory deficits that are reminiscent of those that accompany aging (Geinisman et al., 1995; Moscovitch & Winocur, 1992). For example, bilateral damage to the hippocampal area results in loss of acquisition and recall of declarative memories, particularly for material learned relatively recently. As discussed earlier, impairment of declarative memory is often observed in older people, albeit to a much lesser extent than in those with severely damaged hippocampi. Also, information is forgotten more rapidly with both hippocampal damage and aging. Numerous studies on rodents have shown that spatial learning and memory are greatly impaired in animals with hippocampal lesions; the same is true of humans, particularly when the right hemisphere is damaged. As discussed earlier, spatial learning deficits accompany old age as well.

Given that hippocampal lesions in young adults cause deficits similar to those that are characteristic of older adults, it is reasonable to hypothesize age-related hippocampal damage as having a causal role. Of course, for this hypothesis to be tenable, it must be established that hippocampal damage or dysfunction accompanies healthy aging, at least in individuals who exhibit learning/memory deficits (as discussed in chapter 11, Alzheimer's disease is accompanied by substantial hippocampal pathology, but that is another story). Let us examine the evidence.

The anatomical literature provides some indications of hippocampal vulnerability, with many studies finding histological signs of degeneration and/or cell loss in older subjects. As is usually the case in histological studies counting the number of neurons or synapses, however, considerable variance exists in the literature, due undoubtedly to both methodological variables and true individual differences among the subjects. Geinisman and colleagues (1995) reviewed this literature. Many but not all studies have concluded that aging is accompanied by a loss of hippocampal neurons. Because some of these studies may have suffered from methodological flaws, Geinisman and colleagues (1995) singled out a study by West (1993) as being especially well done. This anatomical study on humans used modern "unbiased" methods (see chapter 3) and demonstrated age-related loss of neurons in only two regions, the hilus (31%) and the subiculum (52%), neither of which plays a major role in learning and memory. This study suggests that the number of neurons in the dentate gyrus and hippocampal subfields CA1 to CA3 (the hippocampus proper) may remain relatively stable as people age.

However, other studies using unbiased counting methods are not in full agreement. A study by Simic, Kostovic, Winblad, and Bogdanovic (1997) observed a loss of tissue volume in the principle hippocampal subdivisions of old subjects, along with a decrease in the number of neurons in the CA1 area and subiculum, but not other regions. This agrees with West (1993) regarding the loss of neurons in the subiculum, but differs in finding a loss in CA1 but not in the hilar region. Simic and colleagues (1997) felt that the differences between the two studies were likely due to individual differences or (less likely) the unknown occurrence of ischemic episodes, which can damage the CA1 region. On the other hand, Harding, Wong, Svoboda, Kril, and Halliday (1997) used unbiased methods and found that hippocampi of chronic alcoholics and control subjects did not exhibit significant correlations between age and tissue volume or neuron number. It appears that, whether the methodology is unbiased or otherwise, there is still a good deal of variability in hippocampal cell loss, with plenty of examples of both normalcy and degeneration.

Some of the variability in the cell-counting literature may depend on individual differences with respect to the age at which hippocampal neurons disappear. An imaging study (MRI and CT scans) by Golomb and colleagues (1993) indicated that more than 80% of healthy individuals age 65 or younger had yet to show serious hippocampal damage. However, the prevalence rose substantially at older ages, so that about 80% of men ages 77 to 88 did exhibit hippocampal atrophy. Women fared better, as only about 40% of the 77- to 88-year-olds exhibited hippocampal atrophy. It would seem that a decade or two of aging can have a real impact on the severity of hippocampal atrophy and that gender can be relevant.

Another potential source of between-subject variance in studies of the hippocampus might be the cognitive status of the subjects, rarely if ever rigorously tested in postmortem subjects prior to their death. People may be healthy and nondemented, but they can differ widely with respect to mnemonic abilities. In the imaging study by Golomb and colleagues (1993), memory tests were administered in conjunction with brain imaging. Subjects with deficits in recent memory were more likely to exhibit hippocampal atrophy. A PET study by Eustache and colleagues (1995) obtained significant negative correlations between hippocampal oxygen metabolism and scores on tests of episodic memory in older subjects. Correlations between learning/memory and hippocampal damage have also been examined in studies comparing old rats differing in their behavioral performance. Several studies have found correlations between learning/performance and histological measures (Brizzee & Ordy, 1979; Issa, Rowe, Gauthier, & Meaney, 1990), although others have not (Geinisman, deToledo-Morrell, & Morrell, 1986; West, Amaral, & Rapp, 1993).

In addition to the research on LTP described earlier that was performed on hippocampal neurons, other physiological studies have identified age effects in the hippocampus that have the potential to contribute to learning/memory deficits. For example, as young animals are trained in a learning task, the activity level of their hippocampal neurons grows. In old rabbits, both behavioral training on a classical conditioning task where delay is introduced and the growth of hippocampal neural activity require more trials than what is required for young rabbits (Woodruff-Pak, Lavond, Logan, & Thompson, 1987). Amplitudes of "slow" excitatory postsynaptic potentials, a response to tetanic stimulation of cholinergic inputs, are smaller in the hippocampus of aged rats (Shen & Barnes, 1996, and others referenced in this paper); these findings suggest that cholinergic circuits involving the hippocampus become impaired with age (see discussion below on the basal forebrain). CA1 hippocampal neurons of old rats exhibit signs of reduced excitability (Potier, Rascol, Jazat, Lamour, & Dutar, 1992). Landfield and Pitler (1984) showed that the calcium-dependent "afterhyperpolarization" response of hippocampal neurons, which exhibits a decrease after conditioning has occurred, was prolonged in old rats. Many other studies have implicated calcium currents in age-related physiological changes in hippocampal neurons (see Campbell et al., 1996; Disterhoft et al., 1994). Altered calcium regulation could both affect the functional properties of hippocampal neurons and render them vulnerable to calcium-induced damage (refer to chapters 3, 4 and 11, 13).

Other indications of age effects in the hippocampus abound. The hippocampus is rich in receptors for glucocorticoids, adrenal hormones secreted during stress, and there is strong evidence that glucocorticoids damage the hippocampus during the course of aging (Landfield, 1980; Sapolsky, 1992; see chapter 10 for a discussion of glucocorticoids and stress; see chapter 13 for a discussion of how this might affect neurotrophins). There have been many demonstrations of age-related changes in markers of cholinergic neurotransmission in the hippocampus and some evidence of changes in other neurotransmitter systems (Morgan & May, 1990; Rogers & Bloom, 1985). Degenerating axons were observed in the hippocampus and associated fiber tracts of old rats (Greene & Naranjo, 1987). Dendritic spines are lost as rats age (Nunzi, Milan, Guidolin, & Toffano, 1987). Phosphorylation of a particular (F1) protein declined in hippocampus but not in other brain regions (Barnes et al., 1988). Microtubule-associated proteins (MAPs) declined in hippocampus, and MAP2, associated with dendrites, was almost completely depleted (Chauhan & Siegel, 1997a). A decrease in the calcium-binding proteins parvalbumin and calbindin was observed in certain hippocampal sites of old rabbits (DeJong et al., 1996). Finally, in some cases dendritic growth can be observed in aging hippocampal neurons (Coleman & Flood, 1987; Pyapali & Turner, 1996).

Conclusions about the hippocampal formation and aging.   The inconsistencies in the anatomical literature are likely to stem, in part, from methodological differences. However, this is not a sufficient explanation. Rather, it is almost certainly the case that hippocampal neuron degeneration really does differ enough to smear the arbitrary age boundaries used to classify subjects as old or middle-aged. The best guess is that some people make it well into old age with little or no loss of hippocampal neurons, whereas others are less fortunate. However, perhaps we are spending too much time on the issue of cell numbers. As noted in chapter 3, the most germane neurogerontological changes during healthy aging are likely to be more subtle than the simple attrition of neurons. Thus, when we look beyond cell counts, there is ample evidence that hippocampal neurons, synapses, and afferent inputs of many older humans and other mammals suffer physiological alterations, listed above. One would think that many of these are likely to detract from optimal learning and memory.

Some fairly compelling correlational evidence has linked dysfunction of hippocampal circuitry to individual differences in spatial and declarative learning/memory deficits. On the other hand, the correlations are always far from perfect, suggesting that the complete aging-learning-memory story cannot be found in the hippocampus alone. Those who escape hippocampal damage are not out of the proverbial woods. As we are about to see, many other brain structures are likely to contribute to the declines in learning and memory that accompany aging.

The Basal Forebrain

The *nucleus basalis of Meynert, medial septal nucleus*, and *diagonal band* are located in the *basal forebrain* region of the brain. They give rise to major cholinergic systems and play important roles in learning and memory. Neurons in the medial septal nucleus and diagonal band innervate the subregions of the hippocampus via the *septo-hippocampal* pathway (Gallagher, Nagahara, & Burwell, 1995). A key role of this pathway in spatial learning and performance has been shown with several behavioral tasks, including the Morris water maze. The nucleus basalis is the primary source of cholinergic input to the cerebral cortex but also has many noncholinergic neurons (Mesulam, 1996).

Various studies have indicated that cholinergic basal forebrain structures can become somewhat altered with age, although as usual, results are mixed and variable according to species, strain, and tissue sampling (Decker, 1987; Finch, 1993; Gallagher et al., 1995; Mesulam, 1996; Murchison & Griffith, 1996). Experimental variability is reduced somewhat by studying old rats shown to be deficient spatial learners. Compared to old but good learners, they are likely to have reduced size, number, and/or cholinergic activity in the basal forebrain, especially in the medial septum and diagonal band (Gallagher et al., 1995). On the other hand, there are indications that even severe deficits in the cholinergic system are not sufficient to interfere with spatial tasks (Gallagher & Rapp, 1997). Monoaminergic circuits (using NE, dopamine, or serotonin) are also found in the basal forebrain structures, and these exhibit age effects as well. Luine and Milio (1990) presented evidence that NE and dopamine turnover rates decreased in old rats, whereas levels of the serotonin metabolite 5-HIAA were elevated, suggesting increased activity of serotonergic neurons.

The nucleus basalis exhibits degeneration in Alzheimer's disease and is thought to contribute to memory loss characteristic of the disease (see chapter 11). However, there is some question with respect to the role of cholinergic processes in memory impairment associated with damage to the nucleus basalis. Research suggests that nucleus basalis damage may primarily disrupt attention, rather than memory (see Zola-Morgan & Squire, 1993). This being the case, degenerative changes in the nucleus basalis associated with Alzheimer's disease may affect learning and memory in an indirect manner, by impairing attention.

The extent to which the nucleus basalis becomes altered and/or contributes to learning and memory impairments in healthy older people has not been clearly established. Anatomical studies of humans are characterized by the usual inconsistencies, with about equal numbers of studies finding either substantial loss of neurons in very old subjects or no loss (Chui, Bondareff, Zarow, & Slager, 1984; Decker, 1987; De Lacalle, Iraiziz, & Gonzalo, 1991; Mann, 1997). The work of Mesulam and colleagues (see Mesulam, 1996) indicates that age effects tend to be modest, with some hypertrophy of neurons around age 60, followed by shrinkage of cells and cell losses at advanced ages. A recent study found that cholinergic neurons in the nucleus basalis and diagonal band of nondemented humans exhibited a marked decrease in immunostaining for calbindin (Wu, Mesulam, & Geula, 1997), suggesting functional changes.

Recent studies on nonhuman species have not clarified the story, but do suggest some age effects. Smith and Booze (1995) used an unbiased counting method and immunostaining for cholinergic and GABAergic neurons to evaluate age-related neuronal loss in the nucleus basalis of Fischer 344 rats. There was an overall neuronal loss of 30% (using Nissl stain, which stains all neurons). Only about 20% of that cell loss could be attributed to a loss of cholinergic neurons, and none to a loss of GABAergic neurons. The findings indicate that the rat nucleus basalis is vulnerable to neuron loss with aging but raise questions as to the neurochemical properties of the affected neurons. In a study of monkeys up to 33 years of age, Voytko and colleagues (1995) found the number of cholinergic neurons to be stable in the nucleus basalis. Hypertrophy of neurons was observed in old monkeys, consistent with the findings of several studies on humans (Mesulam, 1996). Voytko and colleagues were able to behaviorally test some of the monkeys. They obtained significant correlations indicating that animals with fewer neurons in the intermediate region of the nucleus basalis had poorer spatial memory and concurrent discrimination abilities. Thus, differential regional losses within the nucleus basalis may be significant even if the overall number of neurons remains high. Indeed, regional variations in age effects may be characteristic of the nucleus basalis (Decker, 1987).

Looking at the evidence as a whole, functional age effects in the basal forebrain region probably contribute to learning and memory deficits in at least some healthy elders, although cholinergic involvement alone may not be sufficient to account for all learning deficits (Smith & Booze, 1995; see also Gallagher & Rapp, 1997; Lee et al., 1994). The research on rats has demonstrated a reliable relationship between spatial learning ability and the cholinergic septo-hippocampal pathway in old subjects. In the nucleus basalis, functional deficiencies in the cholinergic system appear to occur (Decker, 1987; Sparks et al., 1992). Because the nucleus basalis provides major cholinergic input to the cerebral cortex, it is germane that some robust age effects are observed in cortex for the cholinergic system (see below).

The Diencephalon

The many subdivisions of the thalamus and hypothalamus comprise the diencephalon. Two diencephalic structures, the *mammillary nuclei* and *dorsomedial thalamic nuclei* (and probably some adjacent regions and fiber tracts), are known to play important roles in memory (Zola-Morgan & Squire, 1993). For example, these structures exhibit pathology in *Korsakoff's syndrome*, a disorder associated with chronic alcoholism and thiamine deficiency, characterized by severe memory impairments. Also, damage to the medial thalamus from stroke or injury results in memory impairments, in particular the formation of long-term declarative memory (also true of hippocampal damage). The extent to which these structures become damaged with age and contribute to memory impairment has not been established. A decrease in the number of thalamic neurons and size of neuronal nuclei were observed in older nonalcoholic subjects (Belzunegui, Insausti, Ibanez, & Gonzalo, 1995). These losses were similar to those observed in younger chronic alcoholics. A PET study revealed decreased oxygen metabolism in the thalamus of older subjects, and this was correlated with poorer performance on tests of declarative memory (Eustache et al., 1995).

The Amygdala

The amygdala consists of several subdivisions and is a key limbic structure for behaviors and experiences involving emotions (as discussed in chapter

10). The amygdala plays an essential role in fear conditioning (Davis, 1992; LeDoux, 1995) and also participates in visceral-autonomic learning, such as classical conditioning of heart rate (Powell et al., 1991). The amygdala communicates with many brain regions and appears capable of modulating learning and memory formation in other structures such as the hippocampus and caudate nucleus. The amygdala presumably contributes to aspects of learning and memory that have emotional significance as well. Given its central role in these phenomena, the amygdala would seem to have great potential in contributing to age-related changes in avoidance conditioning and other types of emotionally charged learning and memory.

Degeneration of the amygdala accompanies Alzheimer's disease, and this pathology is believed to contribute to memory losses accompanying the disease (see chapter 11). With respect to healthy aging, the amygdala has not been very well studied, but there is some evidence of age effects. An anatomical study by Herzog and Kemper (1980) found small decreases in neuronal density (especially the medial nucleus) and amygdala volume in human autopsy material, but only studied four old brains. Sarter and Markowitsch (1983) likewise observed a substantial loss of neurons in the medial nucleus but not other amygdaloid nuclei of old Wistar rats. In one MRI study, significant atrophy of the amygdala was observed in cognitively normal and memory-impaired older subjects, compared to young adults (Laakso et al., 1995). Patients with Alzheimer's disease had even worse atrophy. Soininen and colleagues (1994) observed a correlation between amygdala volume and performance of older subjects on visual memory tests, and amygdala volume was especially reduced in subjects identified as having age-associated memory impairment (which may or may not be a sign of early Alzheimer's disease). Iseki and colleagues (1996) described an age-related increase within the amygdala of ubiquitin-positive granular structures, which they felt were derived from degenerating axon terminals. In a study on rats, some loss of cholinergic receptors was observed in the amygdala by Narang (1995).

Although some neurogerontological evidence suggests that the amygdala exhibits age effects, the functional significance of these findings with respect to memory (if any) is not yet clear. As discussed in chapter 10, the emotion of fear does not appear to become consistently diminished with age, as might be expected if the amygdala were to exhibit a general functional decline.

The Cerebellum

The cerebellum participates in some forms of classical conditioning (e.g., the eyeblink response, conditioned heart rate), instrumental learning (e.g., avoidance conditioning), and other types of learning (Mauk, Steele, & Medina, 1997). For example, Thompson and colleagues have done extensive work on the role of the cerebellum in classical conditioning of the eyeblink CR, where the UCS is a puff of air to the cornea and the CS is a tone (Thompson & Krupa, 1994). Whereas the hippocampus influences such conditioning, the key structure is the cerebellum, in particular the *interpositus nucleus,* one of the deep cerebellar nuclei. Thus, lesions of this structure disrupt conditioning of the eyeblink or, if made after learning, abolish the conditioned response (lesioned animals still show the UCR, indicating that sensory and motor processing are not hampered). The cerebellum is required for some other classically conditioned responses as well (e.g., leg withdrawal to a painful stimulus).

Some age-related changes in cerebellum have been found, most notably a loss of *Purkinje cells* of the cerebellar cortex (Duara et al., 1985; Mann, 1997; Powell et al., 1991), which send their axons to synapse on the deep cerebellar nuclei (the latter are influenced by noncerebellar neurons via the Purkinje cell route). Whereas, the evidence for Purkinje cell loss in humans is fairly reliable, this is not true of rats. Studies of two rat strains, the Fischer 344 (Dlugos & Pentney, 1994) and Wistar/Louvain (Bakalian, Corman, Delhaye-Bouchaud, & Mariani, 1991), were careful to avoid biasing pitfalls in their counting methods and observed little or no loss of Purkinje cells in old animals (the latter study used very old rats). On the other hand, more subtle histological age effects have been found in the rat, including decreased volume in the region where cerebellar granule cells and Purkinje cells synapse (Dlugos & Pentney, 1994) and a loss of dendritic spines (Pentney, 1986). Henrique, Monteiro, Rocha, and Marini-Abreu (1997) reported that the nuclei of granule cells decreased in size in old rats.

Some studies have demonstrated age effects for cerebellar neurotransmitters including Ach, GABA, dopamine, and NE (Morgan & May, 1990; Rogers & Bloom, 1985), but the findings are inconsistent and inconclusive. GABAergic inhibition of Purkinje cells is modulated by NE, and several studies have demonstrated that this modulation becomes diminished in old rats. Recent studies have shown that reduced activity of β-adrenergic receptors is particularly important; this is correlated with age-related deficits in motor learning (Bickford, 1993; Gould & Bickford, 1996; Parfitt & Bickford-Wimer, 1990).

Other studies have obtained findings suggestive of degenerative changes in aging cerebellum. Schipper, Yang, and Wang (1994) used immunocytochemistry to identify neurons in the rat brain containing *terminin*, a protein they used as a marker of cellular aging. By 18 months of age, neurons in the deep cerebellar nuclei (but not in the cerebellar cortex) were staining for terminin. By 33 months, staining in the cerebellum was more widespread. Fattoretti, Bertoni-Freddari, Caselli, Paolini, and Meier-Ruge (1996) found that the numerical density of mitochondria decreased in cerebellar neurons of old rats, suggesting that this could be associated with impaired metabolic activity. Other studies used immunostaining of tissue from old rats to demonstrate a decrease of immunoreactivity in Purkinje cells for calbindin (Amenta, Mancini, Naves, Vega, & Zaccheo, 1995) and for the expression of the cytoskeletal component *neurofilament protein*, found in axons in and around Purkinje cells (Vega, Sabbatini, Del Valle, & Amenta, 1994); both findings suggest deleterious age effects. Shimada (1994) found the cerebellar cortex to be atrophy-prone in SAM mice. In a molecular biology study, Chauhan and Siegel (1997b) found evidence suggesting that impairments in cerebellar neuronal physiology (polypeptide turnover; changes in Na,K-ATPase alpha 1- and alpha 3-mRNAs) accompanied aging. Forster and colleagues (1996) obtained evidence of oxidative molecular damage in the cerebellum of old mice; this was correlated with a loss of motor coordination.

To summarize, despite some inconsistencies, evidence of various types indicates that changes in cerebellar physiology are likely to accompany aging. Thus, a causative role of the cerebellum in age-related declines in some types of classical conditioning and other forms of learning is feasible. The most reliable finding, damage to Purkinje cells, might be sufficient to interfere with classical conditioning by virtue of their modulating influence on deep cerebellar nuclei (Powell et al., 1991).

The Basal Ganglia

The basal ganglia are important components of the motor system, and their role in motor behavior is discussed in chapter 9. However, structures in the basal ganglia, including the *caudate nucleus* and *putamen*, collectively called the *striatum*, are key elements in the dopaminergic neural circuits that influence some types of instrumental and somatomotor learning (Knowlton, Mangels, & Squire, 1996; Powell et al., 1991) and probably govern implicit memory processes (Petri & Mishkin, 1994). The striatum receives input from the *substantia nigra* (another of the basal ganglia) and from many areas of the cerebral cortex; via the ventral thalamus, they communicate with the *premotor* and *supplementary motor* cortex, which are active in advance of movements. This circuitry seems well situated to mediate implicit learning and memory such as motor skills, and basal ganglia lesions do indeed produce deficits in these abilities.

Many studies have demonstrated age effects in the basal ganglia, including receptor loss and other alterations in the dopaminergic circuits (Powell et al., 1991). This literature is discussed in chapter 9 in the context of motor behavior. The relevance of the basal ganglia in age-related deficiencies in learning and memory is not clear at present. The basal ganglia contribute to somatomotor classical conditioning (Powell et al., 1991), which becomes impaired with age. On the other hand, these brain regions are implicated in nondeclarative memory, which is typically not greatly diminished with age. Thus, it would seem that those modifications of basal ganglia circuits that do accompany aging are not having widespread impacts on implicit memory.

The Cerebral Cortex

The cerebral cortex presides over most aspects of brain functioning, including learning and memory. Not surprisingly, studies using PET have shown that many cortical regions are active during the acquisition or encoding of memory. Damage restricted to the neocortex results in specific memory deficits in young adults (Kolb & Whishaw, 1996), and injuries to various cortical regions can produce specific long-term memory deficits, such as amnesia for faces or names of objects. However, physiological changes in the cortex can also reflect altered inputs from subcortical regions involved in memory. Indeed, the circuits and structures described earlier in this chapter communicate synaptically with various cortical regions. Thus, one must consider the possibility that age changes in subcortical regions can alter cortical function, as can cortical damage per se.

The frontal lobes—the prefrontal regions in particular—are critically important for some types of mnemonic processes. According to the model of Moscovitch and Winocur (1992), the frontal lobes, in cooperation with the hippocampus, appear to be implicated in "working *with* memory," the "application of remembered events to the organization of behaviors in a current context" (p. 359). Thus, frontal lobe dysfunction would be expected to interfere with some aspects of memory. Accordingly, both patients with frontal lobe damage and healthy older people tend to have difficulty on many of the same neuropsychological tests (Moscovitch & Winocur, 1992). Both groups are challenged when it comes to forming associations between stimuli and responses and in time-related memory (e.g., remembering the order in which items were presented), in tasks where responses must be withheld for a period of time, and in recalling the source of acquired information (see Gallagher & Rapp, 1997).

All of this suggests that many of the learning and memory problems that accompany aging could result if damage were to occur in prefrontal and other cortical regions. In fact, there is considerable evidence indicating that the ability of the cerebral cortex to function normally often becomes diminished with age. PET studies have found the cortex (especially temporal and frontal cortex) to be vulnerable to age-related metabolic deficits (e.g., De Santi et al., 1995; Eustache et el., 1995; Loessner et al., 1995). Several PET studies have evaluated the relationship between brain activity and memory processes in older subjects. Cabeza and associates (1997) obtained PET data suggesting that cortical activity associated with encoding, recognition, and recall differed between young and old subjects. They observed decreases in local regional activity (especially in prefrontal and temporal-occipital regions), which they interpreted to indicate less efficient processing. Increases in activity also occurred, perhaps indicative of inadequate strategies and/or functional compensation. Other PET studies have found age differences in the loci of cortical activity during encoding (Grady et al., 1995) and recall (Schacter, Savage, Alpert, Rauch, & Albert, 1996).

Anatomical research also indicates the occurrence of age-associated changes in the cerebral cortex. MRI studies on humans have found the frontal lobes (in particular, the prefrontal region) to be especially prone to atrophy with age, with other areas also being affected, but to lesser degrees (Coffey et al., 1992; Raz et al., 1997). Many studies have employed Golgi and electron microscopic methods to look for evidence of structural changes in cortical synapses in old humans, monkeys, and rodents. Whereas some synapses and dendrites appear unchanged with age, many cortical neurons exhibit substantial abnormalities and/or loss of dendrites, dendritic spines, and presynaptic terminals (Cotman & Holets, 1985;

Mann, 1997). A quantitative study by Jacobs and colleagues (1997) found a reduction in dendritic spines of about 50% in the prefrontal cortex of older human subjects (interestingly, it appeared that most spine loss occurred by age 40, with little additional loss thereafter).

In the neurochemical literature, some, albeit not all, studies have shown decreases in the synthesis of Ach and GABA in the cerebral cortex of old animals (Rogers & Bloom, 1985). Morgan and May (1990) determined that three quarters of the studies published between 1983 and 1988 found evidence of diminished cholinergic receptors in the rodent cerebral cortex, with the best estimate being that muscarinic receptors typically declined by about 30%. A similar loss of GABA receptors (as indicated by benzodiazepine binding) may occur in the rodent cortex. The fate of other cortical neurotransmitter systems is less clear in rodents, but a few studies have indicated age changes in some of these also. Some evidence points to a role of decreased efficacy of subcortical dopaminergic systems that provide input to the prefrontal cortex (Gallagher & Rapp, 1997). Although evidence of age effects for dopaminergic subcortical systems is variable (refer to chapter 10), there is strong evidence for the occurrence of both dopamine and NE deficits in the prefrontal cortex of old primates (Arnsten, 1993, 1997). Moreover, drugs affecting dopamine and NE modify cognitive performance in old subjects (see chapter 13). Other relevant neurochemical changes may occur in the cortex as well. D'Costa, Xu, Ingram, and Sonntag (1995) found a 20% decline in *in vivo* protein synthesis in the cerebral cortex of old rats but not in the hippocampus, hypothalamus, or cerebellum.

Taking all of the research on aging cortex together, it seems clear that cortical neurons and circuits (especially in the frontal and temporal lobes) often do not function at full capacity or efficiency in elderly individuals. Older adults often experience deficits in medial temporal lobe/hippocampal type learning and memory (e.g., formation of declarative memories, spatial learning), as well as frontal type learning (e.g., temporal tasks; see West, 1996). This suggests deficits in learning and memory that accompany aging involve changes in the cerebral cortex and/or subcortical regions providing them with input.

SUMMARY AND CONCLUSIONS

A formidable amount of evidence essentially establishes correlations among (1) age, (2) deficits in learning and memory, and (3) changes in all sorts of structural and physiological properties in virtually every neural circuit known to play a role in learning and memory. It is not clear if all of this tells us everything or if it tells us nothing with respect to the neural bases of age-related declines in learning and memory. We cannot refute the following hypothesis: To varying extents (according to individual differences, genotype, species, etc.), every relevant circuit and system goes downhill with age; deficiencies in any of these are sufficient to cause some sort of learning/memory deficit. Thus, the magnitude and nature of the deficits depend on the overall constellation of neural age effects. Likewise, we cannot refute this hypothesis: Age-related deficits in learning and memory are largely restricted to the malfeasance of only a small subset of the possible systems and circuits (the remainder being of little gerontological relevance). Such is the nature of correlational data when many events covary with age.

Progress is being made, however, particularly with the growing prevalence of studies that are able to vary behavioral performance within old subject groups. At some point it may be possible, even with correlational analyses, to determine the sufficiency and necessity of changes in each system. If reliable correlations between physiology and behavior occur only for certain neural substrates, the second hypothesis can find support. However, even here, the support is soft because of the perils in interpreting null effects; that is, the failure to find an age effect in some circuit may simply be due to our looking at the wrong thing. A probable example is neuron counting, where a full complement of neurons does not necessarily imply normal function (even though a prominent loss of neurons probably does have significance).

However, it seems unlikely that the problem to be faced by neurogerontologists will be trying to interpret apparent normalcy. As more and more techniques are applied to the study of aging neural tissue, more and more subtle age effects are found. The really difficult task, then, is to determine if and how these changes interfere with neural function in general and with learning and memory in particular. This task is doable, but it will take considerable time and effort.

9
Movement and the Production of Behavior

Many of the most obvious concomitants of aging involve limitations in movements and motor behaviors—the fourth basic function of nervous systems. As people age, changes are typically observed with respect to athletic ability, gait (particularly in the very old), postural adjustments, maintenance of balance (avoiding falls), and precision of manual skills, to name a few. These difficulties are of concern because effective motor behavior is essential to the maintenance of a healthy lifestyle, performance of many jobs and hobbies, getting from place to place, avoiding hazards, and the quality of life in general.

Some motoric limitations are simply a function of muscle atrophy (Harridge & Saltin, 1996; Roos, Rice, & Vandervoort, 1997; Spirduso & MacRae, 1990). Aging is associated with a decrease in muscle mass due to a reduced number of muscle fibers and smaller size of fibers (especially for the fast type). As expected, this is accompanied by a loss of strength. For example, muscle strength (the maximum force or tension a muscle can generate in a contraction) reaches peak values during young adulthood, then begins to decline; people in their 80s can exhibit a 50% or greater loss of strength. Although everyone becomes weaker at some age, the rate and magnitude of decline are quite variable among individuals, depending on physical exercise (a potent factor), general health (e.g., arteriosclerosis may exacerbate degenerative change), and other factors. In addition, the speed of muscle contraction can slow with age, and muscles can fatigue more readily when a force is maintained.

Whereas the condition of muscles accounts for some deterioration of motor behaviors, the most important and interesting stories are found in the workings of the nervous system, with several neurogerontological subplots: The slowing down of motor behaviors, altered posture, balance, and gait, and poorer motor performance are prominent problems. These changes undoubtedly involve suboptimal functioning of neural circuits on two levels: the control of muscle fiber contraction by motor neurons in the spinal cord and the control of the motor neurons by central motor systems. Diseases that affect the motor systems of older people, notably Parkinson's and Huntington's, provide sorrowful examples of central motor dysfunction taken to extremes.

BEHAVIORAL CHANGES

Slowing Down

Many aspects of motor behavior proceed more slowly as people get older. Indeed, the slowing of behavior in general is considered by many gerontologists to be a ubiquitous, fundamental property of aging, even in the healthiest of individuals (e.g., Birren & Fisher, 1995; Birren, Woods, & Williams, 1980; Salthouse, 1985; Woodruff-Pak, 1988). Slowing of motor responses can result from an increase in response initiation time (reaction time), an increase in the duration of movements, and/or a reduced capacity for decelerating movements. The duration of movements, once initiated, often increase by 15% to 30% in older people; the more difficult the movement, the greater the slowing. However, inherent in the slowing down is a speed-accuracy tradeoff, whereby slower movements are performed more accurately (Seidler & Stelmach, 1996).

Much of the research on behavioral speed has focused on what might be called *psychomotor responses*, motor behavior in which a rapid response is made with one or more limbs or digits. A well-studied parameter is *reaction time*, how long it takes to execute a behavior in response to a triggering stimulus. Research studies have shown that reaction time is often slowed by 15% to 30% in older subjects. Both central (premotor) and peripheral (motor time) factors contribute to slowing. However, the greater contribution typically comes from the premotor component (stimulus identification and processing, response selection, and response programming). The central, premotor phase can be especially taxed if an older subject is asked to maintain preparation for a movement before executing it (e.g., wait for several seconds), if the stimulus-response relationship is not simple, if a number of possible response choices are available, and/or if a prepared response must be changed (Seidler & Stelmach, 1996). These variables presumably have little differential effect on the peripheral components of the response (e.g., contraction of muscles).

Reaction time and other aspects of central motor processing have been studied primarily by cognitive psychologists. From an information-processing perspective, the behavior can be viewed as being controlled by a sequence of central processes: stimulus perception, encoding and memory functions, decision making, motor programming, and initiation/execution of the movements (Spirduso & MacRae, 1990). Because these processes involve the integration of a variety of neural systems, motor speed is discussed in more detail in chapter 11. For now, it is sufficient to appreciate that the slowing of central motor processing is a robust aspect of aging.

Control of Posture, Balance, and Gait

A number of age-related problems arise with respect to balance and posture (Horak et al., 1989; Simoneau & Leibowitz, 1996). Falls are more likely to occur because of weakening of muscles, reduced ability of CNS motor systems, and sensory mistakes in posture control or navigating the environment. Older individuals exhibit more sway when standing quietly with eyes either open or closed. Balance and postural deficits may contribute to increased risk of falling (although many falls result from slips or tripping, rather than a loss of static balance). Older people may exhibit altered responses when the upright stance is altered (Gu, Schultz, Shepard, & Alexander, 1996). Although balance problems may appear earlier in men as they age, both sexes exhibit progressive declines sometimes beginning in middle age (Balogun, Akindele, Nihinlola, & Marzouk, 1994).

Gait exhibits progressive change, starting around the sixth decade of life for some (Adams, 1984; Murray, Kory, & Clarkson, 1969; Simoneau & Leibowitz, 1996). In elderly people, walking slows, steps get shorter and more flat-footed, and the legs are placed farther apart—an overall pattern that attempts to improve stability. Slower gait speed and other changes tend to occur even when diseases or physical impairments are controlled for (Winter & Eng, 1995; Woo, Ho, Lau, Chan, & Yuen, 1995). Moreover, it becomes more difficult to control compensatory stepping movements (Maki & McIlroy, 1996; McIlroy & Maki, 1996). Relevant factors include muscle weakness, changes in central motor control, orthopedic problems, and fear of falling. The various problems with balance, posture, and gait may place greater demands on attention as well (Lajoie, Teasdale, Bard, & Fleury, 1996).

Although we focus on the motor systems in this chapter, the essential importance of the sensory systems in regulating balance, posture, and gait must always be taken into account. The vestibular system is required to monitor motion and the position of the head in space; the system is also integral to the vestibulo-ocular reflex, which coordinates eye movements to maintain a stable image on the retina when the head and body are moving. The visual system is needed for proper orientation in space (the location of environmental features with respect to the body) and, of course, navigating through hazards, impediments, and other relevant features of the environment. The somatosensory system provides information about the body such as joint position, muscle activity, and touch/pressure (especially in the feet). The evidence presented in chapter 7 makes it clear that aging is accompanied by diminished capacity in each of these sensory modalities. Thus, the sensory components of postural control systems may be compromised.

As outlined by Horak and colleagues (1989), postural control can be viewed as having several functional motor components that interact with the sensory systems. These include biomechanics, latency to achieve postural responses, coordination of postural movement patterns, scaling the postural response to the stimulus, and motor learning. One or more of these functions are often subpar even in healthy elderly people. The central motor systems regulate each of these components, with the exception of biomechanics (although even here, secondary effects of neural degeneration on the muscles might occur). Clearly, the neurogerontological investigations of the central motor systems are important to understand changes in posture, balance, and gait.

The Properties of Movements

Everyday motor behavior is comprised of different types of movements. Reflexive movements are consistent, automatic responses to stimuli; they are more or less involuntary, but some control is often possible (e.g., swallowing is a reflex but can be controlled to some extent). Ballistic movements are those that, once launched, cannot be corrected; the direction, distance, and magnitude of the movement must be computed by central neural processes prior to the movement. By contrast, guided movements are those that can be adjusted as they are carried out. The control of these types of movements can decline with age (Seidler & Stelmach, 1996). For example, when aiming a movement, there is an accelerating phase and a decelerating phase (homing in on the target, using both sensory information and motor control). Older people spend a greater relative portion of the movement in the decelerating phase. They have a shorter initial ballistic movement toward the target as well. Movements also tend to become more variable as people age, with more ongoing modifications and greater reliance on feedback and visual guidance. Age effects are observed for reach-to-grasp movements, which entail a sequence of alternating agonist and antagonist muscle activity (muscles moving joints in opposite directions). The antagonist activity becomes impaired, and excessive grip forces are often employed. Older people do improve their motor performance with practice (e.g., increasing speed and reducing variability) but usually have a hard time reaching the same level as young adults.

A variety of movement abnormalities may appear in elderly people, most typically in conjunction with neurological conditions in the CNS (see Klawans & Tanner, 1984). *Postural tremor* describes abnormal rhythmic movement of the upper extremities when maintaining posture against gravity and performing tasks such as writing. *Intention tremor* refers to rhythmic involuntary movements superimposed on purposeful action. *Rest tremor* is characteristic of parkinsonism (see below); it disappears when purposeful movement is engaged. There may also be abnormalities of muscle tone, the resistance present in resting muscle. These may take the form of increased tone or rigidity (associated with damage to the basal ganglia), spasticity (associated with the pyramidal tract damage), Gegenhalten (increased resistance to passive movements associated with frontal lobe pathology), and diminished muscle tone (associated with some forms of cerebellar and basal ganglia damage).

The various changes and abnormalities in motor behavior suggest that the motor systems of the CNS are not able to perform so well as individuals age. As we are about to see, there is ample evidence that this is the case for virtually all of the neural structures and circuits that control movements. To review the literature, we will address separately how muscle contractions are controlled and discuss each of the major CNS components of the motor systems, the spinal cord, motor cortical areas, the cerebellum, and basal ganglia. It is, of course, the cooperative interactions of neural circuits in these and other parts of the nervous system that serve to plan, shape, and execute movements appropriate to the behavioral context and goals.

Control of Muscle Fiber Contraction by Motor Neurons

The contraction of muscle fibers is controlled by *motor neurons*. The cell bodies of motor neurons are located in the CNS (the *alpha* motor neurons in the *ventral horn* of the spinal cord and cranial nerve motor neurons of the brainstem). Their axons leave the CNS, make their way to the appropriate muscles, branch, and form specialized cholinergic synapses (the *neuromuscular junction*) at the postsynaptic end plates of striated (skeletal) muscle fibers. Each muscle fiber is innervated by only one motor neuron, although each motor neuron innervates several muscle fibers, via its axonal branches. The synapses controlling the muscles are excitatory only; unlike synapses on CNS neurons, muscle fibers cannot be directly inhibited at the neuromuscular junction. The contractions evoked by motor neuron synapses are brief because the enzyme acetylcholinesterase (AchE), present at the junction, inactivates Ach to end the contraction. Thus, for precise motor function to continue as aging ensues, an appropriate balance between the actions of Ach and AchE must be maintained: Too much AchE or a deficit in Ach will interfere with contraction; too little AchE will prolong contractions. Figure 9.1 provides an overview.

Motor Units

A single motor neuron and all the muscle fibers it controls is called a *motor unit*; action potentials in a motor neuron cause all of its muscle fibers to contract together (see Figure 9.1). Therefore, precise movements, such as those of the hand, require motor units with a low innervation ratio (e.g., each motor neurons innervates only a few muscle fibers), whereas motor units controlling gross movements, such as those used to maintain posture, have high innervation ratios (> 2000 muscle fibers per motor neuron).

All movement involves activation of motor units in various combinations, but they are essentially slave units. The selection of motor neurons

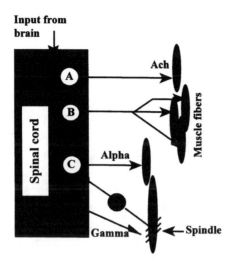

FIGURE 9.1 Schematic of motor units. Alpha motor neurons (A, B, C) in the spinal cord and brainstem send their axons out of the CNS to synapse with the muscles, using Ach as the neurotransmitter. The motor neurons can be controlled by descending input from the brain. Some motor units (A) have a low innervation ratio, synapsing with a small number of muscle fibers, whereas others (B) have a large ratio, innervating many muscle fibers. Thus, firing of motor neuron A contracts only one muscle fiber (allowing for precise control), whereas motor neuron B contracts several at once (poor precision). The spindle organ is shown for motor unit C. When the muscle stretches (relaxes), the spindle fires action potentials to the spinal cord via an afferent neuron (S), which re-excites motor neuron C to maintain muscle tone. The gamma motor neuron can modify this process by controlling the intrafusal muscle fiber of the spindle organ.

to be brought into play and the temporal sequencing of their activation are under the control of synapses from other neurons in the CNS, as discussed below. The force of muscle contractions can be controlled by the CNS in two ways: by varying the firing rate of motor neuron action potentials and by altering the number of motor units activated at a particular time (recruitment). In addition to their innervation ratios, motor units differ with respect to speed and fatigability of their muscle fibers and size of the motor neuron soma. Thus, there are *fast fatigable* motor units (they generate great force but cannot sustain repeated activation; the motor neurons are large), *slow fatigue-resistant* motor units (they take longer to contract; the motor neurons are small), and *fast fatigue-resistant* motor units (intermediate between the other two). The smallest motor neurons, and therefore the slower motor units, are most readily recruited by descending CNS inputs. One consequence of this size principle is that larger motor units are activated less frequently.

Motor units are likely to undergo a variety of age-related changes (reviewed by Galea, 1996; Larsson & Ansved, 1995; Mikiten, 1981; Roos et al., 1997; Spencer & Ochoa, 1981). Various studies have demonstrated some loss of motor neurons with age, although the occurrence of motor neuron loss seems to vary across species and muscles innervated. In our own species, motor neurons become fewer in number, with losses estimated as high as 1% per year beginning as early as the third decade of life and accelerating after age 60. Some motor neurons are more susceptible to attrition than others, with large motor neurons being generally most vulnerable. Regional differences can occur as well. For example, in a study of mice, a significant loss of neurons was observed in the motor nucleus of the facial nerve but not in motor nuclei of the trigeminal nerve (Sturrock, 1996).

Motor neuron loss results not only in fewer motor units but also in other modifications (Larsson & Ansved, 1995; Roos et al., 1997). *Motor unit remodeling* refers to the natural cycle of turnover of synaptic connections at the neuromuscular junction. Some degeneration occurs, and this is followed by sprouting of new axon branches and reinnervation of the muscle. Reinnervation continues to occur in older motor units, although there may be diminished sprouting (Kanda & Hashizume, 1991). There is some evidence that, in older individuals, fast muscle fibers are preferentially denervated, and they are then reinnervated by sprouts from axons from slow motor units. This may result in alteration of the fast motor units, transforming them into slow units (Roos et al., 1997). As remodeling continues during aging, the balance may shift away from sprouting/regeneration toward denervation, although the probable occurrence of compensatory changes can make it difficult to interpret the functional significance of the age-related changes. Indeed, some of the conflicting findings in the literature may reflect both degenerative and compensatory processes going on to greater or lesser extents. In any event, as motor neurons are lost during aging, the denervation-reinnervation process results in larger innervation ratios (with exceptions according to muscles, spinal cord regions, and other factors). This can produce increased amplitude and other modifications in the electrophysiological responses of motor units.

Changes in myelin of motor neuron axons and slowing of action potential conduction velocity have also been found by various studies. Under some force level conditions, the discharge rate of motor units decreases and variability increases with age (Roos et al., 1997).

It is quite evident that changes in the motor units are likely to contribute to slowing, altered grip force control during fine motor tasks, the greater variability in force, and other movement-related deficits.

The Neuromuscular Junction

The neuromuscular junctions undergo continual growth and degeneration in normal muscles of healthy adults. This process continues into old age, but there are age effects. Depending on the species and/or muscles, these can include decreased number but increased length of motor neuron terminals, increased or decreased number of presynaptic vesicles and Ach receptors per junction (the direction of change depending on various factors), decreased Ach in terminals, increased length and complexity of end plates, ultrastructural signs suggestive of altered vesicle turnover, decreased rate of spontaneous Ach release, decreased levels of AchE and choline acetyltranferase (an enzyme involved in making Ach), and changes in the properties of synaptic potentials (Larsson & Ansved, 1995). In some respects, changes in the aging neuromuscular junction resemble those occurring when muscles are partially denervated by damage to motor neuron axons (Rosenheimer, 1990).

Balice-Gordon (1997) described a series of gerontological studies on neuromuscular innervation in mice. She observed a loss of motor axon terminals and underlying Ach receptor-rich areas. During middle age, some junctions appeared to compensate with axonal sprouting and the addition of new synaptic sites; however in old mice, this compensatory processes decreased greatly, and many of the new synaptic sites disappeared within a few weeks. Ultimately, old mice exhibited significant losses of pre- and postsynaptic sites, and physiological activation of synapses failed frequently. These changes likely resulted from an interaction between presynaptic degenerative changes in the motor neurons and reduced sprouting ability, postsynaptic atrophy of the muscle fibers, and/or possible changes in the Schwann cells, which provide myelin and other support for the motor neurons (see chapter 3). Trophic factors associated with all three cell types probably play an important role in all of this as well.

In summary, modifications of the neuromuscular junction occur with age and undoubtedly contribute to the movement difficulties that tend to accompany aging. The exact nature and significance of the various reported synaptic age effects and their functional significance remain to be clarified. The mutual influences among dynamic changes occurring in neuromuscular junctions, muscles, and motor neurons, as well as regional and species differences, add to the complexity of the age-related changes.

The Muscle Spindle Stretch Reflex

The stretch reflex is initiated by the *muscle spindle organs*, whose sensory receptors are triggered by stretching of the muscle. Action potentials generated by this activity are relayed to the spinal cord and synaptically excite the alpha motor neurons controlling the stretched muscles, resulting in an automatic reflex contraction. When the muscle contracts, stretch of the spindle decreases, and its afferent discharges likewise decrease, quieting the reflex. This feedback loop keeps the muscle contractions adjusted and maintains muscle tone. The muscle spindles are also under efferent control by the CNS. The spindles are wrapped around modified (*intrafusal*) muscle fibers, which normally stretch along with the skeletal muscle fibers. However, the intrafusal fibers can be made to contract independently by small *gamma motor neurons* in the spinal cord. Contraction of the intrafusal muscle fibers alters the amount of stretch to which the spindles are subjected, particularly when the muscles are contracted, and modifies the stretch reflex.

Age-related changes in the muscle spindle system, while potentially important, have not been well studied. An anatomical investigation of human muscle spindles showed age-related increase in the thickness of the spindle capsule due to increased collagen, as well as slightly fewer intrafusal muscle fibers per spindle and other signs of pathology (Swash & Fox, 1972). In one physiological study of aging rats, Miwa, Miwa, and Kanda (1995) obtained evidence that the conduction velocity became slower in the afferent axons from spindle organs to motor neurons. However, evidence that the stretch reflex becomes significantly slower in aging humans is not strong, and the literature is equivocal (for references see Hart, 1986; Miwa et al., 1995; Wolfarth et al., 1997). Indeed, Hart (1986) found that older people actually had faster reflex times, a finding attributed to their shorter stature compared to the young subjects; for smaller people, the distance action potentials have to travel to and from the muscle is shorter.

There is some evidence that the sensitivity of the spindles declines with age. In a neurophysiological experiment on old rats, the sensitivity of the muscle spindles appeared to have lessened, in that the peak frequency of neural firing during dynamic stretch was lower than that seen in middle age (Miwa et al., 1995). In a study of humans, Corden and Lippold (1996) also obtained electrophysiological data indicating that the spindles became less sensitive with age. This loss of sensitivity was evident in middle-aged subjects.

CONTROL OF MOTOR NEURONS BY THE CENTRAL NERVOUS SYSTEM

Movement is an extremely difficult endeavor. One must continuously plan ahead from moment to moment, make adjustments constantly using sensory information and feedback from ongoing movements as conditions change, and coordinate many muscles, limbs, and balance. Not surprisingly, a great proportion of the nervous system is devoted to movement—deciding what to do, planning how to do it, and carrying it out by controlling the activity of thousands of motor units. The main components and connections of the central motor systems are shown in Figure 9.2.

The Spinal Cord

Axons descending from the brain to control the activity of the motor neurons travel through several fiber tracts within the spinal cord. The motor neurons in the ventral horn of the spinal cord are controlled by two major sources of descending synaptic input. Axons arising from neurons in the motor cortex, discussed in the following section, directly control the firing of motor units. The *bulbospinal pathway* (medulla oblongata-to-spinal cord) originating from neurons in the raphe nuclei, also influences motor neurons. The raphe system is serotonergic and is thought to modulate both sensory input and motor neuron excitability (the system has ascending pathways as well, as discussed in chapter 10). Johnson and

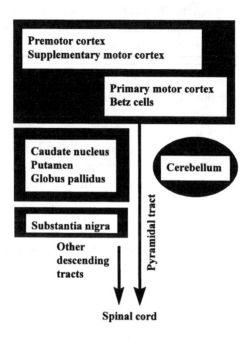

FIGURE 9.2   Main components of the central motor systems. Because the circuits and interconnections are complex, they are not shown here. Several key cortical areas exert control and planning of neural commands. The subcortical basal ganglia structures (caudate nucleus, putamen, globus pallidus, substantia nigra) interact to modify and regulate various aspects of movement, as does the cerebellum. Ultimately, commands descend the spinal cord by the pyramidal and other tracts to control the motor units.

colleagues (1993) evaluated this bulbospinal system in young and old rats. They observed a decrease in the number of normal-looking serotonergic axons especially in the lower (lumbosacral) spinal cord. Signs of degenerating axons were present in this region as well. Changes in neuropeptides associated with the raphe system, substance P and thyrotropin-releasing hormone (which might exert a trophic function on motor neurons), were also observed in the old rats. Assuming that the bulbospinal system normally facilitates motor neuron activity, degeneration of this system would be expected to contribute to age-related motor deficits. Thus, it is of interest that behaviorally, the motor disturbances present in the old rats in this study primarily involved the hind limbs, which are innervated by the lumbosacral motor neurons.

The spinal cord does more than relay motor commands from the brain to the motor neurons. It has a number of neural circuits that support organized movement sequences such as walking, scratching, and sexual reflexes. Although capable of these activities, the neural circuits are generally modulated by the brain. Importantly, various reflexes are inhibited by descending neural pathways, and removal of inhibition by brain damage unleashes these reflexes. For example, the Babinski reflex (stroke sole of foot causes extension of big toe and spread of toes) occurs in infants, but the neural circuitry becomes inhibited in adults; the reappearance of this reflex is a neurological indicator of brain damage. Given that various age effects are observed in the brain, altered descending modulation of spinal cord reflex circuits is a potential neurogerontological concern.

The Motor Cortical Areas

Several regions of the cerebral cortex participate directly in the generation and control of movements. The *primary motor cortex* is the major source of descending axons to the motor neurons. The *pyramidal tract* is the key pathway followed by motor neuron axons as they make their way to control the motor neurons. The motor cortex is topographically organized; a systematic map of the body exists for the location of neurons with respect to the surface of motor cortex and the contralateral body parts they control. The force and direction of movements are encoded by the activity of populations of neurons in this cortical area. Neurons in the primary motor cortex also receive sensory feedback, important for the precise manipulation of objects and other guided movements. The *premotor cortex* and *supplementary motor cortex* are adjacent to the motor cortex, in the frontal lobe. They also have a topographic organization and relay input to both the primary motor cortex and subcortical areas. Premotor cortical neurons are active during preparation for movement, and supplementary motor neurons participate in the planning of complex sequences of movements.

Several studies have described age-related histological changes in *Betz cells*, the large neurons of the primary motor cortex. Using Golgi staining of human tissue, Scheibel and colleagues (Scheibel, 1996; Scheibel et al., 1975; Scheibel, Tomiyasu, & Scheibel, 1977) observed irregular swellings of the somata and large dendrites and a progressive loss of dendritic spines in Betz cells of older brains. Many dendrites appeared to die back, with the smallest twigs being affected earliest; ultimately the large dendritic trunks and soma degenerated as well. Fewer synapses (especially excitatory synapses on dendritic spines) were observed by Adams (1987) in motor cortex of older humans. Tigges, Herndon, and Peters (1990, 1992) performed light- and electron-microscopic examinations on the primary motor cortex of rhesus monkeys. Many Betz cells of old monkeys had pronounced accumulations of lipofuscin, and a small amount of shrinkage occurred. However, in contrast to the findings on humans, no age-related loss of Betz cells or other neurons was observed. There were also no significant age effects with respect to the number of synaptic terminals, their size, or the number of mitochondria they contained. However, degeneration of axons and other signs of pathology in and around the Betz cells were observed in the primary motor cortex of old monkeys.

To summarize, the primary motor cortex of primates does appear to undergo age-related change, whether a loss of Betz cells (as occurs in humans) or the development of other abnormalities irrespective of cell loss. Because the motor neurons play a critical role in descending control of the motor units, it is plausible that these sorts of central changes contribute importantly to movement deficits that accompany aging.

A neurophysiological study of single units in the forelimb regions of the motor cortex of aging rabbits was conducted by Mednikova and Kopytova (1994). Motor cortex neurons of old rabbits exhibited a lower level of spontaneous action potential discharges. When the contralateral forelimb was moved, the firing rate seen in youthful cortical neurons was reduced by half in old rabbits. When the limb was repeatedly stimulated electrically, many neurons of young but not old animals increased their firing rates. These results suggest a general decrease in the excitability of motor cortex neurons in old rabbits. Interestingly, the initiation of movements and reaction times appear to depend on the achievement of an adequate level of activation of motor neurons (Hanes & Schall, 1996). This suggests that reduced excitability of aged motor neurons could be responsible for some geriatric motor deficits.

Several brain waves or voltage shifts can be measured from motor cortical areas about 1 second or less before movements are made. These are thought to represent preparatory processes leading up to the initiation of movement, presumably involving the activity of the supplementary and premotor cortex. Singh, Knight, Woods, Beckley, and Clayworth

(1990) measured these movement-related potentials in young and older human subjects. Neither the topographical distribution of responses, the onset latency, nor the mean amplitude differed as a function of age. This study, then, found no evidence of age-related deficits in presumed electrophysiological correlates of motor programming. However, the researchers noted that evidence of age effects had been reported by earlier studies. At this time, the occurrence or nature of age effects in premotor and supplementary motor cortex remain unclear.

The Cerebellum

Damage to the cerebellum disturbs balance, posture, gait, and the adjustment and coordination of movements, including sequences requiring aiming, timing, and/or accuracy and behaviors in which related movements must work together. As discussed earlier, these are motoric behaviors that exhibit deficits in older people. The cerebellum does not directly control motor units, but interacts with other regions of the motor systems, including premotor and motor cortex, brainstem, and spinal cord. Information about the environment and head/eye/body position, needed to carry out its functions, is received from the relevant sensory systems.

The types of age-related changes that have been observed in the Purkinje cells and other neurons of the cerebellum were discussed in chapter 8. These include histological signs such as a loss of dendrites and spines and changes in neurotransmitter systems. It is not yet possible to definitively relate specific changes in cerebellar physiology to the motor and balance deficits that accompany aging. However, the ample evidence of age effects for both the cerebellum and the motor behaviors it mediates certainly implies a causative relationship.

The Basal Ganglia

The basal ganglia are synaptically interconnected subcortical structures of the forebrain: the substantia nigra, subthalamic nucleus, globus pallidus, caudate nucleus, and putamen (the latter two are lumped together as the striatum or neostriatum). The basal ganglia receive input from diverse regions of the cerebral cortex and from the thalamus. Their action potential output is sent back to premotor and motor cortices and the nonmotor prefrontal cortex via circuits that include the thalamus. The basal ganglia also communicate with the superior colliculus in the midbrain, which controls reflexive eye movements. They seem to be involved in the planning and organization of self-initiated, complex movements, the control of postural adjustments, and other aspects of motor behavior and are very important for motor learning. The basal ganglia may carry out their duties by selecting certain movements while inhibiting others. They are also important in cognitive functions, as suggested by their connections with frontal and other cortical areas. Damage to the basal ganglia results in various disruptions of motor behavior, as evidenced by the motor symptoms of Parkinson's and Huntington's diseases, disorders affecting the basal ganglia discussed below. The consequences of less severe basal ganglia damage as might occur during normal aging are not clear.

Aging of neurotransmitter systems in the basal ganglia (the striatum in particular) has been extensively studied in rodents. Many experiments have shown age-related declines in synthesis, receptor number, functional activity, and other aspects of the cholinergic and dopaminergic systems (Morgan & May, 1990; Rogers & Bloom, 1985). As is always the case, some studies have not found age effects for Ach or dopamine, but the majority of studies indicate that, by and large, these systems tend to decline functionally with age in rats and mice. Whereas fewer studies have evaluated dopamine and the striatum in healthy human subjects, the majority indicate a reduction in dopamine content and decrease in various markers of dopaminergic activity (DeKosky & Palmer, 1994). Several PET and SPECT studies have shown that *dopamine transporters* (membrane proteins that move dopamine into neurons, e.g., for reuptake) are diminished in healthy older people (Bannon & Whitty, 1997; Tissingh et al., 1997; Volkow et al., 1996), another indication of age-related change in this system. The gerontological story is less clear for other neurotransmitter systems that participate in basal ganglia circuits of rodents and humans.

In contrast to the abundance of neurochemical research, relatively few neuroanatomical studies have focused on the basal ganglia in the context of aging. As expected, the available studies differ in their findings. Some researchers have found cell loss in human substantia nigra or putamen, whereas others have not (see Mann, 1997). A thorough study of the substantia nigra was performed by Fearnley and Lees (1991). In normal subjects, a linear 4.8% per decade loss of pigmented neurons was observed in the caudal region of the substantia nigra, and there were regional differences in the severity of loss. This degree of neuronal loss was much less than that necessary to produce symptoms of Parkinson's disease, however (see below).

An age-related loss of neurons staining for AchE in rats was reported by Altavista, Bentivoglio, Crociani, Rossi, and Albanese (1988), whereas Tatton, Greenwood, Salo, and Seniuk (1991) saw a 68% loss of immunolabeled dopaminergic nigrostriatal neurons in aging mice (interestingly, the synthesis of dopamine increased even as neurons became fewer). Levine and colleagues (1986) observed a decrease in the length of dendrites and reduced density of dendritic spines on medium-sized neurons in the caudate nucleus of old cats, which accelerated after age 15 years. Similar findings were obtained in mice by McNeill, Koek, Brown, and Rafols (1990), but only for a subpopulation of old animals that exhibited motor deficits.

Levine, Lloyd, Hull, Fisher, and Buchwald (1987) obtained extracellular recordings of neural activity from neurons in the caudate nucleus of aging cats. Their main finding was that neurons from old cats exhibited reduced excitability in response to electrical stimulation of inputs from the cortex or substantia nigra. The neurons of old cats could not respond as well to repeated stimulation either. The same group of researchers also obtained intracellular recordings from striatal neurons of rats (Cepeda, Lee, Buchwald, Radisavljevic, & Levine, 1992; Cepeda et al., 1989). Here, too, there were indications of reduced excitability, and it was more difficult to evoke excitatory postsynaptic responses in many but not all neurons from old rats. Findings from these studies also suggested that inhibitory responses were not as greatly altered with age.

Ou, Buckwalter, McNeill, and Walsh (1997) used a paired-pulse stimulation paradigm to study age-related changes in the physiological properties of neurons in slice preparations obtained from rats. In the paired-pulse paradigm, the neural responses of striatal neurons evoked by an electrical stimulus pulse are facilitated when paired with a preceding pulse. This facilitation was attenuated in striatal tissue from old rats. The experimenters presented evidence suggesting that the reduced facilitation was not due to changes in inhibitory GABAergic interneurons, but resulted from a diminution of synaptic excitation. This was also associated with a loss of dendritic spines, a site of excitatory synapses. It appears that the release of excitatory neurotransmitters was reduced in the old rats, probably because of a calcium-related mechanism (recall that the entry of Ca^{++} is required for the release of neurotransmitters at synapses) and/

or a diminished pool of presynaptic vesicles capable of releasing their neurotransmitter contents. In any event, the physiological processing of successive inputs was altered in old rats.

To summarize, there is a large body of evidence that cholinergic and dopaminergic systems are likely to become somewhat altered in the aging striatum of rodents and humans. However, this research is not without disparities, and the consistency and extent to which humans and other species exhibit age effects is unknown. The relatively small amount of histological and physiological research does not add much insight, although it does seem to be the case that excitability of striatal neurons decreases in older animals.

PARKINSON'S AND HUNTINGTON'S DISEASES

Parkinson's and Huntington's diseases are not necessarily linked to aging and can strike people well before old age. These diseases are, however, most prevalent in older people. Both diseases attack the basal ganglia and have dramatic effects on movement. Whereas cognitive and psychiatric symptoms often occur as well, the motor deficits are ubiquitous and definitive for both disorders. Therefore, it is appropriate to discuss these diseases here.

Parkinson's Disease

Parkinson's disease is a neurological disorder affecting about 1% of people over the age of 60 in the United States and has been the focus of considerable neurological and other medical research (Feldman, Meyer, & Quenzer, 1997; Klawans & Tanner, 1984). It can be first noticed during the mid-50s but often emerges after age 65. The classic symptoms are motoric: resting tremor, increased muscle tone (rigidity), and difficulty initiating voluntary movements (bradykinesia). The motor aspects of speech are often affected also. Cognitive and emotional symptoms of Parkinson's disease often occur (Bondi & Troster, 1997). These can include depression, memory impairment (especially for recall rather than recognition), visual-spatial perception, and frontal executive behavior (the basal ganglia communicate with the frontal lobes via the thalamus; see chapter 11 for a discussion of frontal lobe function). The prevalence of cases where the severity of cognitive decline rises to the level of dementia is about 20% to 40% of Parkinson's patients.

Other disorders affecting the striatum (not necessarily restricted to older people) can result in similar symptoms. The term *parkinsonism* includes these in addition to Parkinson's disease proper (Bondi & Troster, 1997). Parkinsonism can result from encephalitis, toxic drugs (e.g., the drug MPTP), and other causes.

Parkinson's disease involves the progressive dysfunction and loss of neurons by which the substantia nigra and striatum communicate, the nigrostriatal system (see reviews by Bondi & Troster, 1997; Ebadi et al., 1996; Fearnley & Lees, 1991). Specifically, the dopaminergic pigmented cells in the *pars compacta* region of the substantia nigra are severely impacted. Neuron death may occur rapidly (a time course of less than 5 years) and exponentially, but a relatively high degree of nigral cell loss (> 50%) and reduction in striatal dopamine (80%, which is much of the brain's dopamine) are required for the development of significant Parkinson's symptoms (Fearnley & Lees, 1991; Marsden, 1990). The persistence of normal function in the face of neuronal degeneration suggests that compensatory processes can overcome the deficits up to a point (e.g., increased dopamine turnover, up-regulation of postsynaptic receptors).

Other neurotransmitter systems and brain regions are involved as well. These include the nucleus basalis of Meynert, dorsal vagal nucleus, and noradrenergic neurons of the *locus coeruleus* and serotonergic neurons of the raphe nuclei in the brainstem, both of which have widespread projections throughout the brain (see chapter 10). A characteristic pathology associated with Parkinson's disease is the occurrence of Lewy bodies (chapter 3) in the pigmented neurons of the substantia nigra and locus coeruleus.

The causes of Parkinson's disease remain poorly understood. Risk factors include exposure to environmental toxins (e.g., pesticides and herbicides) and advanced age, although the pathological progression of Parkinson's disease is not reminiscent of "accelerated aging" (Fearnley & Lees, 1991). A family history of neurological disease is another risk factor, although specific genes seem to play only a limited role in the disease (Bondi & Troster, 1997). A good body of evidence has implicated cellular damage due to free radical oxidative damage as a mechanism of neural damage in Parkinson's disease (Ebadi et al., 1996).

Parkinson's disease is treated in several ways that are designed to replenish the depleted levels and activity of dopamine. The drug L-dopa has been used for some time and continues to be administered to Parkinson's patients. Dopamine itself cannot be used as a drug because it does not penetrate the blood-brain barrier. However, its precursor, L-dopa, does pass through the barrier and is converted to dopamine in the brain, restoring dopamine levels that were reduced by neuronal degeneration. Other drugs affecting dopamine levels and/or oxidative damage have been developed as well. Monoamine oxidase B (MAO-B) breaks down dopamine at synapses and may become more active with age, attenuating dopamine activity. The drug selegiline (deprenyl) is an inhibitor of MAO-B and therefore increases dopamine levels. Selegiline facilitates the activity of nigrostriatal dopaminergic neurons and slows the progressive damage to striatal neurons and Parkinson's symptoms (Ebadi et al., 1996). Additional promising treatments are surgical transplantation of dopamine-producing tissue (see chapter 13), surgical alteration or stimulation of the thalamus or globus pallidus, and use of gene therapy (Choi-Lundberg et al., 1997). Although undesirable side effects may result from some of these treatments (particularly L-dopa), they are often very effective in reversing symptoms—a far cry from our inability to ameliorate Alzheimer's and other neurodegenerative diseases.

Huntington's Disease

Huntington's disease is the second major motor disorder that largely affects older people (see Bylsma, 1997; J. B. Martin, 1996, for reviews). The disease typically reveals itself during middle age, producing both motor and cognitive deficits. Motor symptoms include slow, clumsy, jerky, rigid, uncontrolled, involuntary movements (chorea). Huntington's patients have difficulty tracking slowly moving targets with their eyes, and their saccadic eye movements are slow and imprecise. Motor impairments of speech are common. Cognitive disturbances include slow thinking, memory impairment, motor skill learning, difficulty mentally manipulating acquired information, planning, and organizing—deficits typically associated with damage to the frontal lobes (as is the case for Parkinson's disease, these are presumed to reflect the interrelationship between frontal cortex and striatum). Depression and a variety of other psychiatric symptoms frequently occur as well.

The histopathology associated with Huntington's disease has been well described (see Bylsma, 1997). The caudate nucleus and putamen are primarily affected. Spiny neurons in the head of the caudate nucleus are among the earliest to be lost. The frontal cortex also exhibits degenerative changes, although it is unclear if these are primary aspects of the disease or secondary effects of the loss of synaptic input from the striatum. These pathological changes presumably account for motor and cognitive disturbances that are characteristic of this disease.

Huntington's disease is inherited as an autosomal dominant trait; hence, offspring of affected parents have a 50% chance of inheriting the disorder. Carriers of the gene can now be identified by modern genetic tests.

The leading hypothesis to explain cell damage in Huntington's disease implicates excitotoxicity associated with glutamatergic synapses (see chapter 3 for a discussion of excitotoxicity). As reviewed by Bylsma (1997), there are presently no effective treatments to prevent or slow the progression of Huntington's disease. Attempts to counteract excitotoxic damage (e.g., by blocking glutamate synapses) have thus far been disappointing. However, motor and psychiatric symptoms can be treated. Behavioral manipulations of body position and providing a nonstressful environment have been used to control motor symptoms, whereas pharmacological interventions have proven to be of limited value. Standard drugs are used to treat psychiatric symptoms.

SUMMARY AND CONCLUSIONS

Motor deficits of one type or another abound in older adults. Fortunately, the ever-present variability among individuals means that many older people do quite well. Moreover, the growing appreciation that motor performance can be maintained and improved with exercise, physical activity, and other lifestyle factors (see chapter 13) may change the epidemiological landscape with respect to geriatric motor deficits. Whereas much of the achievable improvement involves making the muscles work better, it remains to be seen if effective strategies can be developed to ameliorate the operation of central motor systems. Such strategies often work well for Parkinson's disease.

The overall amount of neurogerontological research addressing motor systems is somewhat disappointing. The many studies on neurotransmission in the rodent striatum can only take us so far, and much of this research has not addressed motor behavior at all; rather, the striatum has been used as a convenient and familiar neurogerontological model (this is not a bad thing, just a limitation in the context of motor research). Of more direct relevance to understanding movement deficits are physiological studies of the motor cortex, basal ganglia, cerebellum, and spinal cord. The few studies done thus far have provided very interesting findings, as discussed earlier. Neurophysiological studies of movement, especially postural adjustments, gait, and other dynamic motor behaviors, are challenging because it is technically difficult to have an animal move while obtaining electrophysiological recordings from its brain. The same can be said of brain-imaging research on humans. Nevertheless, increased neurogerontological research activity in this area would be welcome and fruitful. Until more research of this kind is performed, we will remain relatively uninformed about the neural bases of motoric deficits that accompany healthy aging.

10
Modulation of the Nervous System: Emotion, Arousal, and Circadian Rhythms

A computer operates at the same speed, efficiency, and level of enthusiasm regardless of the time of day, the content of information it is processing, or the length of time it has been working. Humans and other animals do not. Our behavior varies constantly—up and down, this way and that way—in accordance with emotions, arousal, and biological clocks. These phenomena presumably evolved so that survival and reproductive success are more likely, and it is easy to see how this would be so. For example, emotions such as fear serve to facilitate evasive or aggressive actions in dangerous situations, whereas lust makes reproductive behavior more likely. Downward adjustments in the level of arousal serve to preserve energy, whereas upward adjustments energize behaviors when warranted. Circadian (daily) and other biological rhythms allow physiological processes to be synchronized and to function at the appropriate levels with respect to day and night. In this chapter we consider neurogerontological aspects of these modulatory processes.

EMOTIONS

There is no simple definition of *emotion*. What we call emotions are part and parcel of many behaviors, experiences, cognitive processes, internal feelings, and physiological arousal responses. In addition to being important modulators of experiences and behaviors, the expression of one's own emotional state (or masking it) and perception of the emotions of others are salient aspects of communication. It is hard to pin down specific emotions because there are so many of them, ranging from positive to negative, wonderful to terrible, mild to intense. Moreover, the emotional responses of individuals often differ greatly under the same set of circumstances, making it impossible to categorize typical or average behaviors. Needless to say, an understanding of underlying neural mechanisms will be elusive.

In earlier chapters we have established the general properties of age-related changes in behavior or response measures before discussing age effects in the nervous system. It was clear, for example, that sensory, motor, and mnemonic systems exhibit declines with age, allowing us to consider possible neural correlates. This is much less the case with respect to emotions, however, because of the ubiquity of large individual differences irrespective of age. Both young and old adults come in all varieties, anxious or serene, jovial or staid, happy or dour. Who is typical, jolly old St. Nicholas or Scrooge?

Whether or not consistent age effects are concealed in this forest of variance is an open question. For one thing, relatively little psychological research has been directed at aging and emotion. Literature reviews (Filipp, 1996; Levenson, Carstensen, Friesen, & Ekman, 1991) suggest that the intensity of emotions experienced by aging people may sometimes become attenuated, although there is the usual disagreement on this issue. For example, Levenson and colleagues (1991) measured autonomic responses in subjects who were asked to relive emotional experiences. Older subjects exhibited similar patterns of autonomic responses to those found in young adults, but the magnitude of the effects was reduced. Do these and similar findings by other researchers imply that the neural and/or hormonal "generators" of emotional responses are attenuated? Not necessarily. Decreases might result from longevity and experience; a lifetime of exposure to emotional events makes new ones less novel, and people may learn to control their emotions over the years. And, of course, as in all of the other basic nervous system functions, emotions involve many interacting brain regions, systems, and circuits. Essential are sensory systems for the processing of emotional stimuli and contexts, motor systems for the performance of emotional acts and expression, and various brain regions subserving memory. We have already discussed the many ways these faculties can become altered with age. How such changes might influence emotional systems is hard to predict. Sensory deficits could render some emotion-evoking stimuli less salient, whereas unexpected or confusing stimuli could potentiate emotional responses. A loss of motor control might lessen emotional "acting out," result in calm resignation, or agitated frustration. Similarly, altered memory could have any number of effects on the intensity and quality of emotional responses.

In general, the available literature suggests that emotional age effects are usually weak (e.g., Malatesta & Kalnok, 1984). Take, for example, one of the best studied emotions, anxiety. Many psychologists view anxiety from two perspectives: a person's relatively stable proneness to anxiety (trait anxiety) and perceived feelings of tension, apprehension, and heightened autonomic activity (state anxiety), which is responsive to external events (Spielberger, Gorsuch, & Lushene, 1970). Kausler (1990) reviewed the gerontological literature pertaining to both trait and state anxiety and concluded that age effects were not robust. Essentially, the individual differences in anxiety among older adults and measurement problems tend to overwhelm potential age differences. Furthermore, clinical anxiety disorders (panic attacks, phobias, generalized anxiety) do not become more prevalent in older people (Gatz, Kasl-Godley, & Karel, 1996; Schramke, 1997). Of course, the fact that these conditions do not become exacerbated with age does not imply that anxiety does not affect the lives of older people; indeed, many do experience problems in this area, just as young adults do.

Major depressive disorders (i.e., those rising to the level of very serious mental illness) do not increase in noninstitutionalized elderly people and, indeed, become less prevalent (Gatz et al., 1996; Koenig, 1997; Koenig & Blazer, 1996). In contrast to this, the incidence of subclinical depression (i.e., having some symptoms of depression, but falling short of the criteria for full-blown, clinical depression) *does* increase after middle age. Among the biological factors that might contribute to the risk of depression in older people are the neurotransmitter systems thought to underlie depression, primarily NE and serotonin (the effect of antidepressant drugs is to facilitate these neurotransmitter systems, suggesting that depressed people have diminished serotonergic and/or noradrenergic proficiency). Later in this chapter, research is reviewed indicating that NE and serotonin systems may be faulty in older individuals. However, some noradrenergic and serotonergic circuits probably have nothing to do with mood. This plus the possibility of compensatory adjustments make it impossible to determine whether depression would become more likely on the basis of age-related changes in these neurotransmitter systems. Further muddying the waters are the contributions of factors such as medical illnesses, medications, sensory loss (which can increase depression), negative life situations, and personality, to name several. Again, it is difficult to sort out the variables.

AROUSAL AND SLEEP

Arousal level—the amplitude of general behavioral, neural, and autonomic activity—routinely varies along a continuum: sleep-drowsiness-alertness-excitement-agitation. Studies of physiological measures of autonomic activity, such as the galvanic skin response and heart rate, have suggested that older people tend to be underaroused (Prinz et al., 1990; Woodruff-Pak, 1988). EEG studies also indicate that older people are generally less aroused and/or more drowsy during the day, in that properties of certain EEG waves resemble those characteristic of low-vigilance waking states (low arousal). However, the opposite conclusion (overarousal) has also been reached by some researchers, albeit less consistently. Determining age effects for physiological arousal suffers from difficulty in measuring and interpreting basal levels of autonomic activity and the changes associated with acute arousal. For example, there is some support for the view that, whereas tonic levels of arousal may be lower in older subjects, phasic changes during experimental or other events may be magnified. However, tonic and phasic levels are not completely independent. All in all, age effects for waking arousal are hard to delineate.

At the low end of the arousal scale is sleep, and here age effects are strong. Problems with sleep constitute a major complaint among the senior citizenry (Dement et al., 1985; Prinz et al., 1990; Richardson, 1990; Vitiello, 1997). Behaviorally, older people wake up more frequently during the night and generally spend less time asleep. Elder members of other species also tend to sleep less than their younger counterparts. Disrupted sleep might result from maladroit neural or hormonal mechanisms (see below), altered autonomic arousal, and/or the occurrence of sleep apnea (interference with airflow and breathing), which can increase dramatically in some older people. Factors such as change in lifestyle (e.g., retirement), depression, and arthritic pain may influence sleep patterns as well. Whereas reduced sleep time might be expected to contribute to waking drowsiness, some older people may not need as much sleep as young adults to function optimally.

A night in bed finds people cycling through several sleep phases based on EEG activity, eye movements, and muscle activity. Rapid-eye movement (REM) sleep is characterized by movement of the eyes, low-amplitude, fast-frequency EEG waves (paradoxically similar to that observed during wakefulness), and inhibition of motor neurons. Non-REM (NREM) sleep consists of several stages in which the EEG is mostly comprised of increasingly larger amplitude, slower frequency waves. With age, the percentage of total sleep time spent in stage 1 of NREM sleep (onset of sleep) increases, an indication of sleep disturbance. The sleep spindles in the EEG of stage 2 NREM sleep become atypical. The most striking effect is observed for NREM stages 3 and 4 (slow wave sleep). These stages become shorter and the characteristic delta waves exhibit a decline in amplitude with age. The amount of time spent in REM sleep may decrease, but to a lesser extent than slow wave sleep and primarily at very old ages (see Figure 10.1).

Dement and colleagues (1985) noted that, irrespective of age, sleep deprivation has a number of deleterious effects on the CNS, possibly involving the physiological health of neurons, neurotransmitter efficacy, cerebral metabolism, and other variables. They speculated that sleep disturbances might therefore contribute to some of the nervous system damage and dysfunction that accompany aging. Health issues may also derive

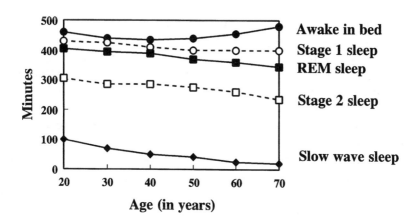

FIGURE 10.1   Age effects for sleep stages. With age, an increase in the total awake time in bed is observed. REM sleep decreases slightly, but slow wave sleep declines substantially. Data were obtained from Dement et al. (1985).

from REM sleep's effects on breathing. As noted earlier, REM sleep is associated with inhibition of muscle activity, including those used for breathing, the intercostal muscles and diaphragm. If there were problems with the pulmonary system to begin with, the interaction with REM sleep paralysis could have deadly potential. Snoring and sleep apnea also interfere with breathing and can present particular problems for older people.

Circadian Rhythms

Circadian rhythms occur for many other functions besides somnolence, such as body temperature, blood pressure, blood chemistry, and hormonal activity. Whereas the literature has been somewhat inconsistent, age effects for both the timing and amplitude of circadian rhythms have been observed in humans and other species (Dement et al., 1985; Mobbs, 1996; Richardson, 1990; Touitou, Bogdan, Haus, & Touitou, 1997). A number of studies have shown that the amplitude of circadian rhythms (the difference between maximum and minimum values) tends to decrease with age. There is also a body of evidence to indicate that the phase of circadian rhythms (the onset of sleep or other daily changes) often occurs earlier as individuals age.

Circadian rhythms are governed by both intrinsic "biological clock" mechanisms and entraining stimuli such as light-dark cycles. If the entraining stimuli are removed, the biological clock still exerts daily rhythms of various physiological processes. However, this "free-running" clock is not as accurate and is subject to drift. Thus, in older individuals altered rhythms could be due to disrupted entrainment secondary to sensory changes and/or changes in the central timing mechanisms. The latter are often altered with age (see below).

The gerontological significance of altered circadian rhythmicity, while not totally clear, has important implications (see Richardson, 1990). Biological rhythms are thought to provide a means for synchronizing various physiological activities, and disruption of circadian rhythms has been shown to shorten life in several species. Altered biological rhythms (e.g., hormones or temperature) might contribute to sleep disorders, which in turn create health problems. Thus, to the extent that circadian rhythms are perturbed in older humans (which remains to be determined), yet another neurogerontological variable presents itself.

NEURAL MECHANISMS

As indicated earlier, emotions and arousal are usually not independent of one another. For example, it is obvious that an intense emotional response is also highly arousing. On the other hand, arousal and emotions are not always in lock step. Slow wave sleep is a period of low behavioral and EEG arousal, yet emotionally charged dream experiences can occur (dreams occur during both REM and NREM sleep). Thus, in discussing the neurobiological mechanisms, we begin with a mechanistic common denominator for emotion and arousal, the autonomic nervous system. Somewhat artificially, this is followed by a discussion of the limbic system, classically linked to emotions, then structures that regulate sleep, general arousal levels, and circadian rhythms.

The Autonomic Nervous System and Stress

The autonomic nervous system and its interactions with the hypothalamus and neuroendocrine system were discussed in chapter 6. Whereas the subject of chapter 6 was the role of these systems in homeostasis and the maintenance of bodily functions, we now turn to their role in arousal. In particular, we focus on the stress response because a good deal of neurobiological and endocrinological research has been directed at this aspect of arousal.

Various stimuli, events, or situations that are actually or potentially threatening, dangerous, or biologically significant (stressors) elicit a pattern of neuroendocrine responses (see Figure 10.2). These can collectively be termed the *stress response*. The stress response involves activation of the sympathetic nervous system and a sequence hormonal reactions: Corticotropin-releasing factor, a product of the hypothalamus, causes the anterior pituitary gland to release adrenocorticotropic hormone (ACTH). ACTH stimulates the adrenal cortex to secrete glucocorticoids (corticosterone, cortisol, hydrocortisone). These adrenocortical hormones have a number of effects on the body, such as mobilizing energy from storage, increasing cardiovascular tone, and inhibiting immune responses. Glucocorticoids, in turn, interact with the brain and pituitary to inhibit this series of events, forming a feedback system. Stress also induces cellular responses (e.g., induction of heat-shock proteins) and inflammatory reactions.

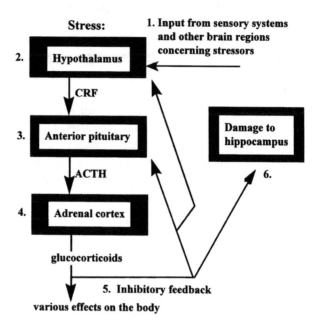

FIGURE 10.2   Stress and the pituitary adrenal axis. Stressors initiate the stress response (1), causing the hypothalamus to release CRF (2). This in turn causes the anterior pituitary to release ACTH (3), which causes the adrenal cortex to release glucocorticoids (4). The glucocorticoids have various effects on the body and also inhibit the stress system (5). A negative effect of glucocorticoids is damage to the hippocampus (6).

Whereas the stress response is adaptive (e.g., it increases the probability of surviving dangerous situations), too much stress is generally considered to be a bad thing. Indeed, psychosomatic illnesses (ulcers, high blood pressure), suppression of the immune system, and exacerbation of diseases are well-known concomitants of stress. Thus, the relationship between stress and aging is potentially important.

As discussed in chapter 6, sympathetic nervous system tone or basal activity (e.g., as reflected by plasma catecholamine levels) generally increases with aging. This may have little to do with stress, but rather may be a function of hormonal/autonomic homeostasis. Indeed, activation of the sympathetic nervous system by stressors may become less potent in older individuals (Mobbs, 1996).

Because of complicated hormonal feedback and metabolic processes, the relationship between sympathetic neural responses and adrenocortical hormone activity is often not straightforward. This is certainly true in the case of aging and stress, as indicated by gerontological studies focusing on glucocorticoids. In aging rats (Tsagarakis & Grossman, 1992), the peak adrenocortical stress response tends to be fairly stable in males but somewhat diminished in females. However, the ability of old rats to terminate the stress response can be greatly impaired, probably due to reduced brain sensitivity to glucocorticoid feedback. In this sense, the stress response is enhanced with age. This does not appear to be the case for normal human aging, however (Sapolsky, 1992; Tsagarakis & Grossman, 1992). A large body of literature indicates that adrenocortical function is relatively normal in older people, and there is little evidence for the enhanced presence of glucocorticoids associated with stress seen in aged rats. However, when very old humans are looked at and/or very sensitive measures are used on them, evidence can be found for subtle effects similar to those seen in rats (see Sapolsky, 1992). These can be especially problematic if depression or dementia is present.

Glucocorticoids, stress, and aging.   Glucocorticoids (in particular, cortisol in primates and corticosterone in rodents) are a key component of the stress response, and their involvement in aging has received considerable attention. The research was reviewed by Mobbs (1996) and may be summarized as follows. Stemming from research in his laboratory, Landfield (1980) proposed that a gradual age-related increase in glucocorticoids was responsible for hippocampal damage in rats (the hippocampus contains glucocorticoid receptors). Furthermore, it was suggested that hippocampal damage in turn lessened inhibition of glucocorticoid secretion, resulting in a recursive cycle. Sapolsky (1992) further elaborated the story, linking damage to an exaggerated stress response (i.e., failure of a negative feedback mechanism), causing down regulation of hippocampal glucocorticoid receptors and potentiating damage to hippocampal neurons—the *glucocorticoid cascade* hypothesis. This hypothesis accounted not only for hippocampal damage (especially in the CA1 and CA3 subfields) but also for other physiological changes that produce age-related changes (i.e., a cause of aging).

There are, however, some issues that need to be resolved with respect to the glucocorticoid cascade hypothesis (Mobbs, 1996; Reagan & McEwen, 1997). For example, glucocorticoids often do not increase with age in humans and some other species; the most compelling evidence of increases is in rats, and even here there are inconsistent findings. Moreover, there is conflicting evidence for decreased sensitivity to glucocorticoids as would be expected with decreased receptor efficacy. Results suggesting increased, decreased, or no change in glucocorticoid receptors have been published. Furthermore, there is research showing that, whereas basal glucocorticoid levels may increase with age, the stress response need not be exaggerated. Complicated feedback mechanisms in which other hormones (mineralocorticoids) interact with the glucocorticoid system further cloud the issue. Thus, whereas glucocorticoid potentiated damage to the hippocampus is undoubtedly important to aging, the impact of stress, cascading processes, and other issues remain to be worked out. An additional issue is how the interaction of glucocorticoids and neurotrophins might affect the hippocampus and aging in general (McLay et al., 1997). Neurotrophins, including their relationship to glucocorticoids and the hippocampus, are discussed in chapter 13.

The Limbic System

Structures collectively called the limbic system have been implicated in various emotional experiences and behaviors such as fear, sexuality, and aggression. These include the hypothalamus, mammillary bodies, septum, amygdala, hippocampus, portions of the thalamus, and the cingulate and other regions of cerebral cortex. A structure heavily studied in rats is the median forebrain bundle, extending from midbrain to hypothalamus. Many sites in the median forebrain structure contain dopaminergic neurons, which have been linked to positive (one assumes pleasurable) emotions.

The amygdala.   Of the many emotions, fear has been especially well studied, because it appears to occur in a variety of species in a form not unlike that observed in humans. Furthermore, fear conditioning is relatively easy to produce, allowing this emotion to be manipulated in animals. At the center of the neural circuitry that mediates fear is the amygdala, a relatively small structure in the temporal lobe region, composed of a half dozen subdivisions. Sensory information about the fearful stimuli and unpleasant events (e.g., pain) are received by the amygdala, and its output is sent to relevant motor and autonomic circuitry. Damage to the amygdala eliminates or attenuates various correlates of fear, such as blood pressure changes or fear behaviors (freezing or potentiated startle reflexes) in response to fearful stimuli (Davis, 1992). The amygdala plays an important role in other emotional contexts as well, such as appreciating the emotional significance of situations and aggressive behavior.

The neurogerontological literature on the amygdala was reviewed in chapter 8, in the context of fear conditioning. As indicated there, not much evidence of consistent age effects has been obtained in healthy elderly people. The amygdala, however, is a structure that is strongly affected by Alzheimer's disease, which is characterized by emotional deficits (refer to chapter 11).

One way of assessing the status of the amygdala in animals (including humans) is to obtain measures of fear. We have done this with old mice using the fear-potentiated startle paradigm, as described in chapter 8. After a tone has been paired with a mild but unpleasant foot shock, the tone, now a conditioned stimulus, elicits fear. This is manifested by a potentiated startle response when the tone is present. As shown in Figure 10.3, fear-potentiated startle effect elicited in old mice is considerably greater than that observed in young mice. Apparently, the emotion of fear and the ability to condition fear are retained—and perhaps enhanced—in old CBA/CaJ mice. This is consistent with the absence of strong age-related declines in amygdaloid function.

The nucleus accumbens and mesolimbic dopaminergic system.   Positive emotions such as pleasure, rewards, and the euphoric effects of some drugs (e.g., opiates, cannabis) have been linked to neural circuits that utilize dopamine, in particular the *mesolimbic dopamine system* (R. A. Wise, 1996). Whereas many structures are probably involved in positive emotions, the *ventral tegmental area* and its efferent target, the *nucleus accumbens*, have received much recent attention. The nucleus accumbens is located in the ventral striatum (below the caudate nucleus and putamen) and is synaptically linked to various components of the limbic system such as the hippocampal formation, midline thalamic nuclei, and hypothalamus, as well as frontal cortex. The system may be particularly important in anticipating rewards (Wickelgren, 1997b), and may also be involved in learning and declarative memory in cooperation with the hippocampus (Setlow, 1997).

There is little evidence that the nucleus accumbens and mesolimbic dopaminergic system are especially susceptible to age-related changes. Studies of dopamine in the mesolimbic system have been mixed, but Morgan and May (1990) estimated that the consensus indicates about a

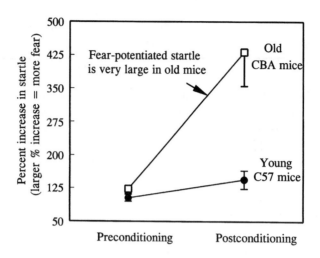

**FIGURE 10.3   Fear-potentiated startle in old CBA mice. The data show
the size of the startle response when a 12-kHz background tone was present
divided by the size of the startle when evoked in quiet, expressed as a percent
(100% means there was no effect of the tone on startle; values greater than
100% indicate that the tone potentiated the startle, a measure of fear). There
were 10 mice in each age group; the error bars are standard errors of the
mean. In the *preconditioning* tests, the 12-kHz tone had little effect on startle
of either young C57 mice or old CBA mice (values were near 100%). After
pairing the 12-kHz tone with a mild but unpleasant foot shock, startle in
the presence of the 12-kHz tone increased significantly in both subject groups
(*postconditioning*). In young C57 mice the increase (i.e., fear-potentiated
startle) was about 30%, and this was statistically significant. In the old CBA
mice, however, fear-potentiated startle was huge: an increase of more than
400%. The data for young C57 mice are from Falls et al. (1997). Those from
old CBA mice are unpublished, obtained by J. Turner, W. Falls, S. Heldt,
S. Carlson, and J. F. Willott.**

10% decline in rodents. Dopamine content was reported to be decreased
in the nucleus accumbens of old male rats (Demarest, Riegle, & Moore,
1980) but not in old females (Demarest, Moore, & Riegle, 1982). Woods,
Ricken, and Druse (1995) found an age-related decline in D1 dopamine
receptors in the nucleus accumbens and frontal cortex of Fischer 344 rats
but Crawford and Levine (1997) found D2 receptors to be especially

vulnerable to age-related change. Whereas this research suggests some age effects in rodents, the same cannot yet be said of humans. Most work on aging and dopamine has focused on the nigrostriatal system (see chapter 9), with little evidence of age effects for the mesolimbic system. An anatomical study of humans failed to obtain significant evidence of age-related loss of neurons in the nucleus accumbens (Huang & Zhao, 1995). However, an earlier study indicated reduced dopaminergic activity in the nucleus accumbens of old subjects (E. G. McGeer & P. L. McGeer, 1976). Thus, the jury is still out with respect to the mesolimbic system. However, given that learning with positive reinforcement is not very much diminished with age (see chapter 8), and age effects for emotions are weak in general, perhaps we should not expect great age-associated changes in this particular dopaminergic circuitry.

Arousal and Sleep

Arousal is determined by the complex interaction of various neural circuits and brain regions (see Figure 10.4). We shall focus here on the brainstem. The reticular formation is a seemingly loosely organized region that occupies the center of the brainstem, extending to its upper levels. Neurons of reticular formation receive input from the sensory systems and project axons both upward into the forebrain and downward into the spinal cord. As neural activity in the reticular formation increases, so does arousal and the characteristic fast, low-voltage, desynchronized EEG pattern observed from electrodes over the cerebral cortex. The reticular formation influences the autonomic nervous system by way of the hypothalamus. Two other brainstem regions that have widespread influence on the brain (because of extensive axonal branching) are the locus coeruleus and raphe nuclei. The locus coeruleus is adrenergic and provides axonal output for a system that is involved in arousal (notably, when memories are being formed) and sleep (particularly REM sleep, during which its descending axons inhibit motor neurons in the spinal cord). The level of activity of the locus coeruleus is directly related to both arousal and REM. The raphe nuclei give rise to a major serotonergic system, which is also important for the regulation of arousal and sleep. Damage to the raphe nuclei results in a great drop in serotonin in the forebrain (to which it projects) and disrupts sleep. It is important to note that, whereas the reticular formation, locus coeruleus, and raphe nuclei have received most of the attention

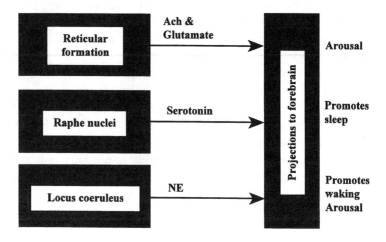

**FIGURE 10.4   Brainstem structures involved in arousal and sleep. The
reticular formation has many functions, among which is the production of
arousal via projections to the forebrain. Ach and glutamate are thought to
be key neurotransmitters. The raphe nuclei project to the forebrain using
serotonin, with one effect being the promotion of sleep. By contrast, forebrain
projections of the locus coeruleus, which utilize NE, promote arousal and
waking.**

with respect to the modulation of arousal and sleep, other structures
also participate, including the medial thalamus, the anterior and preoptic
hypothalamus, and the basal forebrain region.

   Given the participation of all this neural hardware, it is not surprising
that sleep cannot be characterized as a period of neural quiescence, despite
the fact that behavioral arousal is low. During REM sleep in particular,
elevations are observed for neural activity in the cerebral cortex and
elsewhere, metabolic rates in some brain regions, and sympathetic nervous
system activity. On the other hand, during slow wave sleep, the direction
of many changes reverses. This makes it especially difficult to relate
neurobiological age effects to changes in elderly sleep patterns. More can
be said about arousal (whether in the context of sleep or not), but even
here the neurogerontological research has large gaps.

   The reticular formation has not received much attention from neurogerontologists. It is, in general, a difficult region to study due to its diffuse
anatomical organization. There is evidence of age-related degenerative

changes in reticular formation neurons in mice, including dendritic atrophy and loss of spines (Machado-Salas, Scheibel, & Scheibel, 1977). A recent study comparing the reticular formation of young and old cats also found age effects (Zhang, Sampogna, Morales, & Chase, 1997). Immunostaining for a component of neurofilaments was decreased in neurons, especially dendrites, in most regions of the reticular formation. The findings suggest cytoskeletal changes that could negatively affect cellular function.

Because the reticular formation receives considerable sensory input, one might look here for age effects. For example, the "triggering" of its arousal functions might be altered by age-related sensory changes. On the one hand, it might be expected that the reticular formation would be resistant to modulation because of impaired sensory function. On the other hand, neural plasticity within partially denervated sensory systems has the capacity to enhance the salience of some stimuli, as discussed in chapter 7. In the latter scenario, sensory stimuli might be able to modulate reticular formation neurons more effectively. We tested this notion in our laboratory using C57 mice. As discussed in chapter 7, these mice exhibit presbycusis in that their sensitivity for high-frequency sounds is lost as they age. At the same time, this prompts the occurrence of neural plasticity, so that still-audible, lower frequency sounds become more prominently represented in the central auditory system. Carlson and Willott (1998) obtained recordings of action potentials from neurons in the *caudal pontine reticular formation* (PnC) of young and presbycusic C57 mice. PnC neurons are a key component of a neural circuit that mediates startle responses. The response of PnC neurons to a startle-evoking stimulus (e.g., an intense brief sound) can be modulated (inhibited) by a softer tone that precedes the startle stimulus by about 100 msec, the neural analog of the behavioral phenomenon known as *prepulse inhibition*. Carlson and Willott (1998) measured the extent to which prepulse sounds inhibited the responses of PnC neurons evoked by an intense startle stimulus, as shown in Figure 10.5. A high-frequency (24-kHz) prepulse altered the responses of PnC neurons in young mice but was no longer effective in middle-aged mice with presbycusis. By contrast, the lower frequency (4-kHz) prepulse was significantly more effective in modulating the reticular formation neurons in the older mice. As suggested by this study, modulation of the reticular formation by sensory stimuli is influenced by age-related sensory loss, but the direction of the effect can be bidirectional.

A good deal more neurogerontological research has been directed at the locus coeruleus. The literature on humans has been unusually consistent in showing some age-related loss of neurons and other changes in the

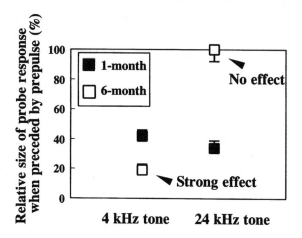

FIGURE 10.5   Neural PPI in the PnC of C57 mice. Action potentials evoked by startle "probe" stimuli (intense brief sounds) were recorded from neurons in the PnC. This procedure was repeated immediately, but now a moderately intense (70-dB) tone preceded the startle stimulus by 100 msec (the PPI paradigm). In young adult mice (1-month-olds), 4-kHz and 24-kHz tone prepulses were effective in inhibiting the responses evoked by the startle stimulus (reduced to about 40% and 30% of the original probe response, respectively). In middle-aged mice with presbycusis (6-month-olds), the 24-kHz tone had no effect on the startle response because of their high-frequency hearing loss. However, the 4-kHz tone had a very strong effect (reduced the response to less than 20% of the original probe response). This reduction was significantly greater than that occurring in young mice. Thus, for the 4-kHz tone prepulse, neural PPI was stronger for mice with high-frequency presbycusis. These data were presented in a different form by Carlson and Willott (1998).

locus coeruleus of healthy older humans (Chan-Palay & Azan, 1989; Mann, 1997; Manaye, McIntire, Mann, & German, 1995; Marcyniuk, Mann, & Yates, 1986, 1989; Vijayashankar & Brody, 1977). Neuron loss may be on the order of 20% to 50%. The loss of neurons is especially pronounced in the rostral region of the locus coeruleus, which projects to the forebrain, compared to the caudal region, which projects to the spinal cord (Chan-Palay & Azan, 1989; Manaye et al., 1995). A study by Ohm, Busch, and Bohl (1997) used unbiased stereological methods and careful screening to eliminate potential early Alzheimer's patients. The researchers failed to find a relationship between neuron number and age in the range of 49 to 98 years; however, data were not presented for younger subjects, so it is not clear if age-related neuron loss might have already occurred in these subjects. The locus coeruleus of rodents has also been found to exhibit cell loss (Collier, Gash, & Sladek, 1987; Sturrock & Rao, 1985), albeit not in all cases (Goldman & Coleman, 1981; Monji et al., 1994a), perhaps due to strain or species differences.

Despite the likely loss of many NE-containing neurons in the locus coeruleus, which contains the largest number of noradrenergic neurons in the brain, some studies have found that NE levels in the human forebrain do not drop with age (see Srivastava, Granholm, & Gerhardt, 1997, for references). A caveat is in order, however, because technical difficulties in measuring NE in human postmortem tissue may cast doubt on some of these findings (Palmer & DeKosky, 1993). Nevertheless, the data suggest that some sort of compensatory mechanism(s) might help to maintain noradrenergic innervation of the synaptic targets of the human locus coeruleus. For example, locus coeruleus neurons from old animals are capable of undergoing axonal sprouting (Srivastava et al., 1997). The potential for compensatory plasticity obviously makes it difficult to interpret the behavioral implications of neuron loss in the locus coeruleus.

Less is known about aging and the raphe system. Several studies of humans failed to find neuron loss in the raphe of older subjects (Mann, 1997). Some neuronal loss, shrinkage, and dendritic degeneration were reported in a study of rats by Lolova and Davidoff (1991), but not by van Luijtelaar (1992). The latter group, however, did observe abnormal fibers in ascending serotonergic fibers of old rats (Van Luijtelaar, Steinbusch, & Tonnaer, 1988; Van Luijtelaar, Wouterlood, Tonnaer, & Steinbusch, 1991). Some studies have found losses of postsynaptic receptors with aging (Morgan & May, 1990). However, more studies than not have failed to find evidence of diminished serotonergic markers in old rats or humans (see Johnson et al., 1993; Palmer & DeKosky, 1993, for references). Indeed, increased synthesis of serotonin by raphe neurons has been observed in older rats (van Luijtelaar, Tonnaer, & Steinbusch, 1992). Furthermore, presynaptic serotonergic markers, which would include terminals of raphe neurons, generally do not exhibit age effects (Morgan & May, 1990). This is the case for several species including humans. Taken together, it is difficult to evaluate the extent to which the raphe system is modified with age. However, the available data suggest that age effects are not particularly consistent or strong.

Circadian Rhythms

As indicated above, circadian rhythms are the product of endogenous biological clock mechanisms plus additional entrainment by daily variations in the environment, signaled by the sensory systems. The suprachiasmatic nucleus (SCN) of the hypothalamus plays a key role in biological rhythms, and more than any other brain structure, warrants the label of the primary "biological clock." Thus, SCN neurons exhibit circadian physiological variations even when isolated from other brain circuits, and damage to the SCN eliminates various circadian rhythms.

Age-related changes in the SCN include altered daily oscillations of neural activity, reduced effectiveness of visual stimuli, and neuronal degeneration (Mobbs, 1996; Richardson, 1990; Wise, 1994; Zhang et al., 1996). A decrease in the number of SCN neurons and other changes have been observed in older humans (Mirmiran et al., 1992; Mobbs, 1996; Swaab et al., 1992; Wise, 1994), especially beyond age 80. SCN neurons containing vasopressin are especially relevant, as these have been shown to exhibit age effects (Richardson, 1990). For example, age-related loss of neurons immunostaining for vasopressin have been demonstrated in both rats (Roozendaal, van Gool, Swaab, Hoogendijk, & Mirmiran, 1987) and humans (Swaab, Fliers, & Partiman, 1985). Moreover, the rhythmic synthesis of vasopressin by the human SCN appears to be attenuated in older brains (Hofman & Swaab, 1994). Signs of neural change (enlarged somata, dendritic degeneration) in the SCN accompany attenuated circadian rhythms in old mice (Peng, Jiang, & Hsu, 1980). Thus, SCN neurons appear to be vulnerable to deleterious age-related changes.

The pineal gland is a second important structure for biological timekeeping. It is situated above and behind the brainstem at the midline (unlike other brain structures that have a left and right version, there is only one pineal). The pineal gland is innervated by the sympathetic superior cervical ganglion, which, in turn, receives innervation from a circuit that includes the SCN. This circuit causes the pineal to produce and release the hormone melatonin in a circadian fashion. Melatonin secretion increases at night, and it has a strong modulatory influence on sleep and other circadian rhythms. The production of melatonin may also exert some feedback control on the SCN, whose neurons possess receptors for melatonin. In seasonally breeding species, the pineal/melatonin system regulates reproductive behavior as well. Sensory information about light levels is accessed by the pineal and plays an important role in pineal physiology and rhythmicity.

Melatonin production decreases gradually with age, ultimately reaching very low levels. There is also an attenuation of the amplitude of rhythmic changes, and combined with low overall levels, the circadian rhythm can be virtually absent in very old individuals (see Reiter, 1995; Touitou et al., 1997, for reviews). Restoration of nightly melatonin levels by ingestion of supplements has beneficial effects on sleeping in many older people. Besides sleep, however, the melatonin rhythm regulates other systems, so age effects could be widespread. Indeed, there is a body of evidence to support the view that the failing melatonin system contributes importantly to the rate and severity of aging in general, both by its modulatory control of physiological processes and the fact that it is a potent antioxidant that can protect cells from free radical damage. Thus, melatonin replacement has potential as an "anti-aging" agent, a topic discussed in chapter 13.

SUMMARY AND CONCLUSIONS

It is apparent that some aspects of nervous system modulation are significantly altered with age. Sleep and circadian rhythms exhibit the clearest age effects, and the responsible neural and hormonal mechanisms are being elucidated. The growing understanding of these processes is even producing therapeutic strategies such as the use of supplemental melatonin. Great strides have also been made with respect to adrenocortical hormone influences on aging and the possible exacerbating role of stress. We certainly know that excessive stress is something to be avoided in a lifestyle designed for successful aging.

Less neurogerontological progress has been made with respect to emotions. This is undoubtedly due, in large part, to the many variables—biological, social, personality, medical, and ecological—that influence individuals in myriad ways. Indeed, this may be an area of inquiry where neurogerontology can help to clarify what is happening behaviorally. Usually, the situation is reversed: Behavioral and clinical observations indicate what gerontological or geriatric problems exist, *then* neurobiological research is brought on line to unravel the underlying mechanisms. With respect to emotion, neurobiological research may be able to show that, beneath all of the extraneous variance, a particular neural system is impaired with aging. We could then work backwards to determine how those variables interact with the biological changes to produce the behavioral age effects. For example, if it were determined that specific serotonergic and/or adrenergic circuits associated with depression were reliably altered in older people, we would be in a much improved position to understand how and why depression becomes more prevalent with age. The focus could shift toward examining how all sorts of variables interact in the context of an altered neural substrate.

11
Cognitive Integration and Disintegration (Dementia)

Integration refers to the broad set of processes by which various sources of input and information (e.g., sensory, intracellular, genetic) interface to determine neural circuit activity and output. This chapter focuses on the rather complex integration associated with cognitive processes, but in actuality we have been discussing integration throughout this book. At a fundamental neuronal level, integration is a function of the spatiotemporal array of excitatory and inhibitory synaptic activity on a dendritic tree. Whether or not the postsynaptic neuron's membrane will be depolarized enough to trigger an action potential depends on the summed events associated with the synaptic inputs.

We saw in chapters 3 to 5 that a variety of age-related goings-on in dendrites, axons, synapses, and cellular physiology can disrupt this integrative process at the single-neuron level. Spinal reflexes are examples of a higher level of integration, involving inputs from sensory systems, descending modulation from the brain, and interneuronal circuits within the spinal cord, all coming together to produce organized motor output. We saw in chapter 9 how this level of integration can become altered with age. A still higher level of integration is exemplified by learning. The relationships between conditioned and unconditioned stimuli in time and space must become linked to new patterns of behavioral output, and this relationship must somehow be shared with other brain areas for storage as memory. Chapter 8 reviewed the various ways these processes become modified with age. It must be the case that perturbation of these "lower" levels of integration will have some effect on the "higher" levels to be discussed in this chapter. However, the field of neurogerontology is far from elucidating these multilevel effects.

Somewhat arbitrarily we shall include several topics under the rubric of cognitive processes: speed of information processing, attention, spatial abilities, the use of language, and intelligence. We shall then (with some trepidation) briefly address the topic of personality, an area for which the neuroscience is sparse. The chapter ends with a discussion of Alzheimer's disease (AD) and other dementias, viewed from the perspective of cognitive and personality disintegration. Needless to say, learning, memory, emotions, perception, and other activities of the nervous system are part and parcel of cognitive processes and personality. These topics, of course, have already been discussed in earlier chapters, and we need only allude to them here.

COGNITIVE PROCESSES

The Speed of Information Processing

One of the more thoroughly researched areas of gerontology is the slowing of behavior and cognition (see Birren & Fisher, 1995, for a recent review). Behavioral/cognitive slowing is a very reliable concomitant of aging and has been proposed as a marker of aging (i.e., a measure that can differentiate chronological age from functional age). Peripheral changes in the sensory and motor systems (reviewed in chapters 7 and 9) generally provide only small contributions to cognitive slowing. Much more salient are the central neural circuits which intervene between stimuli and responses. Thus, for example, the P300 event-related potential, associated with cognitive processing, shows longer latencies with age (Bashore, 1990; Kugler, Taghavy, & Platt, 1993). Latencies of event-related potentials generated by less complex central circuits (e.g., sensory evoked responses) are not prolonged to the same extent with age.

One view holds that there is a general slowing of the CNS, and cognitive slowing reflects the sluggishness of smaller components (sensory, motor, and interconnected central circuits). There is a good deal of research support for this (Birren & Fisher, 1995). The impact of slowing appears to depend somewhat upon tasks, however. Thus, when a task requires the use of knowledge without time constraints, age effects tend to be smaller than those for which speed is of importance. In any event, general age-related slowing or slowing of certain circuit components is likely to have widespread effects on cognition (Birren & Fisher, 1995).

Reaction time (RT) tasks have been used extensively in gerontological studies of slowing. Salthouse (1996) cited three good reasons for this: RTs indicate an individual's neurological status (albeit with interpretive limitations), RTs exhibit robust age effects, and RTs are related to higher cognitive activities. The latter property allows RTs to be used to delve into fairly complex cognitive processes. For example, comparison of *choice RTs* (the subject must choose the correct stimulus) and *simple RTs* (the subject needs to react only to the presence of a stimulus) should reflect the time it takes to discriminate between stimuli. Experiments of this type indicate some slowing of the simple RT (presumably due largely to slowing of sensory and motor processes and their connecting circuitry), but significantly greater slowing for the choice RTs (presumably associated with intervening neural processing). In general, the greater the amount of neural processing, the greater the age effects for speed.

Attention

In an environment filled with stimuli, some degree of selectivity and focus—attention—must be exercised so that optimal behavior occurs in response to important, relevant stimuli at the expense of irrelevant ones. Attentional processes are especially important when the potential stimuli and responses are numerous and complex. Thus, attention is a key element of most cognitive tasks; if one is not "paying attention," one is probably not performing well cognitively. Madden and Allen (1996) reviewed the gerontological literature within the framework of a three-component model of attention: capacity (the processing resources available for task performance), selectivity (ability to control of processing of certain stimuli but not others), and vigilance (the maintained preparatory and orienting component). In general, reliable age effects are obtained for attentional tasks that require substantial effort and tax the subjects' cognitive resources (capacity). In this regard, *divided attention* (performing two simultaneous tasks) exhibits age-associated deficits except for very simple tasks (McDowd & Birren, 1990). Vigilance also depends on the difficulty of the task, with simple tasks being relatively stable across age. Whether or not older people perform more poorly on tasks of *sustained attention* is unclear. Whereas some researchers have obtained age effects (Parasuraman & Giambra, 1991), others have not (Giambra, 1997). Some types of *selective attention* to relevant versus irrelevant information can be performed quite well by older people, with the exception of various tasks requiring the inhibition of irrelevant stimuli. Thus, older people tend to be more easily distracted (McDowd, 1996). It is interesting to recall that inhibitory components of neural circuits are often susceptible to negative age effects (see chapter 5).

General slowing has been viewed as a very important factor in attentional deficits. A review of the literature suggests that this is so, but slowing is not a sufficient explanation for attentional deficits (Hartley, 1992).

Spatial Behavior

Important components of many cognitive processes and behaviors are those associated with spatial relationships. Spatial relationships come in many varieties: the relative locations of features in a photograph, the position of one's own body parts, one's orientation inside a room, the organization of landmarks in the neighborhood, places within geographical expanses.

Most types of spatial behavior are challenged by aging (see Kirasic & Allen, 1985), although relatively simple spatial behaviors such as orienting attention to visual cues may be spared (Baxter & Voytko, 1996). In chapters 7 and 9 we saw that the monitoring of one's bodily orientation and appropriate motor adjustments can be made more difficult by sensory deficits in visual, vestibular, and somatosensory systems. In chapter 8 it became evident that spatial learning can decline in older humans (e.g., learning to navigate a new neighborhood) and rodents (e.g., poorer performance on Morris water maze or radial arm learning tasks). Salthouse (1992) reviewed the literature on spatial abilities in the context of tasks requiring spatial transformations like mental object rotations, paper folding, and cube comparisons. These types of spatial tasks can be viewed as closely related to reasoning tasks, and both exhibit robust age effects. Finally, memory deficits would be expected to result in a loss of key details in thinking about geographic locales.

Language

Many studies have shown that various elements of language production continue relatively unabated with age. These include reading aloud, writing, sound production, and the appropriate use of language in different situations (Obler & Albert, 1996). Problems arise with naming and lexical semantics; the ability to remember the names of nouns, verbs, and proper names declines with age, especially as people reach their 70s. The difficulties lie with accessing information, not with storage per se, as evidenced by greatly improved performance when mnemonic retrieval cues are provided. The lexical deficiencies are probably linked to memory deficits, as discussed in chapter 8. Memory problems may also have an impact on language tasks that make heavy demands on memory (e.g., extended discourse). Similarly, language comprehension may be affected when the material is difficult.

MacKay and Abrams (1996) reviewed the literature on language and aging from the perspective of a *language-memory* hypothesis. This approach views the acquisition, comprehension, and production of words as being intimately linked to the processes underlying memory. One manifestation is word retrieval, with the tip-of-the-tongue (TOT) phenomenon providing a familiar example. TOTs occur when a person is temporarily unable to retrieve a familiar word from long-term memory, and the incidence of TOTs is strongly age-related. The researchers also hypothesize that the ability to form "new connections" by the brain accounts for age-related deficits in fluency (planning what is to be said and how to say it during language production). These deficits include hesitation, false starts, and word repetitions.

The auditory dimension is, of course, important for speech comprehension, and many older people have difficulties with speech perception. Assuming that their hearing loss is not too severe, however, the problems typically arise only when listening conditions are poor (Willott, 1991). Thus, speech may be understood quite well when spoken clearly in a quiet environment, but not when noise is present, speech is degraded (speeded up, distorted), and/or voices are competing (the "cocktail party effect"). Both central and peripheral factors (CEBA and CEPP; see chapter 7) are likely to be involved.

Intelligence

Most intelligence tests evaluate a number of dimensions or abilities, all of which may not have the same rate of change. Schaie (1996) reviewed his and others' longitudinal studies of aging and intelligence. In general, performance on most tests tends to peak around early middle age and remain stable until about age 60 (plus or minus a few years). All in all, age effects tend to be mild until the mid-70s for primary mental abilities, such as verbal meaning, spatial orientation, inductive reasoning, and word fluency. Numeric ability exhibits a relatively early and more precipitous decline, and perceptual speed appears to decrease as early as the 30s. It is important to note that the declines in intellectual abilities are not global. Whereas almost all 60-year-olds decline in one primary mental ability, few decline in more than two. Furthermore, by age 80 most people do not decline in more than three primary abilities.

A distinction worth noting is that of *fluid* versus *crystallized intelligence*, often made in gerontological contexts. Crystallized intelligence, based largely on the store of knowledge, typically increases through much of old age and rarely exhibits large declines. Fluid intelligence, related to flexible skills such as problem solving and the formation of new concepts, tends to exhibit significant declines in later years.

NEURAL MECHANISMS

Slowing

Any number of age-related changes in neuronal physiology might contribute to slowing of neural circuits. Possible sources of slowing, reviewed in earlier chapters, include the following:

1. Slower conduction of action potentials. Thinning of axon diameters with age would slow conduction time because smaller axons conduct action potentials more slowly. Thinning or loss of myelin could have an effect because well-myelinated fibers conduct faster. Because larger neurons generally have larger axons and conduct faster, selective loss of larger neurons could result in slowing. Less efficient membrane biophysics resulting from age effects on ion channel dynamics, membrane composition/permeability, and so on, could increase the time required to generate action potentials. Longer recovery of the resting potential after action potentials, both short term (refractory period) and longer term (regulation with ionic pumps), could interfere with rapid firing of action potentials. Birren and Fisher (1995) noted that neurological disorders affecting white matter (myelinated axon pathways) are associated with slowing. MRI studies have provided some linkage between age-related white matter damage and slowing, albeit not in a simple way.

2. Slower synaptic transmission.   Decreased amounts of neurotransmitter released, fewer postsynaptic receptors, and/or less efficient receptor binding could slow the activation of synapses. Altered effectiveness of enzymes or reuptake mechanisms that terminate synaptic activity could prolong the activation of synapses (either an increase or decrease in the efficacy of transmitter inactivation could affect synapses). Reduced transport of neurotransmitters and related compounds by the cytoskeleton could result in a diminished supply of available neurotransmitters at axon terminals. Altered glial activity might impair glial function in support of synapses and/or affect the microenvironment at synapses. Changes in calcium-related mechanisms (necessary for neurotransmitter action at synapses) could make it more difficult to activate synapses.

3. Slower cellular processes.   Slower second messenger systems might interfere with the efficiency of many synapses. Diminished intracellular metabolism (e.g., associated with mitochondria damage) could conceivably slow various cellular processes. Reduced production of neurotransmitters and/or other critical products in the neuron soma would affect pre- and postsynaptic events. Modified DNA/RNA mechanisms (e.g., associated with DNA damage) could impair the production of essential proteins. The histological structures that accrue, sometimes even during healthy aging (e.g., lipofuscin, Lewy bodies, etc.), might interfere with speedy cellular processes.

4. Neural circuits.   At the circuit level, an imbalance between "competing" excitatory and inhibitory synapses could prevent one or the other from acting quickly. The loss of circuit elements (e.g., neurons, dendrites, axon branches) might affect circuit speed in various ways, such as preventing temporal or spatial summation at synapses. Switching strategies to accomplish a behavioral or cognitive task might result in the use of more complicated (longer acting) circuits. Forms of neural plasticity that alter topographic relationships might make them less efficient by rerouting the flow of information processing.

5. General neural systems.   Diminished arousal could have a general effect on processing speed. A change in emotional tone or motivation might affect various tasks. Reduced cerebral metabolism (blood supply, access to glucose or oxygen via capillaries) would be expected to slow neural activity. Reduced speed of sensory and motor systems undoubtedly contributes to some slowing.

Attention

Many regions of the brain participate in the modulation of attention. Recent research on attention has tended to focus on the cerebral cortex, but brainstem and other subcortical regions of the brain are equally important. For example, arousal and attention are often mutually interactive; arousal often involves the orientation to stimuli, which, in the process, are being attended to. Thus, factors that affect arousal (see chapter 10) have the potential to diminish attention as well. Similarly, impaired sensory systems, both peripheral and central, can interfere with discrimination and encoding of the stimuli that are being attended to, making attention a more difficult task in general. Even the cerebellum appears to play a role in attention (Allen, Buxton, Wong, & Courchesne, 1997); it also exhibits some age-related deficits (see chapter 8). The interaction of various brain functions during aging has been a recurrent theme, and it certainly applies here.

The role of the cerebral cortex has been elucidated anatomically by evaluating attention in cases of cortical damage and by using neurophysiological methods. Physiological correlates of attention can be inferred if it is shown that neural responses evoked by a stimulus change when the stimulus is attended to by the subject. This can be done using microelectrodes surgically implanted in the brain of behaving animals and by using PET or fMRI in human subjects. As reviewed by Kolb and Whishaw (1996), the research suggests that several cerebral cortical regions are especially important in different aspects of attention. These include spatial attention (parietal cortex), selection of object features (visual and posterior temporal cortex), selection of objects per se (inferior temporal cortex), selection of responses and specific movements (prefrontal/frontal cortex), divided attention (anterior cingulate cortex), and preparation for specific tasks (premotor cortex). Taken together, at least three cortical attentional systems may be identified (see also Posner & Peterson, 1990). First, the posterior parietal cortex may be especially important in engaging, disengaging, and shifting attention from one stimulus set to another.

Second, the posterior temporal region may be especially important for focusing attention on features of the engaged object. Third is the frontal and prefrontal cortex, an attentional system related to short-term memory and associated with tasks involving perceptual demands and response selection. The frontal system has been called the executive attentional system and has been proposed as a region that programs mental operations (Posner & Peterson, 1990).

As mentioned earlier, the gerontological literature indicates that various attentional capacities become diminished with age, but significant age effects tend to be seen only with fairly difficult tasks. Such findings suggest that the neural mechanisms underlying attention are likely to exhibit some age-related changes, albeit not devastating ones. This seems to jibe fairly well with the neurogerontological findings. For example, waking arousal mechanisms involving subcortical structures are generally not severely impaired in older subjects (refer to chapter 10). Similarly, suprathreshold auditory and visual sensory capacities (most important for attention) are typically maintained fairly well unless the systems are overly taxed.

With respect to the cerebral cortex, it must always be kept in mind that there are many avenues of communication with other regions of the brain. Thus, age effects in the cortex are likely to reflect both altered input from other brain structures and changes in the cortical tissue per se. We saw in chapter 8 that the ability of the cerebral cortex to function optimally often becomes diminished with age, as shown by PET studies (Cabeza et al., 1997; De Santi et al., 1995; Eustache et el., 1995; Grady et al., 1995; Loessner et al., 1995; Schacter et al., 1996). Furthermore, aging cortical neurons often exhibit histological abnormalities and/or loss of dendrites, dendritic spines, and presynaptic terminals (Cotman & Holets, 1985; Mann, 1997) and some neurochemical changes (Morgan & May, 1990; Rogers & Bloom, 1985). However, these studies also suggest that the magnitude of age-associated physiological changes usually do not reach a level that would be expected to heavily affect basic mechanisms of attention required for relatively easy tasks.

Chao and Knight (1997) obtained behavioral and event-related potential recordings from young and old subjects in auditory delayed match-to-sample tasks (the subjects had to indicate whether an initial and subsequent test sound were identical). The older subjects exhibited reduced electro-physiological attention-related activity in the frontal cortex (see Figure 11.1). Moreover, when distracting sounds were present, their responses

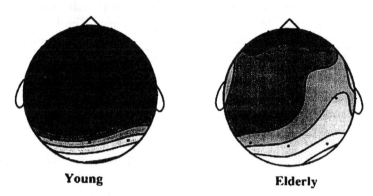

Young   **Elderly**

**FIGURE 11.1   Event-related potential recordings from young and old sub-
jects in auditory delayed match-to-sample tasks. The older subjects exhibited
reduced electrophysiological attention-related activity (sustained frontal neg-
ativity) in the frontal cortex, as indicated by the lighter shading. Reprinted
from Chao, L. L., & Knight, R. T. (1997). Prefrontal deficits in attention
and inhibitory control with aging. *Cerebral Cortex, 7,* 63–69, with permission
from Oxford University Press.**

were stronger to the distractors, compared to the responses of young
subjects (i.e., the young subjects could inhibit responses to the distractors).
The authors interpreted these findings as evidence for reduced ability of
the prefrontal cortex to inhibit responses to irrelevant, distracting stimuli.
As indicated earlier, attentional tasks requiring inhibition are especially
difficult for many older people.

Spatial Abilities

The hippocampus plays a key role in spatial behaviors, presumably in
cooperation with the nearby temporal cortex and other brain regions.
There is a good body of evidence that humans and other species exhibit
deficits in spatial ability when the hippocampus is damaged (Kolb &
Whishaw, 1996). Direct neurophysiological evidence has been obtained
from animal experiments showing that the firing of many hippocampal
neurons is related to spatial stimuli and an animal's location. Indeed,
cognitive maps of space appear to be formed by the activity of populations
of hippocampal neurons. We saw in chapter 8 that a variety of age effects
have been reported for the hippocampus, and that one of the behavioral

manifestations of these appears to be deficits in spatial learning. Given all of this, it is reasonable to conclude that age-related deficits in spatial behaviors are linked to altered hippocampal function.

Recordings of action potentials can be obtained from neurons using microelectrodes implanted in the hippocampi of behaving animals while they engage in spatial behaviors. When this is done, it can be shown that the action potential firing patterns of hippocampal pyramidal neurons are correlated with the animal's spatial location and spatial cues within the test environment (O'Keefe & Nadel, 1978), defining neuronal "place fields." These spatially sensitive neurons are called *place cells* and are presumably critical to spatial learning and other spatial behaviors, collectively producing cognitive maps of space.

Some age-related changes have been observed in the way place cells respond to the spatial environment. Tanila, Shapiro, Gallagher, and Eichenbaum (1997) recorded from young and old rats while manipulating environmental spatial cues. They found, as have others, that the place fields of hippocampal neurons were in many ways similar in old and young rats. There was, however, an age-related decline in the scope of spatial information (different types of cues) that were coded by the neurons of old rats with spatial memory impairment. Hippocampal neurons of these rats were also less able to alter their spatial representations with continued experience (i.e., neural plasticity was attenuated). The same group of researchers (Tanila, Sipila, Shapiro, & Eichenbaum, 1997) found that the hippocampal place fields of old rats did not adapt well to changes in the spatial cues associated with a novel environment. Also, in old rats with poor spatial memory, the spatial selectivity of place fields was diminished.

Another study observed deficits in the plasticity of place fields in hippocampal neurons of old rats that were poor spatial learners (Shen, Barnes, McNaughton, Skaggs, & Weaver, 1997). Hippocampal neuronal activity was monitored in the rats as they ran a rectangular track. As young rats began traversing the track, their hippocampal place fields became larger (for rather arcane reasons, this appears to enhance the quality of spatial information available to the brain); however, this normal expansion of place fields did not occur in the old rats. These data suggest that the old rats were not able to exhibit a type of experience-dependent plasticity likely to improve spatial behavior.

Yet another study found that the place fields of old rats were not stable from test session to test session, although within a test session the place fields maintained consistency (Barnes et al., 1997). Said differently, the old rats could not retrieve the proper cognitive map of space if a period of time had passed.

Taken together, these studies suggest that the ability of hippocampal neurons to process spatial information becomes altered in old rats, especially those with demonstrable spatial learning deficits. However, under some conditions or testing paradigms, the hippocampal neurons of old rats perform their spatial coding tasks quite nicely.

Other cortical regions also contribute to spatial abilities (Kolb & Whishaw, 1996). The parietal lobe is involved in directing movement to a visual target in space. The frontal cortex is important for spatial discriminations and memory. It is also the case that damage to the right hemisphere tends to cause more severe spatial deficits than damage to the left hemisphere.Thus, in addition to looking to the hippocampus and temporal lobe for age effects on spatial behaviors, other brain regions should not be overlooked (recall also that "mental" spatial maneuvers are akin to reasoning). Some of the same physiological changes in cortex discussed earlier could also have an impact on spatial behaviors.

Language and Hemispheric Lateralization

The left hemisphere of most people is specialized for verbal, sequential, and analytical processes. Particularly important for language are *Broca's area* in the left frontal lobe (language production and use of complex grammar) and *Wernicke's area* in the left temporal lobe (comprehension and content of language), although various cortical regions participate in language skills. The right hemisphere is less important for most aspects of language but is quite important with respect to the interpretation and expression of emotion in speech. It is also adept with complex visual patterns, including spatial relationships—more simultaneous or holistic processing rather than sequential.

The cortical neurons of the two hemispheres communicate with one another via their axons, which traverse the corpus callosum. In order to use information in the right hemisphere for the comprehension or production of language, the corpus callosum is required for transfer to the left hemisphere. As discussed in chapter 5, a number of studies have found evidence that the interhemispheric transfer of information across the corpus callosum is often slowed or diminished with age. Thus, less efficient interhemispheric transfer is a potential contributor to those language deficits that do accompany aging.

The various age-related changes in cortical anatomy and physiology, referred to elsewhere, presumably have the potential to interfere with optimal language use. However, as mentioned earlier, many basic language abilities remain relatively unfazed in older people unless strong demands are made upon memory retrieval. Thus, it seems likely that Wernicke's, Broca's, and other cortical areas that are essential for language are not especially vulnerable to age-related declines.

Evidence has been presented by various investigators suggesting that the right hemisphere is more prone to age-related declines than the left (see Nebes, 1990). For example, performance of elders on certain cognitive tests (e.g., object assembly task in the Wechsler IQ test) tend to show changes reminiscent of patients with right hemisphere damage (e.g., spatial skills), whereas verbal (left hemisphere) abilities are less affected. However, such evidence is rather indirect and potentially confounded by differences in the difficulty of tasks and other factors. More direct tests of left-right hemispheric processing, such as reaction times for verbal and spatial stimuli presented to the left or right visual field, have not supported a differential age effect (Nebes, 1990). A recent MRI study by Raz and colleagues (1997) found no evidence of differential left-right hemispheric aging. Thus, there does not seem to be a strong case for asymmetrical aging of the two hemispheres.

Strokes affecting the left hemisphere often produce *aphasia*, a serious disruption or loss of language production and/or comprehension. Because strokes become increasingly common in the elderly population, aphasia has an especially strong impact on this group. Furthermore, when aphasia is acquired by older people, it tends to be severe (Beeson & Bayles, 1997). Whereas aphasia is not an age-related disorder per se, it is a significant gerontological concern.

Intelligence

At this time we know little about the neural basis of intelligence in general, and even less about the neurogerontological aspects. As mentioned above, intelligence is typically viewed as being comprised of a number of different abilities. Because intelligence is multifaceted, the underlying neural mechanisms undoubtedly involve the integration of many different brain functions. Some of the abilities that can become diminished with age are likely to affect certain components of intelligence profiles. An obvious example is deficient learning and declarative memory. By the same token, relatively intact implicit memory systems are likely to stabilize certain components of intelligence.

Whereas many brain regions and neural networks must be involved in intelligence, the frontal cortex may play a particularly important role in the context of aging. There is some evidence that frontal lobe damage has strong negative effects on fluid intelligence (Duncan, 1995), the type of intelligence that declines with age. As indicated earlier, the frontal lobes are particularly vulnerable to age-associated dysfunction, suggesting that the diminution of fluid intelligence with aging might be a function of frontal lobe impairment.

PERSONALITY

Personality can be viewed in the context of integration as an interaction among neural circuits subserving cognitive, emotional, perceptual, and many other functions related to personal behavior and behavioral tendencies. Most research and theory concerning personality has not interfaced with neuroscience, and we can say very little about any neurogerontological correlates. Nevertheless, personality is a defining concept with respect to individual differences in behavior and presumably plays an important role in the overall aging process. Thus, a brief discussion and some speculation are warranted.

Ruth (1996) discussed three theoretical approaches to the study of personality that have gerontological implications. First is the *personality traits* approach. Fairly specific personality traits can be defined and measured by various psychological tests. When this approach is taken, it seems that most traits tend to remain stable during adulthood. On the other hand, when traits are defined as dimensions or motives (e.g., achievement, affiliation, power), there is evidence that their relative weights change with age. Second is the *developmental* approach, which views personality in terms of stages or phases across the life span. Thus, for example, there may be a transition from young adulthood to middle age and another from middle age to old age. These often involve evaluations of one's past accomplishments and progress and future directions and prospects. The most famous stage theory is that of Erik Erikson (1963), who postulated eight stages based on biological, psychological, and sociocultural processes, each of which involves a basic "crisis." The dominant crisis of old age is *integrity versus despair*, with resolution leading to wisdom, which includes a philosophical view about one's life, humanity, and death. The third approach is the *experiential-contextual model*, in which personality change is mapped as a function of social, historical, and individual variables—a transactional process with continual change across the life span.

How can we begin to approach something as varied, complicated, and biologically elusive as personality from the perspective of neurogerontology? At this time, perhaps all we can do is to conceptualize how a biological approach might work. To do so, let us take the three approaches to personality just outlined and apply them to a more tangible entity, say, personal participation and interest in sports. It is not too difficult to see how biological and environmental variables combine to produce sports participation patterns across the life span and, by analogy, how personality might be modulated as well.

Traits.   The sports a person likes to take part in or follow as a spectator can be seen as traits, and these are likely to remain relatively stable across time (subject to physical limitations). The original trait sports resulted from the person's biological abilities (speed, size, coordination, emotional reactions to playing them) and exposure to specific sports as a youngster. Presumably, personality traits form along similar lines, and there is no a priori reason for either to change drastically as a person ages. On the other hand, one's motives for playing these sports (winning vs. just having fun) may change dramatically over the years. The winning motive in sports, one assumes, is closely related to aggressiveness. In males, this is probably linked to testosterone and other mechanisms that peak during young adulthood (see chapter 12). As these hormonal-aggressive mechanisms wane with age, sport motives are likely to follow suit. The basic trait sports may still be followed, but the motives for playing them vary in accord with biological change. It seems reasonable that motives driving certain personality traits could be affected in an analogous manner as people age, and thus be accessible to neurogerontological research approaches.

Development.   Within the array of sports one enjoys, there is likely to be a transition favoring high-energy activity during young adulthood, to medium energy during middle age, to low energy during old age. There is likely to be an increased interest in the strategic or intellectual aspects of the game as well. For example, this might be manifested as playing different roles in one sport (singles player vs. doubles player vs. coach).

The notion of developmental stages in sports participation is presumably closely tied to the relevant physical and psychological factors that change across the life span. In sports these are likely to involve sensory and motor abilities, which have a peak stage devolving into stages of lesser proficiency. At the same time the finer details of the game become more central as one becomes older. These stages are derivatives of an array of biological changes and learned material, upon which roughly defined boundaries can be imposed. Just as these biological stages influence sports participation, it is reasonable that changes in a whole array of neural and other variables could promote a developmental progression through personality stages.

Experiential-contextual model. The sports one has grown up with, the opportunity to continue with these or learn new ones, and the age-appropriateness of various sports determine which sports are played as one ages. The experiential-contextual factors basically modulate the manifestation of the traits and motives, either facilitating or inhibiting them according to age-appropriate variables. This is, in some ways, another way of viewing the always-occurring interactions among genetic and environmental factors. Presumably, most age-related changes in both sports participation and personality are influenced by the nuances of experience, life situations, and context overlaying an individual's biological status.

When viewed through the lens of an analogy like this, it is reasonable to assume that personality—and the way it is or is not modified with age—is modulated by neurobiological variables. Indeed, several theorists have proposed neurobiological models of personality that might serve as a framework for neurogerontological studies (see Starratt & Peterson, 1997). Furthermore, some neurodegenerative diseases affecting older people result in clear changes in personality (see below), suggesting that less severe changes associated with normal aging might have subtle effects. We may be very far from elucidating the neural bases of personality variables and aging, but such an endeavor seems conceptually feasible.

ALZHEIMER'S DISEASE: THE DISINTEGRATION OF COGNITION

The notion that higher levels of integration of cognitive processes reflect the effectiveness of integration at the neuronal level is tragically validated by AD. Patients in the advanced stages of AD have a myriad of neuronal pathologies that disable many brain circuits, and this is accompanied by a multifaceted demise of cognition, emotion, and personality. Both the severity of AD symptoms and the growing number of people stricken with the disease (nearly 4 million Americans, a number that could double in 20 years) have moved AD to the forefront of neurogerontological research efforts. Research on AD has been the focus of intense effort supported by the National Institute on Aging and other research-funding bodies. With new findings surfacing weekly to build on an already huge body of research, we cannot begin to do justice to this topic in this book. Thus, we review some of the highlights, particularly those that fit within the themes developed thus far. Recent books and chapters have reviewed the latest work in this area (e.g., Albert & Knoefel, 1994; Cohen, 1988; Khachaturian & Radenbaugh, 1996; Mann, 1997; Salmon & Bondi, 1997; Terry, Katzman, & Bick, 1994), and much of this review is drawn from these detailed compilations of research on AD.

AD probably includes several related disorders that differ with respect to etiology, age of onset, and other factors. The onset of Alzheimer's disease is often subtle, being first manifested by mood changes, faulty judgment, memory impairment, disorientation in time and space, and depression. These can progress, possibly being joined by bouts of irritability or anxiety, disruption of sleep, loss of communication skills, and impairment in the performance of routine tasks, abstract thinking, learning, and the ability to carry out mathematical calculations. Changes in personality occur. The disease may progress to include severe neurological complications, apathy, loss of responsiveness to stimuli, institutionalization, and, ultimately, death. The time from onset to death can range from 2 to 20 years.

From the time it was discovered by Dr. Alois Alzheimer in 1907, AD has been definitively diagnosed using postmortem histological criteria, the presence of neuritic plaques and neurofibrillary tangles in the brain (see below). Premortem diagnosis has always presented problems, because other disorders (and even normal aging) share some symptoms of early AD, with memory impairment being the most obvious of these. Until relatively recently, there were large error rates with respect to diagnosis of AD and other types of dementia, often as a misdiagnosis of depression. However, newer mental status tests and questionnaires have much improved diagnostic accuracy. Key elements are sensitive tests of episodic memory, one of the first capacities to become diminished in AD (see

Salmon & Bondi, 1997). Modern criteria for probable AD appear to be quite accurate when confirmed by autopsy. Other methods are being brought into the diagnostic arsenal as well. Sophisticated analyses of EEG patterns (Besthorn et al., 1997) and ERPs like the P300 (Kugler et al., 1993) are likely to prove useful. Modern neuroimaging techniques, including CT, MRI, PET (see Figure 2.2), and SPECT, are being increasingly used to assess pathologic signs of AD in living patients, such as enhanced localized brain atrophy (Davis et al., 1994). Figure 11.2 (de Toledo-Morrell et al.; 1997) presents MRIs from a normal (left) and a clinically diagnosed AD patient with moderate dementia (right). In the AD patient, cortical sulci and ventricles (the spaces in and around the brain) are enlarged, indicative of atrophy. The hippocampus (seen on each side in the lower portion of the images) is severely degenerated. Still, AD can be confused with multiple cerebral infarcts or some other types of cerebrovascular events, and postmortem histology remains, for now, the definitive criterion for a determination of the disease.

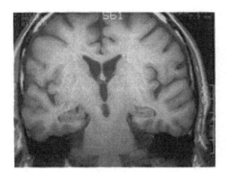 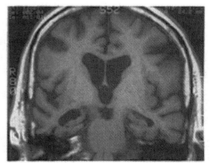

FIGURE 11.2   MRIs from a normal (left) and a clinically diagnosed AD patient with moderate dementia (right). In the AD patient, cortical sulci and ventricles are enlarged, and the hippocampus (seen on each side in the lower portion of the images) is severely degenerated. Reprinted from De Toledo-Morrell, L., Sullivan, M. P., Morell, F., Wilson, R. S., Bennett, D. A., & Spencer, S. (1997). Alzheimer's disease: In vivo detection of differential vulnerability of brain regions. *Neurobiology of Aging, 18,* 463–468, with permission from Elsevier Sciences, Inc.

Risk Factors and Causes

Three major risk factors for AD have been identified (Khachaturian & Radenbaugh, 1996). First is age. The prevalence of AD increases exponentially with age, and the percentage doubles every decade beyond age 65. Some 25% to 35% of those over 85 are affected by some form of dementia. Second is family history (genetic predisposition). The occurrence of AD in a parent or sibling increases risk by 3 or 4 times. As many as five genes have been linked to AD, including *APP*, *Presenilin 1*, *Presenilin 2*, *ApoE4*, and *A2M* (Marks, 1998). Third, a history of severe head injury that leads to loss of consciousness doubles the risk of developing AD. On the other hand, some factors decrease risk. These include educational and occupational success, and possibly postmenopausal estrogen replacement and long-term use of anti-inflammatory drugs. Evidence has indicated that cigarette smoking can decrease the risk of AD (nicotine is a cholinergic drug, which might ameliorate the degeneration of cholinergic neurons; see below). However, a recent study of a large population in Rotterdam concluded just the opposite: Smoking was associated with a doubling of the risk of AD and other dementias (Ott et al., 1998).

The reasons that various abnormalities arise in the brains of AD patients are not yet clear, but both environmental and genetic factors undoubtedly play key roles. Indeed, because AD apparently includes a number of related disorders, a variety of causes are feasible, and these are not mutually exclusive. Some leading contenders are genetic defects (e.g., Rubinsztein, 1997), including the genes mentioned earlier (the allele ApoE-4 and its relationship to AD is discussed later in the chapter); mitochondrial dysfunction and associated cellular energy crisis; free radical damage to cells (e.g., Harman, 1995b); deformed capillaries and/or impaired blood-brain barrier; faulty protein synthesis by cells (van Leeuwen et al., 1998); glutamate excitotoxicity and/or altered calcium homeostasis (see chapter 3); the toxic effects of β-amyloid protein, a major component of the plaques that are characteristic of AD (some research has suggested that the protein itself might be a cause of the pathology associated with AD and that its occurrence can be associated with genetic abnormalities). The accumulation of aluminum can produce tanglelike structures or other damage in the brains of experimental animals, and there have been reports of increased aluminum content in AD patients; however, strong evidence for a causative role of aluminum or other trace elements has not been provided. Aluminum, however, may accumulate in degenerating neurons and might exacerbate degeneration, as might mercury, zinc, iron, and certain other elements (Markesbery, 1996).

Changes in the Brain

The brains of AD patients exhibit a variety of degenerative changes, including the loss of dendrites and synapses, neuron death, abnormal capillaries, senile plaques, and neurofibrillary tangles (Giannakopoulos, Hof, Michel, Guimon, & Bouras, 1997; Khachaturian & Radenbaugh, 1996; Mann, 1997; Terry et al., 1994). Senile plaques and tangles are the histopathological hallmarks of AD.

Senile plaques.   Senile plaques are found in the brain tissue. They are composed of various glial and neuronal cellular elements surrounding or intermixed with β-amyloid protein. Although these are seen in older brains of many non-AD patients, they increase greatly in number in those afflicted with AD. The deposition of amyloid is probably the first event in the formation of plaques, which can evolve into more complex forms over the years. The β-amyloid is not produced directly from a gene but is derived from *amyloid precursor protein*, which is coded by a gene. β-amyloid is thought to be toxic to brain and other tissue, probably causing or contributing to neural damage. The toxicity may involve the induction of apoptosis or necrosis following oxidative stress, Ca^{++}-mediated excitotoxicity, or other mechanisms. However, whether there is a direct role of β-amyloid is still not clear (e.g., a substance or process that produces β-amyloid may be the real culprit). The deposition of β-amyloid is influenced by apolipoprotein E (ApoE), and a variant of the gene coding ApoE has been linked to some forms of AD (see Figure 11.3, colorplate following page 268).

Neurofibrillary tangles.   These thick, twisted fibrils are found within neurons, where they occupy the cell body and even extend into axons and dendrites. The fibrils are actually pairs of aligned filaments that are wound about one another to form a helix, and the term *paired helical filament* is often used instead of neurofibrillary tangle. Sometimes tangles are seen in the neuropil without a host neuron, presumably because the neuron has disappeared, leaving the "ghost" tangles behind. Neurofibrillary tangles come in a variety of forms depending on which type of neuron they occupy. The principal constituent of neurofibrillary tangles is the microtubule-associated protein *tau*, at least some of which exists in an abnormal (overphosphorylated) state. Presumably, disruption of the microtubule component of the cytoskeleton would interfere with neuronal cell functions such as the transport of substances between soma and axon terminal (see chapter 3) and other cellular functions—events likely to prove fatal to the neuron (growing evidence is indicating that changes in tau can cause damage to neurons in several forms of neurodegenerative disease [Vogel, 1998]). Neurofibrillary tangles are observed in the brains of many nondemented older people, but in much lower numbers than in patients with AD. In healthy elderly people, tangles are most likely to occur in the hippocampal complex (especially the CA1 field), nearby entorhinal cortex, and amygdala, but they occasionally show up elsewhere as well. Tangles are prevalent in these areas and elsewhere in AD patients but at much higher concentrations.

Deficits in cerebral metabolism and blood supply. Insufficiency of cerebral blood supply and oxidative metabolism have been implicated in AD (Blass, 1996; De la Torre, 1997). It is well known (e.g., from aviation literature) that impaired cerebral oxidative metabolism produces cognitive changes similar to those seen in AD. The development of PET and other physiological imaging techniques has shown that parts of the brain involved in cognitive functions do not use glucose normally in AD patients (see chapter 2, Figure 2.2), lending credence to this view. And, of course, severe oxygen deprivation spells doom for neurons.

Many studies have observed pathological changes in the blood vessels and capillaries of AD brains, and this has been proposed as playing a causative role in AD pathology (de la Torre, 1997). Capillaries of AD patients exhibit deformities such as twisting and kinking, especially in the hippocampus. The capillaries also become thicker, the endothelial cell lining (the substrate of the blood-brain barrier) becomes altered, and amyloid is deposited in the vessel walls. Such changes would be expected to deprive the brain of basic nutrients (glucose, oxygen), affecting cell metabolism. Furthermore, impairment of the blood-brain barrier could make it difficult to eliminate metabolic waste products and expose neural tissue to toxins.

There is also evidence accumulating to indicate that impairments of oxidative metabolism occur within the neurons of AD patients (Blass, 1996). Because the mitochondria are the metabolic engines of cells, they are probably involved here, and damage to mitochondria has been identified in AD brains. Recent work has indicated that mutations in mitochondrial DNA may contribute to AD in some patients (Barinaga, 1997).

Brain Regions Affected in AD

AD is a heterogeneous disease in that it affects various brain regions and to various extents. However, the common thread is the loss and dysfunction of neurons and disrupted connections. In particular, the significant loss of synapses in the cerebral cortex is thought to be a primary factor in the behavioral and cognitive symptoms of AD (see Jones & Harris, 1995).

A good deal of early evidence indicated that cholinergic neurotransmitter systems were impaired in AD patients, particularly those involving the basal forebrain (Bartus, Dean, Beer, & Lippa, 1982; Coyle, Price, & DeLong, 1983). Since Ach has long been known to be important in cognitive functioning, impairment of this transmitter made sense. However, a preeminent role of cholinergic mechanisms of AD has proven to be less compelling than was first believed. Indeed, other neurotransmitter systems and noncholinergic brain regions are also severely affected in AD.

Many anatomical studies of AD brains have reported degenerative changes, diminution of synapses, and neuronal losses, often in excess of 50% (Giannakopoulos et al., 1997; T. L. Kemper, 1994; Mann, 1997; Scheibel, 1996). Whereas, brain atrophy can be widespread (refer back to Figure 11.2), some regions of the brain are affected more than others.

1. The cerebral cortex.   The cerebral cortex of AD patients is generally reduced in volume, and this is associated with the loss and degeneration of cortical neurons. Especially vulnerable are the large pyramidal cells in areas of frontal, parietal, and temporal lobes, areas of special importance for a variety of cognitive processes. The cingulate cortex, involved in certain attentional and emotional functions, is also prone to damage in AD. Various areas of the cerebral cortex also exhibit a large decrease in the density of synapses, indicating severe disruption of neural circuitry and, presumably, neural coding and the processing of information.

The several layers of cortex exhibit different degrees of histopathology in AD, and the cortical layers that are most affected differ across brain regions (Giannakopoulos et al., 1997). In the entorhinal cortex, layers 1 and 5 tend to have the greatest concentration of neurofibrillary tangles. These layers contain neurons whose axons project to the hippocampus, amygdala, and other regions of the cortex, suggesting that AD might produce a sort of disconnection syndrome, analogous to conditions where projecting axons are severed or interrupted, preventing normal communication among brain regions.

2. The basal forebrain. As discussed in chapter 8, the basal forebrain region (nucleus basalis of Meynert, medial septal nucleus, and diagonal band) is a major source of cholinergic and noncholinergic innervation of the cerebral cortex and hippocampus. Numerous studies have demonstrated extensive loss of neurons and/or other degenerative changes in the basal forebrain (especially the nucleus basalis) of AD patients. For example, Mann (1997) listed 20 research articles showing such effects. These circuits play key roles in spatial and other types of learning and memory as well as attention, and damage to the basal forebrain has serious consequences for these capacities. Thus, it is generally accepted that this neuropathology contributes to the attentional and cognitive changes that accompany AD.

3. The hippocampus, amygdala, and associated circuitry. The CA1 area, subiculum, and entorhinal cortex are especially susceptible to damage in AD. In the amygdala, as much as a 50% to 70% loss of neurons may occur in AD patients (Herzog & Kemper, 1980; Vereecken, Vogels, & Nieuwenhuys, 1994), and it is an area where plaque and tangle formation are pronounced. Presumably, hippocampal damage contributes to learning, memory, and spatial orientation deficits observed in AD patients, whereas dysfunction of the amygdala can help explain emotional and learning changes.

4. The locus coeruleus. A good-sized body of research has demonstrated severe loss of locus coeruleus neurons in AD patients. A recent study using unbiased stereological methods found the locus coeruleus of AD patients to have 50% fewer neurons than like-aged, non-AD patients (Busch, Bohl, & Ohm, 1997). An early sign of AD pathology is the appearance of neurofibrillary tangles, especially in those regions of the locus coeruleous projecting to the cerebral cortex and hippocampus (vs. regions projecting to the cerebellum or spinal cord). As discussed in chapter 10, the noradrenergic neurons of the locus coeruleus innervate many other areas of the brain and play an important role in arousal, sleep, and other functions that are disrupted in AD.

5. Other regions.   Damage to a number of other brain regions (loss of neurons or accumulation of tangles) has been reported as well. These include the dopaminergic mesolimbic system, serotonergic raphe nuclei, and parts of the thalamus, basal ganglia, and hypothalamus. There are also some regional differences in vulnerability within certain brain structures (e.g., the neurons of the locus coeruleus projecting to the forebrain more than those projecting to the spinal cord). Areas that are typically only mildly to moderately affected include the cerebellum and substantia nigra. Some areas are generally spared, such as brainstem nuclei in the pons and the mammillary bodies adjacent to the hypothalamus. One generalization supported by much of the literature is that subcortical neurons that project to the cerebral cortex are likely to be deleteriously affected in AD.

Other Dementias

Several other less common syndromes can severely impair integrative functions in the elderly. Frontotemporal dementias such as *Pick's disease* have clinical similarities to AD, but greater changes in personality, inappropriate social behavior, and altered (usually blunted) emotionality, perseverative behavior, and language impairment characterize these dementias (Usman, 1997). Pick's disease is actually most common between ages 40 and 60—more a disease of middle age rather than old age. Pick's disease and related disorders are associated with neuronal degeneration primarily in frontal and temporal lobes, although subcortical structures (e.g., amygdala, hippocampus) may be involved as well. Round-shaped filamentous inclusions called *Pick bodies* are found in neurons of Pick's disease patients and probably represent degeneration of the neuronal cytoskeleton. Other pathological changes, such as neurofibrillary tangles, are present as well.

Multi-infarct dementias are caused by small infarcts (lesions caused by the occlusion of capillaries or blood vessels) that may occur at any age but are increasingly common after 65 or when the patient has a history

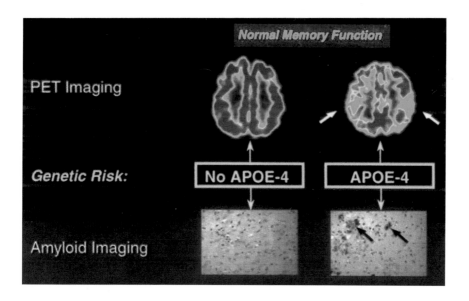

FIGURE 11.3 Imaging genetic risk for AD. Even before cognitive impairment is significant, PET imaging differentiates the patient at risk for AD and normal brain. Courtesy of Gary W. Small, MD, Department of Psychiatry and Biobehavioral Sciences, and Department of Molecular and Medical Pharmacology, Crump Institute for Biological Imaging, University of California, Los Angeles.

of strokes. Multi-infarct dementias have a sudden onset, and the particular type of dementia that results depends on the regions of the brain that are involved. Progression of symptoms may occur in a stepwise fashion as additional infarcts occur. The more general term *vascular dementias* is used to include dementias associated with blood supply interruption not only from infarcts but also from hemorrhage or other causes (McPherson & Cummings, 1997).

There can also be apparent combinations of different neurodegenerative disorders (Mirra & Markesbery, 1996). Patients can have both AD and vascular dementia at the same time, for example. A number of patients also have signs of both AD and Parkinson's disease—Lewy bodies and degeneration of the substantia nigra (see chapter 9). The presence of Lewy bodies in the cerebral cortex has been associated with cognitive impairments similar to those accompanying AD, and there may be several Lewy body diseases that range from Parkinson's disease to some variant of AD.

SUMMARY AND IMPLICATIONS

It is clear that many of the brain regions affected by AD and other neurodegenerative diseases can also exhibit some age-related degeneration in healthy people, albeit to a much lesser extent. And, as mentioned elsewhere, plaques, tangles, and other inclusions can be observed in small numbers in the brains of nondemented people. These qualitative similarities/quantitative differences can be interpreted from two different perspectives. On the one hand, they might suggest that AD reflects an exaggeration of "normal" age-related changes. Assume that AD-like neuropathology ranges from minimal to severe in the general elderly population; those with minimal pathology are considered the healthy elderly, whereas those at the other end of the scale are diagnosed as having AD. The distribution of symptom severity would be a complex function of genetic and environmental factors which facilitate or retard aging of the brain. On the other hand, it might be that only people who are virtually free of AD pathology constitute the healthy elderly. Then, individuals with small magnitudes of neural degeneration, plaques, or tangles would represent preclinical AD patients who would presumably develop full-blown AD if they survived (those features presently being detectable only after death). According to this view, the occurrence of a few plaques and tangles is not "normal aging"; rather, it is the presymptomatic beginning of a disease process.

There is yet a third interpretation, however, and it simply borrows from both perspectives. That is, minimal AD-like neurodegenerative features can occur in healthy brains and, in fortunate individuals, never become significantly worse as they age; such people are not preclinical, because AD will not develop. Another, much less fortunate group develops minimal pathology at some point in life, but this ultimately does progress to full-blown AD; the early stages are indeed preclinical. What determines whether an individual has no AD-like symptoms, minimal nonprogressive symptoms, or symptoms progressing to AD may be a function of the various causes and risk factors outlined earlier. To use an analogy, some generally healthy people may never get a chest cold, some may get minor chest colds that never become severe, whereas for others, a chest cold might progress to pneumonia. The early signs (chest cold) may or may not be preclinical symptoms of pneumonia; that depends on a host of variables.

Although these somewhat subtle distinctions among perspectives might not seem important to the family of a person stricken with AD, they may have implications for the future with respect to how AD is diagnosed, managed, and treated. It seems likely that the most promising future treatment strategies for AD will lie in early diagnosis and retardation of the progression of pathology. This is, of course, true of cancer and many other progressive diseases as well. It is also likely that in the near future, methods will be developed to identify definitive early AD signs *in vivo*. When this becomes feasible, it will be very important to know if the occurrence of these signs does, in fact, represent minimal, "normal" age-related change, or preclinical AD (it might be one or the other for different people). Such a determination would dictate the appropriate course of action (see Mann, 1997, for a good discussion of this issue). Indeed, promising methods are already appearing, as indicated by Figure 11.3. The upper images show PET scans in two people in their mid-sixties with normal performance on neuropsychological tests; the subject with a genetic risk for Alzheimer's disease (the ApoE-4 gene) shows the beginnings of hypometabolism in the parietal lobe (arrows). The lower images show greater amyloid staining (arrows) in a subject with Alzheimer's disease and the ApoE-4 allele compared to one without ApoE-4 allele.

Hopefully, neurogerontological research on the relationships among risk factors, environmental agents, specific gene actions, histopathology, behavioral diagnostic symptoms, and normal aging will someday all come together to interface with new, effective therapeutic strategies for slowing or stopping the elaboration of AD.

12
Sex and Reproduction

Although reproduction is, biologically speaking, the most important of the seven basic functions of nervous systems, we will not have too much to say in this relatively brief chapter. There are two reasons for this. First, reproduction occupies a unique place in gerontology, in that this activity is designed to be carried out prior to old age. After menopause, women are no longer capable of bearing children, and fatherhood is rare (although some men remain fertile beyond age 90). Thus, a good portion of gerontological research addresses the decline of reproductive capacity during middle age. A second reason for the brevity of this chapter is that only a limited amount of research has focused on the involvement of the nervous system in the decline of reproductive capacity. Although the brain has an important role to play, changes in the gonads and their hormones have been the focus of most research on aging and reproductive systems.

It should be emphasized at the outset that, in our species, a loss of fertility with age does not go hand in hand with a parallel cessation of sexual behavior (see Morley, 1992; Weg, 1996). Whereas a variety of studies have shown there to be a decrease in sexual activity with advancing age, quite a few older women and men have active sex lives. Studies have differed in their findings but have reported that anywhere from about 10% to more than 30% of women in their 70s and 80s engage in sexual intercourse. Studies have also shown that the attitudes many older people have about sexual activity are quite positive, and sex is an important aspect of their lives. These data undoubtedly reflect the fact that human sexual behavior is not a simple function of hormonally driven biological mechanisms. The sex hormones, in particular, testosterone, do indeed facilitate and activate sexual behavior, but other factors are important as well. These include physical and emotional pleasure, maintenance of interpersonal relationships, and sociocultural practices and expectations.

In any event, it seems clear that the neural circuitry necessary for sexual desire and/or motivation remains intact in many older people.

Although many elderly people have active sex lives, this is not to say that aging of the nervous system does not place limits on sexual capacities. As is the case with virtually every other behavior we have discussed in this book, sexual behavior is a complex function of many interacting brain circuits and regions. Sensory stimuli are important for sexual arousal and performance, so it would be expected that declines in sensory systems would take a toll. The autonomic nervous system has a major influence on penile erections and other bodily sexual responses, and we know from chapter 6 that autonomic changes occur (and impotence is a problem for some older men). The same can be said of the cardiovascular system, whose limitations are also relevant to the physical exertion attendant to sex. The various other functions of the nervous system presumably come into play as well. The spirit may be willing, but the nervous system may not always be up to the task.

HORMONES AND SEXUAL ACTIVITY

In women, hormones of the hypothalamus, pituitary gland, and ovaries interact to regulate the menstrual cycle and ovulation (see Kalat, 1998; Rosenzweig et al., 1996). Two key hormones are released by the anterior pituitary. The first is follicle stimulating hormone (FSH), which promotes the growth of ovarian follicles to produce ova (egg cells) and the secretion of estrogen (in particular, estradiol) by the ovaries. This is followed by a surge in the second anterior pituitary hormone luteinizing hormone (LH). The LH surge leads to the release of an ovum, followed by the secretion of the ovarian hormone progesterone by the follicle remnant (the corpus luteum). If the ovum is not fertilized, menstruation occurs and the cycle begins anew. The whole process is regulated by various feedback interactions among hormones, some of which are discussed later.

The male anterior pituitary also produces FSH and LH. LH stimulates the *Leydig cells* of the testes to produce testosterone and other steroid hormones. The main effect of FSH is to support the function of the *seminiferous tubules*, which play a key role in the production of sperm. Testosterone, in turn, has a variety of effects and participates in a negative feedback loop to inhibit LH secretion by hypothalamus-pituitary activity.

The hormone inhibin is synthesized in the ovaries and testes. The action of inhibin is to suppress FSH secretion in a feedback loop.

For both males and females, anterior pituitary hormone release is under the control of a hormone produced by the hypothalamus, gonadotropin-releasing hormone (GnRH), also known as luteinizing hormone-releasing hormone (LHRH). The hypothalamic-releasing hormone causes the pituitary to secrete LH and FSH into the bloodstream. GnRH release by hypothalamic neurons is suppressed by the gonadal hormones (testosterone and estrogen) in a negative feedback arrangement. The hypothalamic-pituitary-gonadal relationships are shown in Figure 12.1.

AGE-RELATED CHANGES IN WOMEN: MENOPAUSE

Menopause occurs reliably during middle age, and a good deal of research has addressed this topic (Bellantoni & Blackman, 1996; Harman & Talbert,

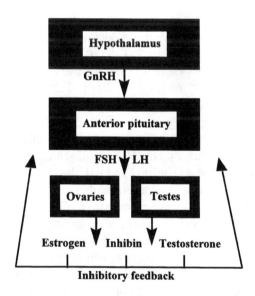

FIGURE 12.1 The hypothalamic-pituitary-gonadal axes. Stimulation of the anterior pituitary by the hypothalamus, under the control of GnRH, causes the anterior pituitary to release hormones. The hormones FSH and LH act on the gonads, which secrete their respective sex hormones. Estrogen and testosterone have a variety of effects on reproductive and other tissue, and there is a negative feedback influence as well.

1985; Mobbs, 1996; Morley, Korenman, & Kaiser, 1992; Nowak & Mooradian, 1996; Wise, Krajnak, & Kashon, 1996). Failure of the ovaries is responsible for the cessation of menses and loss of fertility, as well as a drastic reduction in estrogen. The transition to menopause usually takes from 2 to 7 years (obviously, a wide range of individual differences), with the average age in the United States being about 50 years (range: 40 to 60 years). There is a progressive loss of ovarian follicles in women of ovulating age, and the onset of menopause is associated with a reduction in their number to a critical level. The length of the menstrual cycle decreases with age from about 35 days at age 15 to 28 days at age 35. As menopause approaches, the cycles may become irregular and hormone secretions are altered in amount and timing. In addition to the loss of fertility, menopause can be accompanied by negative health effects associated with diminished estrogen (see below).

Hormonal Changes

A variety of hormonal changes are associated with menopause (Bellantoni & Blackman, 1996; Harman & Talbert, 1985; Mobbs, 1996; Morley et al., 1992; Nowak & Mooradian, 1996; Wise et al., 1996). Most notably, secretion of estrogen by the ovaries drops dramatically. Progesterone secretion also falls. As estrogen levels drop, levels of FSH and LH increase (with LH increases occurring later). The increases in FSH and LH are presumably a result of the loss of negative feedback influences of estrogen on the hypothalamic-pituitary GnRH system, which modulates these gonadotropins (increased levels of FSH and LH also occur in ovariectomized young women). A decrease in ovarian inhibin may also contribute to the rise in FSH, which begins even before estrogen levels are greatly altered. Postmenopausal FSH levels increase to a greater extent than LH, but neither continues to change much thereafter.

The ovaries also produce androgens (which can be converted to estrogen), and these are reduced, but to a lesser extent, with menopause. Besides the gonads, other sources of hormones exist, such as adipose tissue (estrogen) and the adrenal glands (the androgen dehydroepiandosterone, or DHEA, and small amounts of progesterone). However, their output is reduced with age as well. Growth hormone (GH) activity is attenuated with menopause as well.

The occurrence of menopause and the accompanying reduction in estrogen are of considerable importance to older women. In addition to its role in reproductive physiology, estrogen affects a variety of other functions. These include nutrient absorption, bone and mineral metabolism, cardiovascular function, regulation of circadian rhythms, memory, and other aspects of cognition. Thus, menopause may have far-ranging age effects. Consequently, estrogen replacement therapy is often prescribed for postmenopausal women. Indeed, there is a rapidly growing body of evidence that estrogen can attenuate or retard the onset of Alzheimer's disease and associated cognitive deficits (Wickelgren, 1997a).

AGE-RELATED CHANGES IN THE MALE REPRODUCTIVE SYSTEM

Men do not experience a cessation of fertility comparable to menopause (Mobbs, 1996; Nowak & Mooradian, 1996; Tenover, 1992). Rather, changes occur gradually and over a long period of time. The term *male climacteric* is often used to describe the decline in testosterone production and associated symptoms that have similarities to menopause, but a constellation of severe changes is not typical of healthy aging men.

Age-related changes in testicular function are characterized by a great deal of individual variance. The changes can include small reductions of tissue involved in spermatogenesis (and therefore a decline in sperm production), Leydig cell number or output, and testicular size. Circulating levels of testosterone decline in most but not all older men. Circadian fluctuations in testosterone levels become blunted. The clearance rate of testosterone does not become increased and may even decrease with age, leading to the conclusion that it is the production of testosterone that is affected.

Testosterone can be converted to estrogen (estradiol), and a low level of this "female" hormone is present in men. Because of reduced levels of testosterone and/or greater levels of estrogen (e.g., from reduced clearance), the estrogen-testosterone ratio is typically higher in older men.

As the functional capacities of the testes decline with age, an increase in the serum level of LH and FSH is often observed. This is likely to reflect a decrease in testicular function, including reduced production of inhibin. Changes in the hypothalamus-pituitary production of gonadotropins may occur as well. The frequency and amplitude of the pulsed release of LH may decrease, and there may be a lower reserve of LH in the older pituitary. The interactions among hormone production, hormonal feedback influences, and hypothalamic-pituitary function are complex, and much remains to be learned with respect to the mechanisms underlying age-related changes in men (see Mobbs, 1996; Nowak & Mooradian, 1996; Tenover, 1992).

Testosterone and aggressive behavior.   Various lines of research have linked aggressive male behavior to testosterone (see Rosenzweig et al., 1996). For example, the emergence of aggressive behavior during human adolescence is partly attributable to rising levels of testosterone; in seasonally breeding animals, annual increases in testosterone levels drive intermale aggression; and castration of male animals markedly reduces aggressive behavior, whereas replacement with injections of testosterone restores it.

As we have seen, testosterone levels gradually decrease with age, begging the question of whether this would affect aggressive behavior. Such a relationship is certainly feasible. The rate of participation in violent crime increases during adolescence, peaks at about age 18, and declines steadily during adulthood. After age 50, violent crime rates are very low (Flynn, 1996). This pattern roughly follows the rise and fall of testosterone activity across the life span.

So is the age-related decline in testosterone a major contributor to reduced violent and aggressive behavior exhibited by older men? It seems that very little research has addressed this question. The paucity of gerontological research is perhaps understandable, since the factors underlying aggressive behavior in humans are many and diverse. Obviously, many social, personality, cultural, physical, law enforcement, and other factors contribute to the level of aggressive behaviors exhibited. Moreover, the literature attempting to relate testosterone levels within individual human males to their aggressive or violent behaviors have been mixed and controversial (see Rosenzweig et al., 1996). Nevertheless, it seems feasible that declining testosterone levels would have some gentling effect on at least some older men. This might be manifested not only with respect to physical aggression but also with respect to personality traits such as intermale competitiveness. Although the rarity of violent behavior diminishes its importance as a practical gerontological issue, research on this question might provide important insights into the neurobiology of aggression.

THE HYPOTHALAMUS

It is clear that the events associated with menopause involve hormones of the ovaries (estrogen, progesterone, inhibin), as well as those of the anterior pituitary (FSH, LH) and hypothalamus (GnRH). There has been some debate about the extent to which ovarian hormonal changes trigger menopause, as opposed to being secondary effects of hypothalamic aging (Wise et al., 1996). One view holds that ovarian decline triggers the hypothalamic-pituitary changes of menopause. The other, not mutually exclusive, view holds that changes in the central nervous system drive the menopausal transition. In other words, ovarian changes are a consequence of neural changes. The feasibility of a direct role of the hypothalamus stems from observations that attenuation of GnRH secretion by the hypothalamus could potentially explain both LH and FSH changes that occur as menopause approaches. GnRH secretion is regulated by a number of hypothalamic neurotransmitters and neuropeptide modulators. Research on rodents indicates that hypothalamic control of these systems becomes disrupted during middle age, early enough to be a cause, rather than effect, of ovarian change. Changes include reduced secretion, changes in gene expression within GnRH producing neurons, altered sensitivity to hormonal feedback, and altered synaptic efficacy (Nowak & Mooradian, 1996; Mobbs, 1996; Wise et al., 1996).

Whether or not hypothalamic changes represent cause and/or effect, there is evidence that the regulation of GnRH secretion becomes altered with age in both females and males. For example: (1) Hypothalamic neurons utilizing neuropeptide Y (NPY) are involved in GnRH → LH production; an increase in NPY secretion is an antecedent for the preovulatory LH surge. Sahu and Kalra (1998) examined NPY levels in the median eminence, arcuate nucleus, and other hypothalamic nuclei in young and middle-aged female rats. Unlike young rats, there was no cyclical increase of NPY in these two hypothalamic regions in middle-aged rats. An earlier study demonstrated declines in NPY levels in the hypothalamus of older male rats (Sahu, Kalra, Crowley, & Kalra, 1988). (2) The response of neurons in the median eminence and arcuate nucleus to agonists of the neurotransmitter glutamate were found to be diminished in middle-aged rats (Zuo, Mahesh, Zamorano, & Brann, 1996). This finding suggests that synaptic activation of GnRH neurons by glutamatergic inputs may be reduced in middle-aged rats. (3) In male rats, age-related decreases were observed for the number of neurons in the medial preoptic area expressing the gene for GnRH, and the content of GnRH was lower in neurons of the arcuate nucleus (Gruenewald & Matsumoto, 1991). (4) NPY neurons and reproductive behavior were studied in male rats by Clark (1994). NPY levels were generally lower in the medial preoptic area and arcuate nucleus only in middle-aged rats, which had ceased ejaculating.

Estrogen receptors.   Various areas of the brain contain neurons with receptors for estrogen, including the preoptic, suprachiasmatic, and arcuate nuclei. Estrogen receptors act within the cells by altering gene expression. Thus, the ovarian secretion of estrogen into the bloodstream has the potential to modulate neural activity in these hypothalamic regions.

Some age-related hypothalamic changes are likely to involve declining estrogen secretion by the ovaries. There is evidence in the literature to indicate a loss of estrogen receptors and/or their efficacy with age in neurons of the hypothalamus. For example, in rodents the ovaries can be removed and the animals given estrogen supplements, allowing the neuroendocrine mechanisms to be studied while controlling estrogen levels as the animals age. Under these conditions, a decrease in the ability of estrogen to inhibit LH secretion (a negative feedback loop) can be demonstrated in middle-aged rats. This appears to be due to an age-associated loss of estrogen receptors in hypothalamic neurons (Mobbs, 1996).

The arcuate (or infundibular) nucleus is at the base of the hypothalamus above the pituitary gland. As its location suggests, the arcuate nucleus contains cells that have a strong influence on the hypothalamic-pituitary-gonadal axis, including cells that produce GnRH. A number of neurotransmitters and peptide neuromodulators are found in this nucleus. In post-menopausal women, some neurons in the arcuate nucleus exhibit increased size (hypertrophy), and there is evidence of increased neuronal activity (see Rance, 1992). The hypertrophied neurons were those containing estrogen receptors, and these neurons were about twice as large as comparable neurons of premenopausal women. However, neurons secreting GnRH did not possess estrogen receptors and did not become hypertrophic. All of this supports the hypothesis that, in menopausal women, the reduction of ovarian estrogen eliminates the normal negative feedback on certain neurons (those that become hypertrophic). These hypothalamic neurons do not themselves produce GnRH, but normally activate GnRH-producing neurons via synapses (probably involving the neuropeptides neurokinin B and substance P). This would explain how reduced estrogen results in more GnRH and therefore increased levels of FSH and LH (Rance, 1992).

Why might estrogen receptors become diminished with age? There might be negative, long-term effects of estrogen on estrogen receptors (e.g., their ability to affect gene expression). Another hypothesis is that estrogen is actually toxic to certain neurons in the hypothalamus. Some neurons of the arcuate nucleus are especially vulnerable to estrogen-induced damage, perhaps implying a connection (Mobbs, 1996). In any event, it is apparent that hypothalamic neurons, including those that control the release of gonadotropins by the pituitary, can be influenced, perhaps indirectly, by reduced estrogen levels.

Biological rhythms. Biological rhythms are part and parcel of hormonal regulation. As discussed in chapter 10, the suprachiasmatic nucleus (SCN) is the primary biological clock of the brain, and aging is often associated with impaired function of the SCN and its timekeeping abilities. Thus, a key to the changes in hypothalamic control of hormonal activity is likely to involve disruption of circadian activity, particularly with respect to the SCN. Deterioration of biological clock mechanisms could trigger the irregularity and ultimate loss of normal hormonal cycles which characterize menopause (Wise et al., 1996). For example, NE is a modulator of GnRH release in the medial preoptic hypothalamus. NE receptor activity exhibits rhythmic changes (presumably under the control of the SCN) associated with the normal preovulatory surge of LH. This rhythmic activity is lost in both the medial preoptic nucleus and SCN of middle-aged rats (Weiland & Wise, 1990; Wise, 1994).

The sexually dimorphic nucleus of the preoptic area. This hypothalamic structure is important for sexual behavior, especially in males, where it is much larger than in females (hence the term *sexually dimorphic*). Damage to the region results in a decrease in some or all sexual activity in young adult males, depending on species. Thus, it may be important that the number of neurons in this area declines with age in both men and women (Hofman & Swaab, 1989). A decrease of 3% per year occurs during middle age in men, with no further decrease after age 60. By contrast, women exhibit the greatest loss in cell number after 70 years of age. Whether this late loss of neurons is a cause or effect of ovarian changes is not clear at this time.

SUMMARY AND IMPLICATIONS

It seems clear that gonadal, hypothalamic, and pituitary changes contribute to the decline in reproductive physiology and behavior that accompanies aging. Because these regulatory components interact with one another in various ways, a primary change in any one component could presumably alter the whole system. It seems reasonable that primary age effects might occur in more than one of these components, without the necessity of a single master trigger of all sequelae associated with menopause or male reproductive decline (see Wise et al., 1996, for a discussion of this issue). Is the brain one of the triggers? A good deal of evidence has shown various middle-age effects in the hypothalamus that might cause some of the events associated with reproductive senescence. A caveat is in order, however; most of the research on the hypothalamus and GnRH regulation has used rodents, and there are some differences between rodents and humans in this regard. Firm conclusions about the role of the hypothalamus in aging of the human reproductive systems await additional research.

At this point, we have discussed all seven basic functions of the nervous system and how they fare with age. This leads us to the next and final chapter, the ways and means by which various age-related changes can be retarded or advanced.

13
Modification of Age-Related Changes in the Brain, Behavior, and Cognition

Earlier chapters have detailed the many changes that occur in the nervous system as people age. The sad fact is, most of these changes range from undesirable to dreaded. In this final chapter, topics are addressed that bear directly on how negative aspects of aging might be minimized or reversed.

This is no mean feat. The maintenance of a healthy nervous system over the years is fraught with challenges, even when serious diseases have been avoided. We have seen many examples of "normal" age-related changes in the nervous system throughout this book, and no elderly person can be free of at least some of these. Moreover, even if one's nervous system reaches old age in superb condition, new challenges await. For example, older neurons may be more susceptible to certain toxins and to excitotoxicity by amino acid neurotransmitters (e.g., Dawson & Wallace, 1992; Zawia, Arendash, & Wecker, 1992). Thus, neurochemical events that may not have serious effects on young brains may be dangerous to old brains. Also contributing to the challenge is the fact that age-related changes occurring in other physiological systems can take a toll on the nervous system. For example, altered efficacy of the immune system is a common correlate of aging (Schneider & Reed, 1985), and there is evidence that changes in the brain's immune system can contribute to neural degeneration (E. G. McGeer & P. L. McGeer, 1997; P. L. McGeer & E. G. McGeer, 1996). The same can be said of the cardiovascular and other systems as well.

Given all of this, it goes without saying that general health is a key factor in determining how all physiological systems fare with age, including the nervous system. Thus, avoidance of general health risks and adoption of a healthy lifestyle constitute the most basic and practical strategies for maintenance of a healthy nervous system. Familiar risk factors that reduce the likelihood of healthy aging include smoking, high blood pressure, and a sedentary lifestyle. Health-promoting behaviors such as physical exercise are associated with a variety of effects on the physiology of middle-aged and elderly people, such as improved cardiovascular, endocrine, and metabolic functions (Buskirk, 1985; Goldberg et al., 1996; Goldberg & Hagberg, 1990). Psychosocial factors contribute to general health in a variety of ways as well (Rowe & Kahn, 1987). These positive health outcomes are presumably beneficial to the nervous system.

Whereas myriad variables have the potential to modulate the course of aging, this chapter focuses on topics that are directly associated with the aging nervous system and, more specifically, the possibilities for slowing or attenuating age-related declines in neural functioning and improving or reversing deficits that have already occurred. Before getting on with this task, however, it is germane to first assess the potential for neurons and neural circuits to be modified in nervous systems of old individuals—the capacity for neural plasticity.

PLASTICITY OF SYNAPSES AND DENDRITES IN THE AGING NERVOUS SYSTEM

Neurons in older brains retain much of the capacity for synaptic plasticity that is so evident in developing organisms. Research has made it quite clear that new synapses can form in older brains in response to injury or environmental manipulations and that dendrites continue to be modifiable, as is the case with young brains (see Cotman, 1990; Cotman & Holets, 1985; Kaas, 1991; Willott, 1996a). The ability of the adult nervous system to engage mechanisms of synaptic plasticity has at least two important implications for neurogerontology. First, degenerative tendencies may be counteracted by replacement of damaged synapses and repair of neural circuits. Second, the nervous system can continue to manifest the normal, adaptive types of synaptic plasticity exhibited by young individuals. The latter aspect of plasticity has been addressed in other chapters in various contexts, each of which indicates continued proficiency for adaptive neural plasticity, albeit with limitations in some instances. Examples include the reorganization of central representational maps in response to peripheral sensory losses, long-term potentiation, and learning in general. These types of adaptive plasticity persist in older brains. As we are about to see, the same can be said for plasticity with respect to repair and replacement of synapses.

Repair and Replacement of Synapses

When neurons in the brain are damaged or degenerate, the neurons targeted by their axons become denervated. This situation often results in the sprouting of branches from intact, nearby axons that can then replace the missing synaptic inputs. The formation of new synapses in response to trauma, metabolic disturbances, or other stimuli (including those associated with axon sprouting) is called *reactive synaptogenesis*. The nervous system's capacity for sprouting and reactive synaptogenesis persists with age. This provides the potential to compensate for loss of dendrites and other neuronal damage that may accompany aging, as described in other chapters. However, the rate and, in some studies, the magnitude of sprouting have been found to be diminished in old brains (see Cotman, 1990, for a review). Such age effects have been primarily demonstrated in the hippocampus after damage to its inputs (Cotman & Holets, 1985). One variable that may contribute to the slower reinnervation is an increase in the time required for the initial clearance of degenerated material, but other events appear to be involved as well (Anderson, Scheff, & DeKosky, 1986). For instance, a study by Schauwecker, Cheng, Serquinia, Mori, and McNeill (1995) observed reduced sprouting in partially deafferented hippocampi of old rats and linked this to a diminution of growth associated protein-43 (GAP-43), a factor known to stimulate neuron growth.

An aptitude for neuronal repair is also observed in the aging peripheral nervous system (Spencer & Ochoa, 1981). In the peripheral nervous system, where damaged axons have the ability to regrow (the axon regenerates outward from the stump), this continues with age. In old animals, however, regeneration may be delayed by a sort of latent period prior to regeneration. Also, the magnitude of regeneration may be attenuated, with fewer axons regenerating after a period of recovery time has passed (Vaughan, 1992).

Although sprouting and synaptogenesis may help to compensate for minor degenerative changes during aging, there may be a down side as well. Evidence has been obtained to indicate that localized degeneration in Alzheimer's disease (AD) stimulates aberrant sprouting and plaque formation, and this can make matters even worse (Cotman, 1990). What is more, as degeneration progresses, even more aberrant sprouting is stimulated—a vicious circle.

Another aspect of synaptic plasticity that might have either positive or negative consequences is the enlargement of individual synapses observed in some brain regions. Evidence suggests that age-related decreases in the number of synapses per neuron may be compensated for by enlargement of the remaining synapses in the hippocampus and elsewhere (Bertoni-Freddari et al., 1996). This has been observed in early AD (DeKosky & Scheff, 1990). Such plasticity might help to maintain synaptic function in the face of lost inputs. However, there is disagreement in the literature with respect to the compensation hypothesis, and the cause and functional consequences of synaptic enlargement are not clear. The occurrence of larger of synapses might actually represent a negative functional event, such as selective loss of smaller perforated synapses thought to be involved with adaptive neural plasticity (Jones & Harris, 1995).

Besides creating new synapses, neural circuits may also be maintained or modified by elaboration of dendrites. Dendritic spines and branches are constantly modified throughout life, showing growth, regression, and the formation of new connections. In some brain regions dendrites continue to grow in size and complexity even late in life, although the rate of change may slow somewhat (Buell & Coleman, 1979; Flood, 1993). As mentioned below, procedures shown to improve cognitive performance in rats also induced dendritic growth in the cerebral cortex. However, even when dendritic growth is observed, it can be difficult to determine the functional significance. In one study, increased dendritic length and complexity were observed in the CA1 region of hippocampus of old rats (Pyapali & Turner, 1996). However, there was no significant correlation with the animal's performance (time trials) on spatial behavior in a water maze. Nonetheless, it seems likely that the ability to grow dendritic branches and spines confers considerable benefits on the aging brain.

To summarize, synapses and dendrites continue to be repaired and replaced in the old brain. There is, however, a familiar refrain: The process generally takes longer and may not reach the magnitude typical of younger brains.

MODULATION OF CHANGES IN THE AGING NERVOUS SYSTEM

The dynamic properties of the aging nervous system set the stage for various strategies aimed at modulating the direction or severity of negative age-related changes. A number of approaches are being investigated by neurogerontological researchers. In one way or another, most approaches attempt to enhance neural functioning by promoting the activity of various neurotransmitters or other physiologically important substances that protect neurons from age-related damage (e.g., by free radicals) and/or improve neural functioning per se. This can be done by introducing biological or chemical agents as drugs or dietary components and/or stimulating declining endogenous activity by manipulation of the environment, chronic restriction of calories in the diet, and neural transplantation.

Diet, Vitamins, and Health-Promoting Supplements

Diet and nutrition are clearly linked to general health and the occurrence and severity of many chronic diseases affecting older people (Blumberg, 1996). Of especial importance here, a considerable body of evidence has linked good nutritional status to cognitive competence (Rosenberg & Miller, 1992). Once again, it is obvious that diets that promote the general health of cardiovascular and other systems are also good for the nervous system.

Besides the general benefits of an all-around healthy diet, some dietary components may have particular value for the older brain. For example, aged garlic extract has been shown to improve acquisition and retention of avoidance conditioning and performance on the Morris water maze in senescence-accelerated (SAM) mice (Moriguchi, Saito, & Nishiyama, 1996; Moriguchi, Takashina, Chu, Saito, & Nishiyama, 1994). The effects of specific nutrients on the aging brain are not always unidirectional, however. Some research has shown that high glucose intake is associated with better performance on verbal memory tests in young subjects, but worse performance in elderly subjects (see Messier, Gagnon, & Knott, 1997). Indeed, it appears that the effects of glucose levels on memory or other cognitive processes interact with age, sex, level of glucose, the nature of the cognitive task, and probably other factors. The intake of glucose and resulting increases in blood glucose values can affect memory, but the age effects are complicated. This may also be the case with cholesterol, as suggested by the work of Joseph, Villalobos-Molinas, Denisova, Erat, and Strain (1997). Cholesterol may accumulate in neuronal membranes with age, altering their structural and functional properties. However, the process may also protect the neurons from oxidative damage.

It is perhaps not surprising that the effects of dietary composition on the aging brain are not turning out to be simple or easy to determine.

This may also be the case with respect to some popular dietary supplements discussed in the following paragraphs. Although we shall emphasize research obtaining positive results, epidemiological research presented regularly in the news media often paints a picture of inconclusive or conflicting findings with respect to benefits or negative side effects of various dietary supplements. Caution and guidance by available medical information are always warranted in deciding whether to use a particular health product.

Vitamins and other antioxidants.   The likely involvement of free radical damage in various aspects of neural aging has been alluded to frequently in other chapters. Continuous oxidative bombardment, coupled with a decline in cellular protective mechanisms, undoubtedly has negative consequences for neuronal membranes and other neuronal constituents (e.g. Joseph, 1992; Mo, Hom, & Andersen, 1995). Antioxidants, which counteract free radicals, can have beneficial effects on various kinds of tissue, and research has shown that some antioxidant regimens can extend longevity in various laboratory animals (Harman, 1995a; Schneider & Reed, 1985). Consistent anti-aging properties of vitamin antioxidants have yet to be shown in humans, and there is controversy with respect to the efficacy of gerontological vitamin supplements (e.g., Bunker, 1992; Diplock, 1997; Ward, 1998). Nonetheless, some evidence has been obtained to link vitamin intake with age-associated cognitive changes. Healthy older subjects with low levels of certain vitamins were found to score more poorly on tests of memory and other cognitive tests (Goodwin, Goodwin, & Garry, 1983; Tucker et al., 1990). Vitamin deficiencies may also exacerbate AD and other neurodegenerative diseases (Blumberg, 1996). Conversely, older people with superior vitamin status appear to perform better cognitively. For example, in a longitudinal study of elderly subjects in Switzerland, significant positive correlations were obtained between cognitive performance (especially semantic memory on the Wechsler intelligence test) and plasma levels of ascorbic acid (vitamin C) and beta-carotene (Perrig, Perrig, & Stahelin, 1997). A Dutch study found a significant correlation between beta-carotene intake (but not vitamins C and E) and scores on the Mini-Mental-State Examination (Jama et al., 1996). Another longitudinal study (LaRue et al., 1997) also obtained some significant, albeit weak, correlations among cognitive tests and past or current intake of a variety of vitamins.

Do the epidemiological data reflect the general health benefits of vitamins or a direct effect on neural tissue? Although we cannot answer this question at present, assessments of antioxidant effects on neurons have been made using animal models, with some positive results. For instance, Socci, Crandall, and Arendash (1995) treated aging rats with a spin-trapping antioxidant (PBN) and observed improved performance on the Morris water maze. An earlier study by Carney and colleagues (1991) showed improvement of old gerbils on a radial arm maze after daily administration of PBN. The same antioxidant was used in an *in vitro* slice preparation by Joseph, Denisova, Villalobos-Molina, Erat, and Strain (1996) to demonstrate benefits at the cellular level, including better release of dopamine. Mixed results were found in a study of vitamin E supplements by Monji, Morimoto, Okuyama, Yamashita, and Tashiro (1994b). Supplements were associated with a reduction in lipofuscin content in several brain regions of middle-aged rats but not in old rats. These and other animal studies (e.g., Asanuma, Tamauchi, Koga, & Katayama, 1995) suggest that antioxidants might have potential ameliorative effects on aging neurons. However, we are far from understanding if and how the aging human nervous system is affected by dietary antioxidants, and whether supplementary vitamins can protect aging neurons. In the mean time, given the epidemiological data it seems safe to conclude that a diet rich in natural sources of vitamins (e.g., fruits and vegetables) is likely to be beneficial for human physiological systems and therefore beneficial to the nervous system as well.

Melatonin. Melatonin is a hormone produced by the pineal gland. As mentioned in chapter 12, the pineal gland and melatonin are key to mechanisms of biological rhythms, including sleep and reproductive cycles. The putative effects of melatonin ingestion on sleep are well known, and over-the-counter melatonin is widely used to re-entrain circadian rhythms after jet lag. It is also commonly used as a sleep enhancer and is successful in some older people (Avery, Lenz, & Landis, 1998). The hormone is also important in reproductive behavior, with some gerontological implications. Studies on old rodents have shown that the administration of melatonin or the grafting of pineal glands from young into old animals have ameliorative effects on neural and gonadal aspects of reproductive function (Pierpaoli et al., 1997).

Melatonin's potential extends even further with respect to neurogerontological issues. Melatonin is a very effective free radical scavenger and may also augment immune responses (Brzezinski, 1997; Mobbs, 1996), indicating that its anti-aging role may be quite broad. Of particular interest here, a number of studies have provided evidence that melatonin can protect neurons from free radical damage and apoptosis (Giusti, Lipartiti, Gusella, Floreani, & Manev, 1997; Manev, Uz, & Giusti, 1997; Reiter, Guerrero, Escames, Pappolla, & Acuna-Castroviero, 1997). Given that there has been little evidence of toxic side effects of melatonin ingestion thus far (although long-term studies have not been completed), the use of melatonin supplements is the subject of much current interest (e.g., Huether, 1996).

DHEA. Dehydroepiandrosterone (DHEA) is an androgen present in abundance in humans, as is DHEA sulphate, which is converted to DHEA. It is produced by the adrenal glands, testes, and ovaries and is present in the brain as well (see Barrou, Charru, & Lidy, 1997; Schneider & Reed, 1985, for reviews). DHEA levels reach a maximum in young adulthood, then continuously decline to very low levels by age 70 or so; thus, falling DHEA levels have been suggested as a cause of various age-associated disorders such as atherosclerosis and osteoporosis.

DHEA is sold commercially as an anti-aging compound and appears to have several favorable physiological effects on nonneural systems. Little research has addressed its neurophysiological properties in humans, but animal studies have reported that DHEA and/or DHEA sulphate may have several effects in the CNS. These include antagonistic action at GABA receptors (Majewska, Demirgoren, Spivak, & London, 1990), protection of hippocampal neurons from glutamate excitotoxicity (Kimonides, Khatibi, Svendsen, Sofroniew, & Herbert, 1998), attenuation of age-related decreases in corticotropin-releasing hormone in the hypothalamus (Givalois, Li, & Pelletier, 1997), and stimulation of gonadotrophin-releasing hormone in old rats (Li, Givalois, & Pelletier, 1997). In addition, there is some indication that DHEA can enhance memory in old mice (Flood & Roberts, 1988). DHEA is therefore another biochemical with significant anti-aging possibilities whose benefits may extend to the nervous system. As is the case for melatonin, however, long-term human studies of possible side effects have yet to be completed.

Ginko biloba and ginseng. Ginko biloba and ginseng are key ingredients in traditional Asian health- and vitality-enhancing concoctions and have become popular in Western cultures. Ginko biloba extract (EGb 761) has proven to be an effective free radical scavenger with a variety of beneficial effects in aging laboratory animals and humans. These effects include increased density of serotonin receptors in the cerebral cortex of old rats (Huguet, Drieu, & Piriou, 1994), protection of hippocampal neurons in aging mice (Barkats, Venault, Christen, & Cohen-Salmon, 1995), protection of neuronal membranes from free radical damage, possible mitigation of neuronal apoptosis, and improved cognitive performance (Droy-Lefaix, 1997; Stoll, Scheuer, Pohl, & Muller, 1996). Improved cognitive performance in response to Ginko biloba has been demonstrated in various tasks as diverse as enhanced delayed nonmatching task behavior in rats (Winter, 1998) to shortened latency for the P300 event-related potential in humans (Semlitsch, Anderer, Saletu, Binder, & Decker, 1995). Research has also provided evidence that ginseng possesses cognition-enhancing properties. For example, Panax (Korean) ginseng extract was reported to result in improved performance of old Fischer 344 rats on a radial arm maze (Nitta et al., 1995), although performance on an operant discrimination task was not affected. A diet supplemented with the traditional Chinese prescription DX-9386, which contains ginseng, resulted in improved spatial memory in senescence accelerated mice (Nishiyama, Zhou, & Saito, 1994). Finally, a combination of extracts from Ginko biloba and Panax ginseng at certain doses was associated with improved learning in old rats (Petkov et al., 1993).

Drugs as Modulators of Age-Related Changes in the Brain

Before addressing the issue of using drugs to deliberately alter neural and/or cognitive performance in older people, a general comment with respect to drug use in the elderly population is worth making. Older people are easily the heaviest per capita users of drugs (see Gomberg, 1996). Most of these drugs are used to treat various medical and geriatric conditions, and many affect the nervous system directly or indirectly by acting on various receptors. The neural effects can be desired targeted outcomes or side effects. Because age-associated receptor changes can include up regulation or down regulation, and these vary greatly from brain region to brain region, the terrain upon which drugs are seeking receptors can be quite different and variable in older people. This means that special problems often arise with respect to dosing and drug administration regimens. Although these are medical and pharmacological concerns beyond the scope of this book, they are obviously linked to many neurogerontological issues. Certainly, neurogerontological research has contributed much to geriatric pharmacology and will continue to do so. We cannot hope to understand age-related influences on drug effects unless we understand the aging nervous system.

Now, on to our discussion of drugs that can affect aging of the brain and cognition. It has become evident throughout this book that many synaptic modifications in brain circuits utilizing a variety of neurotransmitters accompany aging. Moreover, these changes have much to do with the behavioral and cognitive concomitants of aging. Thus, it is inherently reasonable that drugs affecting synaptic activity—*agonists* (drugs that facilitate or mimic a particular neurotransmitter) and *antagonists* (drugs that block or attenuate a neurotransmitter)—have the potential to alter the negative behavioral and cognitive changes. Indeed, a good deal of research has been directed at this potential. Our discussion of drugs will focus on their use as enhancers of cognitive and behavioral changes associated with age, the primary focus of the pharmacological aging research. There are, however, some classes of neuroactive drugs that are designed to treat psychiatric or other disorders, yet can also affect cognitive processes. The cognitive effects of such pharmaceuticals may be inconsistent from drug to drug, and their mechanisms are unclear. Antidepressants that are not highly specific for a given neurotransmitter (e.g., tricyclics) illustrate the point. Rowe and colleagues (1997) administered the antidepressant drug desipramine to cognitively impaired old rats and found a beneficial effect—amelioration of the negative effects of glucocorticoids on the hippocampus, as discussed in chapter 11. On the other hand, some antidepressant drugs have negative effects on cognition in older people, and still others have no effect (Knegtering, Eijck, & Huijsman, 1994).

In order to tie the discussion of pharmacology to the various neurogerontological topics discussed elsewhere in this book, we shall focus on drugs affecting various neurotransmitter/neuromodulator systems that have appeared in those discussions: Ach, GABA, glutamate/calcium, the catecholamines dopamine, and, to a lesser extent, NE, serotonin, and neuropeptides.

It should be kept in mind, however, that neural circuits using different neurotransmitters and neuromodulators interact in complex ways (see chapter 4). An agonist or antagonist for one neurotransmitter can have indirect effects on circuits using another neurotransmitter, which may be more directly related to the behavior or cognitive process being tested. Moreover, drugs often have more than one mode of action. Thus, it is often difficult to determine exactly how drugs work with respect to cognition. For example, administration of the compound FR121196 ameliorated memory deficits in old rats (Yamazaki et al., 1995). This was attributed by the researchers to action on cholinergic input to the hippocampus, but a role of serotonergic modulation was implicated as well. Another case in point is acetyl levocarnitine, which occurs naturally in mitochondria and is involved in energy metabolism. Used as a drug, it has been shown to possess properties that can slow neurodegeneration and have benefits for AD patients, including improved cognitive function (Carta & Calvani, 1991; Pettegrew, Klunk, Panchalingan, Kanter, & McClure, 1995; Sano et al., 1992). In addition to its effects on cellular energy metabolism acetyl levocarnitine appears to influence Ach and other neurotransmitter systems (Ghirardi, Giuliani, Caprioli, Ramacci, & Angelucci, 1992), making it difficult to pin down its mode of action on cognition.

Another example of drugs with poorly understood pharmacological mechanisms is the group of compounds classified as *nootropic* drugs, noted for their cognition-enhancing properties. The main group of such drugs are derivatives of pyrrolidone and include piracetam and nefiracetam. These have been shown to improve memory in old or cognitively impaired subjects, but how they do so is unclear, and several neurotransmitter systems (perhaps interacting) have been implicated, including Ach, glutamate, and GABA (Giovannini, Casamenti, Bartolini, & Pepeu, 1997; Stoll, Shubert, & Muller, 1991; Woodruff-Pak, 1997; Yoshii, Watabe, Sakaurai, & Shiotani, 1997).

A final example is phosphatidylserine, an important component of neuronal membranes. Phosphatidylserine may exhibit age-related change (Schroeder, 1984). Thus, administration of phosphatidylserine has been tried as a drug to attenuate cognitive deficits in elderly patients, and some improvements in cognitive function have been reported (Giovannini et al., 1997). An effect on cholinergic function has been implicated, since treatment of old mice with phosphatidylserine appears to increase the availability of muscarinic Ach receptors (Gelbmann & Muller, 1991), and phosphatidylserine administration has been shown to increase the release of Ach from *in vitro* cortical slices (Pedata, Giovannelli, Spignoli, Giovannini, & Pepu, 1985). The effects of phosphatidylserine are not restricted to cholinergic systems, however. Chronic treatment of old mice increased the density of NMDA receptors (Cohen & Muller, 1992), and phosphatidylserine may prevent the loss of dendritic spines in hippocampal neurons of old rats (Nunzi et al., 1987).

To summarize, the effects of drugs on cognition and behavior are typically complicated, often multifaceted, and always hard to unravel.

This confusing situation is exacerbated when age-related changes are thrown into the equation. Whereas the use of drugs that are more or less specific for given neurotransmitters provide some clarity, the waters remain muddy, as will be evident often in the ensuing discussions.

Drugs affecting Ach.   The role of cholinergic circuits in the age-related decline of cognitive abilities has received a great deal of attention, both in the context of normal aging and even more so with respect to AD (e.g., see chapters 8 and 11). There is much research literature implicating cholinergic involvement in cognitive deficits of AD (Bartus et al., 1982). Thus, various gerontologically oriented research groups have evaluated the cognitive and behavioral effects of drugs that modulate cholinergic function. The most obvious approach, attempting to enhance performance of healthy old subjects and AD patients by using Ach precursors (e.g., lecithin, choline), has generally proven ineffective (Bartus et al., 1982). Providing more raw material for the synthesis of Ach is apparently not the answer. Drugs that mimic Ach have fared somewhat better. Some studies on rodents have obtained positive results when aging animals were given cholinergic receptor agonists and tested for cognitive performance on various learning/memory tasks. Drugs affecting both muscarinic receptors (e.g., Gelbmann & Muller, 1991; Stoll et al., 1991) and nicotinic receptors (e.g., Arendash, Sengstock, Sanberg, & Kem, 1995) have resulted in some gains. In general, however, the cognition-enhancing effects of Ach-mimicking drugs have been disappointing, especially with respect to AD patients (Bartus et al., 1982; Ingram et al., 1994; Thal, 1996).

The use of drugs that inhibit AchE, which terminates the action of Ach at the synapse and therefore amplify diminished Ach activity, have shown some promise, albeit with limited success in the early going (Ingram et al., 1996; Thal, 1996). The first of such drugs to be approved for clinical use in treating AD was tacrine, and this had positive but mixed results and some negative side effects (e.g., kidney toxicity, nausea, diarrhea). The second drug to be approved, donepezil, had modest benefits for AD patients and fewer side effects. Various other cholinesterase-inhibiting drugs are being developed with the hope of improved clinical efficacy. For example, the cholinesterase inhibitor metrifonate is longer acting than other drugs and has been shown to facilitate acquisition and retention of eyeblink trace conditioning in old rabbits (sensitive to hippocampal activity) and improve cognitive performance in AD patients, while having relatively mild side effects (see Kronforst-Collins, Moriearty, Schmidt, & Disterhoft, 1997).

Given that AD is associated with disruption of other neurotransmitter systems besides Ach (see chapter 11), it is likely that cholinergic drugs alone will have only limited effects on cognitive performance, even if new generations of improved drugs are developed. Thus, the use of cholinergic drugs combined with drugs affecting other neurotransmitters is being evaluated (Giacobini, 1996). Hopefully, such approaches can maximize whatever benefits AD patients might obtain from enhanced cholinergic activity. Whether or not cholinergic therapies will be useful for the improvement of cognition in nondemented elderly people, with only bothersome memory deficits, remains to be seen.

Drugs affecting GABA. GABAergic drugs have not received much attention as cognitive enhancers, although some potential of antagonists of the benzodiazepine receptor (associated with the GABA receptor complex) to slow age-related change has been shown (Marczynski, 1995). Sarter and Bruno (1997) have noted that GABAergic circuits modulate cholinergic systems involved in cognition, suggesting that drugs affecting GABA might be used to enhance cognitive function. Benzodiazepine receptor "inverse agonists," which act like antagonists but have less profound effects, have been shown to enhance cholinergic activity associated with cognitive activity, in particular attentional processes. Sarter and Bruno (1997) argued that modifying cholinergic cortical activity indirectly (by altering noncholinergic subcortical modulators) may be particularly well suited for enhancement of cognitive processes that rely on complex interacting neural circuits. By comparison, direct replacement or mimicry at cholinergic synapses (e.g., the strategy used to treat Parkinson's disease with L-dopa) may disrupt the interplay among such circuits. One potential difficulty with the gerontological use of antagonists for GABA is that decreased GABAergic activity occurs in some brain regions (e.g., the inferior colliculus; see chapter 5). Decreased GABAergic activity probably has deleterious consequences which could be made even worse by GABA antagonists.

Drugs affecting glutamate. The glutamate receptors, in particular, the NMDA receptor, play key roles in LTP and many other synaptic functions that undoubtedly modulate cognitive processes (refer to chapters 3, 8, and elsewhere). Old rats appear to be more sensitive to NMDA antagonists, suggesting a deficit in NMDA functioning (Ingram et al., 1994) and indicating that glutamate agonists might help to reverse the deficit. One problem with stimulating NMDA receptors pharmacologically is the risk of overstimulation resulting in exicitotixic damage. Thus, drugs such as milacemide, which affect the NMDA receptor in a manner that will not produce excessive opening of calcium channels (e.g., by facilitating certain sites of the NMDA receptor complex) have been investigated, and several studies have reported memory improvement in rodents and humans (Ingram et al., 1994, 1996). McGahon, Clements, and Lynch (1997) used a diet rich in arachidonic acid, which enhanced glucose release in old rats and improved LTP. Useful glutamatergic drugs may not be confined to those reacting with the NMDA receptor. Granger and colleagues (1996) used a drug to enhance AMPA glutamate receptors and observed improved memory in old rats.

The calcium blocker, nimodipine. Whereas a deficiency in glutamatergic receptors can interfere with LTP or other neural functions, too much activity can cause excitotoxicity associated with the influx of calcium (see chapters 3, 4, and 8). Thus, some research groups have evaluated the effects of drugs that block calcium channels. Nimodipine is a calcium channel blocker (in particular, the L-type calcium channel) that readily passes the blood-brain barrier. It has been shown to have beneficial effects on the brain, including better responses to brain damage, ischemia, and neurodegenerative conditions (Fanelli, McCarthy, & Chisholm, 1994; Schuurman & Traber, 1994). The drug also appears to have the ability to slow or improve age-related neural, behavioral, and cognitive deficits. Chronic nimodipine treatment was correlated with slowed deterioration of sensorimotor behavior in aging rats (Schuurman & Traber, 1994). A study by DeJong and colleagues (1992) reported that a decrease in synaptic density observed in the dentate gyrus of aging control rats was prevented by long-term treatment with nimodipine. Chronic administration of nimodipine to senescence-accelerated (SAM) mice attenuated several neurochemical changes associated with rapid aging in this strain (Kabuto, Yokoi, Mori, Murakami, & Sawada, 1995). These and other findings indicate that chronic treatment with nimodipine can have ameliorative effects on aging of the hippocampus and other brain regions.

Disterhoft and colleagues have shown short-term administration of nimodipine to have favorable effects on the hippocampus and on learning in aged rats. Deyo, Straube, and Disterhoft (1989) administered the drug to young and old rabbits prior to classical conditioning of the eyeblink, using a trace conditioning paradigm. An age-related deficit in conditioning was observed for old rabbits that did not receive nimodipine. Learning was facilitated in both young and old subjects that received nimodipine, with old rabbits performing as well as young control animals.

Why would a calcium blocker improve hippocampal physiology? It appears that the attenuation of certain physiological events associated with hippocampal neuronal activity can facilitate learning-related mechanisms (Disterhoft, Moyer, Thompson, & Kowalska, 1993; Moyer, Thompson, Black, & Disterhoft, 1992). The excitation of hippocampal neurons is accompanied by an after-hyperpolarization response that counteracts further excitation. In learning paradigms such as eyeblink conditioning, the firing rate of hippocampal neurons increases, and this is likely caused by a reduction of the after-hyperpolarization. The after-hyperpolarization response is mediated by calcium channels. Thus, by blocking these channels, nimodipine should also block the after-polarization, thereby allowing for greater excitability of the hippocampal neurons. This is especially true in old animals, since the after-hyperpolarization tends to increase with age. Thus, in addition to its long-term neuroprotective effect, nimodipine may also enhance hippocampally mediated learning directly via this (and other) means.

Drugs affecting catecholamines. The prefrontal cortex of old monkeys and humans exhibits consistent and substantial declines in dopamine and NE (see chapter 8), and this is thought to be largely responsible for age-related cognitive deficits mediated by the prefrontal cortex (Arnsten, 1993, 1997). Catecholamine agonists, therefore, would seem to have potential to improve frontal lobe function, and this appears to be the case. At certain doses, the dopamine-enhancing drugs clonidine and guanfacine were shown to facilitate learning of delayed response tasks in old rhesus monkeys, despite producing some interfering side effects including sedation (Arnsten, 1993, 1997). These and other findings support a role for catecholamine agonists for enhancing cognition in primates.

Studies have been performed with rats as well. A dopamine agonist, pergolide, was shown by Felten and colleagues (1992) to prevent age-related degenerative changes in neurons of the nigrostriatal system of rats when given orally for an extend period of time. In another study, the D_1 receptor agonists SKF 38393 and SKF 81297 were found to improve performance in old, memory-impaired rats (Hersi, Rowe, Gaudreau, & Quirion, 1995).

The drug L-deprenyl (selegine) is an inhibitor of monoamine oxidase-B (MAO-B), an enzyme that degrades dopamine; thus L-deprenyl treatments result in enhanced dopaminergic activity. As mentioned in chapter 11, this drug is used to treat Parkinson's disease. It may also enhance cognitive performance in aging animals as well as human AD patients, and even extends the life span of rodents (Ivy et al., 1994). There is also evidence that long-term oral administration of L-deprenyl attenuates certain age-related neuronal changes in the rat frontal cortex and hippocampus, such as neuron loss, hypertrophy of astrocytes, and the buildup of lipofuscin (Amenta et al., 1994). The effects are apparently due to the drug's effects on MAO-B, as well as other mechanisms (e.g., free radical scavenging).

Drugs affecting serotonin. The relationship between serotonergic systems and cognition is confusing, with inconsistencies in the literature (McEntee & Crook, 1991). Some of the confusion undoubtedly arises from serotonin's various modulatory actions with other neurotransmitter systems (e.g., Ach, NE), setting the stage for a variety of indirect effects of serotonergic drugs on other systems. Nevertheless, research suggests that serotonin has a predominantly inhibitory effect on learning and memory (McEntee & Crook, 1991), indicating a potential ameliorative effect of serotonin antagonists. Several studies have shown that serotonin 5-HT$_3$ receptor antagonists have cognitive-enhancing properties in old animals. For example, Arnsten, Lin, Van Dyck, and Stanhope (1997) administered the antagonists ondansetron and SEC-579 to old rhesus monkeys and observed improvement on a visual object discrimination task (although two other tasks were not affected). Chronic treatment of rats with the 5-HT$_3$ antagonist itasetron resulted in improved retention (Pitsikas & Borsini, 1996). In a study of humans, however, ondansetron did not affect cognitive performance (Little et al., 1995). Overall, the research provides evidence for some modest positive effects of 5-HT$_3$ antagonists in older humans, at least for certain tasks (Riedel & Jolles, 1996). The story is never a simple one, however. Improved water maze performance has also been obtained in old rats given the serotonin precursor tryptophan, which should facilitate serotonin activity (Levkovitz, Richter-Levin, & Segal, 1994).

Drugs affecting neuropeptides. Numerous neuropeptides have functional importance in many facets of neural and neuroendocrine function.

A number of these can influence learning, memory, attention, and other cognitive processes, and when administered as drugs, may modulate such activity (Bennett, Ballard, Watson, & Fone, 1997; De Wied, 1997; McGaugh & Cahill, 1997; Moore & Black, 1991). Examples include the opioid peptides (e.g., β-endorphin, enkephalins), releasing hormones (e.g., corticotrophin-releasing hormone, thyrotrophin-releasing hormone, somatostatin), and others such as vasopressin, substance P, and neuropeptide Y. Given the number of neuropeptides and their widespread, often indirect effects on the various neural functions, the neurogerontological story with respect to cognitive enhancement is yet to be told. Nonetheless, there are indications of their potential for gerontological use. For example, vasopressin was shown to improve cognitive performance in old monkeys (Bartus, Dean, & Beer, 1982). The drug JTP-4819 facilitates several neuropeptides (substance P, vasopressin, thyrotrophin-releasing hormone) and has beneficial effects on cholinergic transmission as well as learning and memory (Toide, Iwamoto, Fujiwara, & Abe, 1995). Some neuropeptides, such as galanin, may have negative effects on cognitive performance, suggesting some potential for antagonists (McDonald & Crawley, 1997).

The outlook. Many drugs and treatment strategies are being developed for their potential as cognitive enhancers with hopes of improving the quality of life for healthy elderly people and for treating and managing dementia. We have been able to outline only some of the findings and mention only some of the drugs. Thus far, the effects of various drugs have been mixed, with the holy grail, dramatic cognitive improvements, remaining elusive. This is indeed a challenging area of research. Learning, memory, attention, language, and other cognitive processes undoubtedly make use of extensive and complex neural circuits often involving the proper balance and interaction of excitatory, inhibitory neurotransmitters and neuromodulators, as well as long-term changes in neurons. Pharmacologically altering the relative salience of one or more participating circuits in a facilitative manner (particularly when superimposed on an aged or pathological neural substrate) will be difficult, to say the least. Indeed, some studies have shown inverted U-shaped dose-effect relationships, whereby too much or too little of a drug is ineffective or even detrimental (e.g., Arnsten, 1996). Moreover, there may be little that drugs can do for a brain ravaged by AD or other neurodegenerative diseases. Nevertheless, this remains an exciting area of research. Even moderate improvements are welcome for AD patients and their families, and the potential payoff of finding that holy grail is huge.

Neurotrophic Factors

Neurotrophic factors comprise a class of polypeptides that are essential for the maintenance, growth, and survival of neurons both during development and in adults. Two families of neurotrophic factors are *neurotrophins*, which include brain-derived neurotrophic factor (BDNF) and nerve growth factor (NGF), and *fibroblast growth factors* (FGF). These growth factors are expressed in brain tissue and have been shown to promote the growth and well-being of neurons, with NGF being especially important for cholinergic neurons (Cotman, 1990; Cotman & Neeper, 1996). For example, neurotrophin infusion was found to increase transmitter production in cholinergic neurons; additionally, neurotrophic factors can protect cultured neurons from the effects of hypoglycemia and excitotoxicity, and they may increase activity of free radical scavengers. Furthermore, the production of neurotrophic factors by denervated neurons and/or nearby astrocytes probably encourages axonal sprouting and synaptic replacement.

Whether or not NGF activity is diminished in the aging brain appears to depend on variables such as brain region, gender, and strain (e.g., Crutcher & Weingartner, 1991; Gomez-Pinilla, Cotman, & Nieto-Sampedro, 1989; Nishizuka et al., 1991). Indeed, the literature on age effects on neurotrophins is quite variable, perhaps because these factors react to a variety of stimuli and conditions (McLay et al., 1997).

Nevertheless, neurotrophic factors have intriguing potential as modulators of age-related plasticity and cognitive processes, and a number of studies have found that infusions can improve cognitive and memory deficits in aged rats (see Cotman, 1990; Cotman & Neeper, 1996). In a study by Chen and colleagues (1995), NGF was administered via cannulae into the ventricles to aged, maze-impaired rats for 4 weeks. They exhibited a significant increase in the density of synapses (immunopositive for synaptophysin) in the frontal cortex, compared to controls that were not given NGF. Moreover, this increase correlated with improvement on the Morris water maze. Other brain regions did not show the increase in synaptic density.

These and earlier findings (e.g., Fischer et al., 1987) suggest that NGF mediates trophic processes, which might facilitate sprouting. Backman and colleagues (1996) used a technique whereby NGF could be transported across the blood-brain barrier. NGF delivered in this manner was associated with increased neuron size in cholinergic neurons of the basal forebrain and improved spatial learning in old rats that had performed poorly prior to treatment. In rats that were not deficient performers to begin with, NGF administration disrupted learning, perhaps by promoting excessive, counterproductive sprouting. Fong, Neff, and Hadjiconstantinou (1997) administered GM1 gangliosides to old rats who performed poorly on the Morris water maze. GM1 gangliosides are thought to modulate neurotrophic factors and/or have neurotrophic properties. The treated rats improved both acquisition and retention of place navigation and were superior to control rats of the same age. Young rats' performance was not affected by the same treatment. In another study, Bergado, Fernandez, Gomez-Soria, and Gonzalez (1997) infused NGF into the ventricles of old, cognitively impaired rats and observed improved LTP in the hippocampal formation.

Neurotrophins also can interact with glucocorticoids, perhaps influencing the negative effects of stress on the hippocampus (see chapter 11). As outlined by McLay and colleagues (1997), NGF is secreted into the blood in response to stress. NGF, in turn, can facilitate the release of ACTH, with glucocorticoids then being released by the adrenal glands. Glucocorticoids can affect NGF mechanisms and reduce their effectiveness. All of this suggests that NGF and glucocorticoids may form a feedback loop to modify the stress response. McLay and colleagues (1997) proposed that alterations in the regulation of both glucocorticoids and neurotrophins—and their interaction—modulate age-related impairment of the hippocampus.

Neurotrophic factors are able to modify neuronal damage. When axons projecting to the hippocampus are cut, they exhibit typical retrograde (toward the cell body) degeneration. Administration of NGF or FGF has been shown to retard or prevent such degeneration (Cotman, 1990). Furthermore, infusion of NGF can prevent shrinkage of cholinergic neurons in the basal forebrain which is typically observed with age (Fischer et al., 1987). It appears that neurotrophic factors may have a variety of potentially beneficial effects on the aging nervous system, including defense against apoptosis, excitotoxicity, the ability to up-regulate free radical scavengers, and neuronal repair (McLay et al., 1997).

Dietary Restriction

A large body of gerontological literature on rodents has shown that calorically restricted diets can extend longevity, slow certain age-related physiological declines, and decrease tumors and diseases (e.g., Ausman & Russell, 1990; Bronson & Lipman, 1991; Schneider & Reed, 1985; Weindruch, Walford, Fligiel, & Guthrie, 1986). Although much of this research has focused on nonneural systems, there is ample evidence that dietary restriction modulates aging of the brain. Effects of dietary restriction on some of the general concomitants of neural aging, such as lipofuscin accumulation, glial responses, and loss of dendritic spines, have been reported. Moore, Davey, Weindruch, Walford, and Ivy (1995) measured lipofuscin content in granule cells of the dentate gyrus of the hippocampal formation of mice. Mice maintained on a relatively severe regimen of dietary restriction had reduced accumulation of lipofuscin compared to like-aged mice fed *ad libitum* or a moderately restricted diet. The same group (Moore & Ivy, 1995) observed that, in old mice fed a typical diet, the variability of lipofuscin content from cell to cell was high compared to that of old, calorically restricted mice. They speculated that, if intercellular variability in metabolism (as reflected by lipofuscin buildup) were to have deleterious effects during aging, these data might suggest a benefit of caloric restriction. A study by Castiglioni, Legare, Busbee, and Tiffany-Castiglioni (1991) found that age-related hypertrophy of astrocytes in the hippocampal complex of mice was prevented or reversed in calorically restricted animals. Similar effects in the cerebral cortex appeared in young middle-aged, but not in old, mice. Moroi-Fetters, Mervis, London, and Ingram (1989) reported that 30-month-old rats maintained on a restricted diet exhibited spine densities similar to those of 6-month-old control subjects.

Various neurotransmitter systems have been scrutinized in dietary restriction studies. Yeung and Friedman (1991) provided evidence that age-related changes in serotonergic neurons in the cerebral cortex of rats were attenuated by caloric restriction, whereas Diao, Bickford, Stevens, Cline, and Gerhardt (1997) showed an ameliorative effect on dopaminergic function in old rats. A study by Gould, Bowenkamp, Larson, Zahniser, and Bickford (1995) assessed the effect of dietary restriction on both motor learning and the ability of β-adrenergic receptors to modulate GABA responses in the cerebellum (a response assumed to be relevant to cerebellar activity during learning). Rats maintained on a restricted diet outperformed control rats in motor learning and exhibited signs of improved noradrenergic functioning in the cerebellum.

Other behavioral studies have obtained positive results as well. Algeri, Biagini, Manfridi, and Pitsikas (1991) performed a longitudinal behavioral study of spatial ability using the Morris water maze and found some beneficial effects of caloric restriction. For example, at age 30 months, calorically restricted rats did not exhibit deficits in their ability to benefit from practice, characteristic of control subjects. Dietary restriction was also shown to improve maze performance in rats by Goodrick (1984).

Much of the dietary restriction work on rats has used the Fischer-344 strain. Until various ameliorative effects are replicated in other genetic strains, a caveat may be in order. In our own research on dietary restriction and age-related degeneration of the cochlea, we have found that the consequences of a low-calorie diet vary considerably across mouse genotypes (Willott, Erway, Archer, & Harrison, 1995). We evaluated the effects of a calorically restricted diet on age-related hearing loss in 15 inbred and F1 hybrid mouse strains that were maintained from a young age on either a typical (high-energy) or calorically restricted (low-energy) diet. In most strains, little or no evidence was found to indicate that diet affected hearing loss, determined at 16 and 23 months of age using the auditory brainstem response threshold or the degree of cochlear pathology at the time of death. In several strains that exhibited increased longevity with the restricted diet, cochlear pathology appeared to continue to progress at a rate predictable according to the linear regression curve derived from the shorter-lived high-energy mice. In four strains, however, evidence was obtained to indicate that the restricted diet ameliorated age-related hearing loss as indicated by ABR thresholds and/or cochlear pathology. Thus, dietary restriction reduced age-related changes in some strains but not in others, a conclusion consistent with other research on mice (Henry, 1986; Park, Cook, & Verde, 1990; Sweet, Price, & Henry, 1988). Examples of some different outcomes of dietary restriction are shown in Figure 13.1.

The findings on mice suggest that dietary restriction has the capacity to slow or mitigate the progression of peripheral neural degeneration. However, this appears to be tied to genotype, suggesting that ultimate application of some sort of long-term approach to humans may have to deal with substantial individual differences. The same is likely to be true for the effects of dietary restriction on the CNS as well.

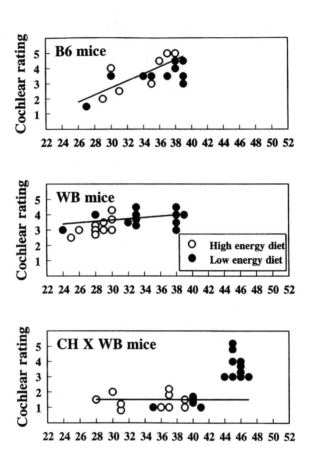

FIGURE 13.1 Some effects of dietary restriction on age-related cochlear pathology. The ordinate indicates the degree of cochlear pathology from normal *(1)* to severe *(5)*; the abscissa indicate the age at natural death. In B6 mice (C57BL/6J), dietary restriction (low-energy diet) had a small effect on longevity, but the degree of cochlear pathology was generally less than that of mice maintained on a typical high-energy diet (regression line = predicted values for low-energy mice using equation derived from high-energy mice). Dietary restriction appeared to ameliorate cochlear pathology. In WB mice, dietary restriction prolonged life but had no apparent effect on the degree of cochlear pathology (regression line was derived from low-energy mice). In the CH (CBA) × WB hybrids, dietary restriction prolonged life, but old mice exhibited cochlear pathology much more severe than that predicted from the regression equation derived from high-energy mice. Reprinted from Willott, J. F., Erway, L. C., Archer, J. R., & Harrison, D. E. (1995). Genetics of age-related hearing loss in mice II: Strain differences and effects of caloric restriction on cochlear pathology and evoked response thresholds. *Hearing Research, 65,* 125–132, with permission from Elsevier Science, Inc.

Environmental Enrichment and Exercise

Pioneering work by Diamond and colleagues (Diamond, 1988; Diamond, Johnson, Protti, Otte, & Kajisa, 1985) indicated that relatively simple environmental manipulations can affect the brain of old rats. Their experiments entailed exposing young and old rats to an "enriched" environment (e.g., 10 rats per cage, large space, toys). Enriched subjects from both young and old age groups exhibited a thicker cerebral cortex, especially in the occipital area, compared to like-aged nonenriched rats. Enhancement of dendritic growth and complexity were also demonstrated in this work and in other studies of environmental enrichment (Flood, 1993). Additional evidence indicates that enriched environments can promote the production or survival of synapses. Greenough, McDonald, Parnisari, and Camel (1986) found that old rats maintained in a complex environment had more dendritic spines on Purkinje neurons of the cerebellum, and Saito and colleagues (1994) showed preservation of youthful synaptic density in the cerebral cortex and hippocampus of old rats reared in an enriched environment.

Cotman and Neeper (1996) presented a scenario whereby physical and mental exercise could ameliorate some of the age-associated declines in cognitive and other brain functions by enhancing the activity of neurotrophic factors. Epidemiological studies on humans, as well as animal studies in the laboratory, indicate that physical activity and exercise are associated with superior cognitive and psychological performance in older subjects (Dustman, Shearer, & Emmerson, 1993). Wheel-running experiments with rats have shown that exercise increases BDNF and NGF activity in the hippocampus and cortex. Taken together, this research suggests that exercise can promote growth factors in the brain. Additionally, it is not just physical activity that might be used. There is evidence showing that CNS expression of BDNF, NGF, and FGF is regulated by neuronal activity. In other words, promoting appropriate neural activity ("mental exercise") may up-regulate growth factors, thereby unleashing their supportive effects.

Neurotrophic factors might also represent the link between environmental enrichment and improved cognitive performance. Environmental enrichment results in increased expression of NGF (Cotman & Neeper, 1996), as well as the formation of new synapses and dendrites mentioned earlier. Thus, it could be that enriched environments or behaviors are associated with increased neural activity, which results in an up-regulation of nerve growth factors, which in turn leads to enhanced neuronal survival, growth, and plasticity.

Recent experiments from our laboratory indicate that exposing C57 mice, which develop presbycusis (see chapter 7), to an augmented acoustic environment (AAE) allays the loss of auditory function (Turner & Willott, 1998a). Recall that C57 mice exhibit progressive cochlear sensorineural hearing loss, with thresholds for high frequencies becoming greatly elevated after about 3 months of age and becoming severe by middle age (6 to 12 months). We evaluated the effects of an AAE on this process by exposing mice to a regimen of 70-dB SPL noise bursts for 12 hours per night (when they are normally active) beginning at age 25 days. One of the tests used to assess auditory behavior was prepulse inhibition (PPI). As discussed in chapter 10, when a moderately intense (70-dB SPL) tone "prepulse" (S1) is presented 100 msec before an intense startle-eliciting sound (S2), the amplitude of the startle response evoked by S2 is reduced (inhibited). The degree of PPI provides a measure of the behavioral salience of S1. As shown in Figure 13.2, when the S1 was a 16-kHz tone,

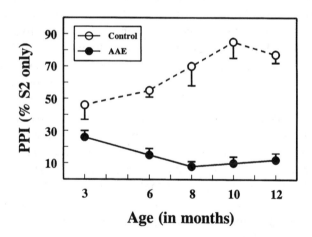

FIGURE 13.2   Effects of an augmented acoustic environment (AAE) on prepulse inhibition in aging C57 mice. In control mice, PPI became progressively worse with age for the 16-kHz prepulses, indicating diminished behavioral salience of these sounds. Mice exposed to an AAE beginning at age 25 days exhibited greatly superior PPI for other prepulse frequencies as well. From J. G. Turner and J. F. Willott, Association for Research in Otolaryngology, St. Petersburg Beach, FL, 1998.

PPI waned progressively as the mice aged and lost sensitivity to these tones. In marked contrast, PPI improved in AAE-exposed mice and showed no signs of declining through 12 months of age. ABR thresholds (not shown here) also remained much lower in the AAE-exposed mice. It is clear that the AAE resulted in dramatic amelioration of progressive hearing loss in C57. Other work from our laboratory has shown similar results with DBA/2J mice, which show earlier and more severe hearing loss, indicating some generality of this phenomenon with respect to genotype and the age/time frame of progressive hearing loss (Turner & Willott, 1998b; Willott, Turner, & Bross, 1997). One important manifestation of the AAE effect in DBA mice was a reduced loss of neurons in the cochlear nucleus, which typically accompanies progressive hearing loss in this strain.

To summarize, environmental enrichment, physical exercise, and an enhanced acoustic environment have all been shown to have ameliorative effects on the aging nervous system. Because methods such as these do not involve the introduction of drugs or other exogenous agents (with potential side effects or complications), they are attractive as potential anti-aging strategies. Future research should delimit the extent to which such manipulations can modify the aging nervous system and hopefully determine how to maximize the benefits.

Neural Transplantation

Sometimes age-related damage to neurons is too severe to be managed by reactive synaptogenesis, neurotrophins, or environmental manipulations. This is especially true of neurodegenerative diseases. In such cases, transplantation or grafting of new neurons into the damaged site might prove to be a feasible approach (see Cotman, 1990; Gage & Bjorklund, 1986; Gash, Collier, & Sladek, 1985). The main problems are survival of the graft and, more importantly, appropriate rewiring of circuitry with the host brain. There is a tendency of the grafted tissue to make contacts appropriate for their neurotransmitters and circuits, although this depends on brain region and other variables. One factor in the success of a neural graft is competition between transplant and host neurons for vacated synaptic sites. If reactive synaptogenesis of the host's neurons outcompete the grafted neurons, the graft may not become successfully integrated. Thus, it may be that partial loss of synapses in older host brains might actually give the graft a competitive edge, increasing the likelihood of an integrated graft.

The possibility of replacing brain tissue lost to aging—thereby restoring function—is an exciting possibility. As mentioned in chapter 9, modest improvements have been obtained by grafting tissue from the adrenal gland or fetal substantia nigra into Parkinson's patients (Feldman et al., 1997), although the results of some studies have been controversial. Encouraging results have been obtained from animal research in other brain regions as well, and several studies have shown that fetal brain tissue can be successfully transplanted into the brains of aged rodents. One series of experiments attempted to reverse the symptoms of reproductive senescence in female rats (Matsumoto, Kobayashi, Maralsami, & Arai, 1984). Typically, by about 10 months of age, the female's estrus cycle becomes irregular and undergoes changes, and reproductive impairment results (see chapter 12). When young hypothalamic tissue was transplanted into old rats, significant increases in the weight of the ovaries and uterus resulted, and the reproductive decline was halted or partially reversed. A different group of researchers transplanted fetal tissue from the locus coeruleus into old rats (Gash et al., 1985). After 6 weeks, the aged animals showed improvement on a test measuring retention of a learning task. Other research showed that fetal transplants of SCN tissue into aged hamsters restored aspects of circadian function (Van Reeth, Zhang, Zee, & Turek, 1994). A study by Martinez-Serrano, Fischer, and Bjorklund (1995) obtained increased NGF levels in the basal forebrain of rats by transplanting cells from a cultured line of NGF-secreting cells. In old, spatial learning–impaired rats, the transplants resulted in a reversal of their learning impairment and increased size of cholinergic neurons to normal size. Finally, behavioral improvements have been demonstrated in old rats with poor maze performance after grafts affecting input to the hippocampus were made (Gage & Bjorklund, 1986).

The research on neural transplants in humans and animal models indicates that the approach is feasible. A big issue is the extent to which the complex behaviors and cognitive processes of humans can benefit. It is one thing to enhance dopamine activity in Parkinson's patients and another to replace intricate neural circuitry underlying cognitive processes. The latter may never be attainable. For now, the utility of neural grafts is likely to be found in their capacity to generate growth factors and other beneficial substances, or boost the activity of certain circuits by replenishing neurotransmitters.

SUMMARY AND CONCLUSIONS

In chapter 1 it was emphasized that the great variance among individuals that characterizes aging is a function of the interaction among genes and environment. Whereas the future may allow us to use genetic engineering to produce infants destined to age optimally, for now we must settle for the genotype we are born with. We can regulate the expression of certain genes, control aspects of the environment, optimize benefits obtained from education, experience, and health care, and alter the body's physiological activity with drugs, diet, and other manipulations—a diverse arsenal of weapons to fight aging. As the research outlined in this chapter shows, such manipulations have the demonstrated ability or potential to modify the old or aging nervous system in beneficial ways. Neurogerontological research is clearly finding new ways to attain *successful aging*, the concept used by Rowe and Kahn (1987) to identify the healthiest and happiest segment of the elderly population. Although we have a long way to go, this last chapter should leave us with an optimistic attitude about aging and the nervous system.

References

Abramson, M., & Lovas, P. M. (Eds.). (1988). *Aging and sensory change: An annotated bibliography.* Washington, DC: Gerontological Society of America.

Adams, I. (1987). Comparison of synaptic changes in the precentral and postcentral cerebral cortex of aging humans: A quantitative ultrastructural study. *Neurobiology of Aging, 8,* 203–212.

Adams, R. D. (1984). Aging and human locomotion. In M. L. Albert (Ed.), *Clinical neurology of aging* (pp. 381–386). New York: Oxford University Press.

Ahmad, A., & Spear, P. D. (1993). Effects of aging on the size, density, and number of rhesus monkey lateral geniculate neurons. *Journal of Comparative Neurology, 334,* 631–643.

Albert, M. L., & Knoefel, J. E. (Eds.). (1994). *Clinical neurology of aging* (2nd ed.). New York: Oxford University Press.

Algeri, S., Biagini, L., Manfridi, A., & Pitsikas, N. (1991). Age-related ability of rats kept on a life-long hypocaloric diet in a spatial memory test: Longitudinal observations. *Neurobiology of Aging, 12,* 277–282.

Allen, G., Buxton, R. B., Wong, E. C., & Courchesne, E. (1997). Attentional activation of the cerebellum independent of motor involvement. *Science, 275,* 1940–1943.

Altavista, M. C., Bentivoglio, A. R., Crociani, P., Rossi, P., & Albanese, A. (1988). Age-dependent loss of cholinergic neurones in basal ganglia of rats. *Brain Research, 455,* 177–181.

Amenta, F., Bongrani, S., Cadel, S., Ricci, A., Valsecchi, B., & Zeng, Y. C. (1994). Neuroanatomy of aging brain: Influence of treatment with L-deprenyl. *Annals of the New York Academy of Sciences, 717,* 33–44.

Amenta, F., Mancini, M., Naves, F. J., Vega, J. A., & Zaccheo, D. (1995). Effect of treatment with the dihydropyridine-type calcium antagonist darodipine (PY 108-068) on the expression of calbindin D28l immunoreactivity in the cerebellar cortex of aged rats. *Mechanisms of Ageing and Development, 77,* 149–157.

Anderson, B., & Rutledge, V. (1996). Age and hemisphere effects on dendritic structure. *Brain, 119,* 1983–1990.

Anderson, K. J., Scheff, S. W., & DeKosky, S. T. (1986). Reactive synaptogenesis in hippocampal area CA1 of aged and young adult rats. *Journal of Comparative Neurology, 252,* 374–384.

Anderton, B. H., Brion, J.-P., Flament-Durand, J., Haugh, M., Kahn, J., Miller, C. C., Probst, A., & Ulrich, J. (1986). Changes in the neuronal cytoskeleton in aging and disease. In M. Bergener, M. Ermini, & H. B. Stahelin (Eds.), *Dimensions in aging* (pp. 69–90). New York: Academic Press.

Andrews, T. J. (1996). Autonomic nervous system as a model of neuronal aging: The role of target tissues and neurotrophic factors. *Microscopy Research and Technique, 35*, 2–19.

Andrews, T. J., Li, D., Halliwell, J., & Cowen, T. (1994). The effect of age on dendrites in the rat superior cervical ganglion. *Journal of Anatomy, 184,* 111–117.

Ankarcrona, M., Dypbukt, J. M., Bonfoco, E., Zhivotovsky, B., Orrenius, S., Lipton, S. A., & Nicotera, P. (1995). Glutamate-induced neuronal death: A succession of necrosis or apoptosis depending on mitochondrial function. *Neuron, 15,* 961–973.

Araki, T., Kato, H., Fujiwara, T., & Itoyama, Y. (1995). Age-related changes in binding of second messengers in the rat brain. *Brain Research, 704,* 227–232.

Arendash, G. W., Sengstock, G. J., Sanberg, P. R., & Kem, W. R. (1995). Improved learning and memory in aged rats with chronic administration of the nicotinic receptor agonist GTS-21. *Brain Research, 674,* 252–259.

Arnsten, A. F. T. (1993). Catecholamine mechanisms in age-related cognitive decline. *Neurobiology of Aging, 14,* 639–641.

Arnsten, A. F. (1997). Catecholamine regulation of the prefrontal cortex. *Journal of Psychopharmacology, 11,* 151–162.

Arnsten, A. F., Lin, C. H., Van Dyck, C. H., & Stanhope, K. J. (1997). The effects of 5-HT3 receptor antagonists on cognitive performance in aged monkeys. *Neurobiology of Aging, 18,* 21–28.

Asanuma, A., Tamauchi, Y., Koga, T., & Katayama, I. (1995). Suppression of age-related changes in mouse hippocampal CA3 nerve cells by a free radical scavenger. *Mechanisms of Ageing and Development, 83,* 55–64.

Ausman, L. M., & Russell, R. M. (1990). Nutrition and aging. In E. L. Schneider & J. W. Rowe (Eds.), *Handbook of the biology of aging* (3rd ed., pp. 384–406). San Diego: Academic Press.

Avery, D., Lenz, M., & Landis, C. (1998). Guidelines for prescribing melatonin. *Annals of Medicine, 30,* 122–130.

Backman, C., Rose, G. M., Hoffer, B. J., Henry, M. A., Bartus, R. T., Friden, P., & Granholm, A. C. (1996). Systemic administration of a nerve growth factor conjugate reverses age-related cognitive dysfunction and prevents cholinergic neuron atrophy. *Journal of Neuroscience, 16,* 5437–5442.

Bakalian, A., Corman, B., Delhaye-Bouchaud, N., & Mariani, J. (1991). Quantitative analysis of the Purkinje cell population during extreme ageing in the cerebellum of the Wistar/Louvain rat. *Neurobiology of Aging, 12,* 425–430.

Baker, H., Franzen, L., Stone, D., Cho, J. Y., & Margolis, F. L. (1995). Expression of tyrosine hydroxylase in the aging, rodent olfactory system. *Neurobiology of Aging, 16,* 119–128.

Balice-Gordon, R. J. (1997). Age-related changes in neuromuscular innervation. *Muscle & Nerve*(Suppl. 5), S83–S87.

Balogun, J. A., Akindele, K. A., Nihinlola, J. O., & Marzouk, D. K. (1994). Age-related changes in balance performance. *Disability and Rehabilitation, 16*, 58–62.

Bannon, M. J., & Whitty, C. J. (1997). Age-related and regional differences in dopamine transporter mRNA expression in human midbrain. *Neurology, 48*, 969–977.

Barinaga, M. (1997). A mitochondrial Alzheimer's gene? *Science, 276*, 682.

Barkats, M., Venault, P., Christen, Y., & Cohen-Salmon, C. (1995). Effect of long-term treatment with EGb 761 on age-dependent structural changes in the hippocampi of three inbred mouse strains. *Life Sciences, 56*, 213–222.

Barnes, C. A., & McNaughton, B. L. (1985). An age comparison of the rates of acquisition and forgetting of spatial information in relation to long-term enhancement of hippocampal synapses. *Behavioral Neuroscience, 99*, 1040–1048.

Barnes, C. A., Mizumori, S. J. Y., Lovinger, D. M., Sheu, F.-S., Murakami, K., Chan, S. Y., Linden, D. J., Nelson, R. B., & Routtenberg, A. (1988). Selective decline in protein F1 phosphorylation in hippocampus of senescent rats. *Neurobiology of Aging, 9*, 393–398.

Barnes, C. A., Rao, G., & Shen, J. (1997). Age-related decrease in the N-methyl-D-aspartate$_R$–mediated excitatory postsynaptic potential in hippocampal region CA1. *Neurobiology of Aging, 18*, 445–452.

Barnes, C. A., Suster, M. S., Shen, J., & McNaughton, B. L. (1997). Multistability of cognitive maps in the hippocampus of old rats. *Nature, 388*, 272–275.

Barringer, D. L., & Bunag, R. D. (1991). Autonomic regulation of reflex bradycardia in rats declines with age. *Experimental Gerontology, 26*, 65–75.

Barrou, Z., Charru, P., & Lidy, C. (1997). Dehydroepiandrosterone (DHEA) and aging. *Archives of Gerontology and Geriatrics, 24*, 233–241.

Bartoshuk, L. M., & Weiffenbach, J. M. (1990). Chemical senses and aging. In E. L. Schneider & J. W. Rowe (Eds.), *Handbook of the biology of aging* (3rd ed., pp. 429–443). San Diego: Academic Press.

Bartus, R. T., Dean, R. L., & Beer, B. (1982). Neuropeptide effects on memory in aged monkeys. *Neurobiology of Aging, 3*, 61–68.

Bartus, R. T., Dean, R. L., Beer, B., & Lippa, A. S. (1982). The cholinergic hypothesis of geriatric memory dysfunction. *Science, 217*, 408–417.

Bashore, T. R. (1990). Age-related changes in mental processing revealed by analysis of event-related brain potentials. In J. W. Rohrbaugh, R. Parasuraman, & R. Johnson (Eds.), *Event-related brain potentials* (pp. 242–275). New York: Oxford University Press.

Baxter, M. G., & Voytko, M. L. (1996). Spatial orienting of attention in adult and aged rhesus monkeys. *Behavioral Neuroscience, 110*, 898–904.

Beach, T. G., Walker, R., & McGeer, E. G. (1989). Patterns of gliosis in Alzheimer's disease and aging cerebrum. *Glia, 2*, 420–436.

Beeson, P. M., & Bayles, K. A. (1997). Aphasia. In P. D. Nussbaum (Ed.), *Handbook of neuropsychology and aging* (pp. 298–314). New York: Plenum.

Bellantoni, M. F., & Blackman, M. R. (1996). Menopause and its consequences. In E. L. Schneider & J. W. Rowe (Eds.), *Handbook of the biology of aging* (4th ed., pp. 415–430). San Diego: Academic Press.

Belzunegui, T., Insausti, R., Ibanez, J., & Gonzalo, L. M. (1995). Effect of chronic alcoholism on neuronal nuclear size and neuronal population in the mammillary body and the anterior thalamic complex of man. *Histology and Histopathology, 10*, 633–638.

Benes, F. M., Majocha, R. E., & Marotta, C. A. (1988). A modular arrangement of neuronal processes in human cortex: Disruption with aging and in Alzheimer's disease. *Journal of Geriatric Psychiatry and Neurology, 1*, 3–10.

Bennett, G. W., Ballard, T. M., Watson, C. D., & Fone, K. C. (1997). Effect of neuropeptides on cognitive function. *Experimental Gerontology, 32*, 451–469.

Bergado, J. A., Fernandez, C. I., Gomez-Soria, A., & Gonzalez, O. (1997). Chronic intraventricular infusion with NGF improves LTP in old cognitively impaired rats. *Brain Research, 770*, 1–9.

Bernardis, L. L., & Davis, P. L. (1996). Aging and the hypothalamus: Research perspectives. *Physiology and Behavior, 59*, 523–536.

Bertoni-Freddari, C., Fattoretti, P., Paoloni, R., Caselli, U., Galeazzi, L., & Meier-Ruge, W. (1996). Synaptic structural dynamics and aging. *Gerontology, 42*, 170–180.

Besthorn, C., Zerfass, R., Geiger-Kabisch, C., Sattel, H., Daniel, S., Schreiter-Gasser, U., & Forstl, H. (1997). Discrimination of Alzheimer's disease and normal aging by EEG data. *Electroencephalography and Clinical Neurophysiology, 103*, 241–248.

Bhatnagar, K. P., Kennedy, R. C., Baron, G., & Greenberg, R. A. (1987). Number of mitral cells and the bulb volume in the aging human olfactory bulb: A quantitative morphological study. *Anatomical Record, 218*, 73–87.

Bickford, P. (1993). Motor learning deficits in aged rats are correlated with loss of cerebellar noradrenergic function. *Brain Research, 620*, 133–138.

Bigham, M. H., & Lidow, M. S. (1995). Adrenergic and serotonergic receptors in aged monkey neocortex. *Neurobiology of Aging, 16*, 91–104.

Birch, D. G., & Anderson, J. L. (1992). Standardized full-field electroretinography: Normal values and their variation with age. *Archives of Opthalmology, 110*, 1571–1576.

Birren, J. E. (Ed.). (1996). *Encyclopedia of gerontology*. San Diego: Academic Press.

Birren, J. E., & Fisher, L. M. (1995). Aging and speed of behavior: Possible consequences for psychological functioning. *Annual Review of Psychology, 46*, 329–353.

Birren, J. E., Woods, A. M., & Williams, M. V. (1980). Behavioral slowing with age: Causes, organization, and consequences. In L. W. Poon (Ed.), *Aging in the 1980's: Psychological issues* (pp. 293–308). Washington, DC: American Psychological Association.

Bitsios, P., Prettyman, R., & Szabadi, E. (1996). Changes in autonomic function with age: A study of pupillary kinetics in healthy young and old people. *Age and Ageing, 25,* 432–438.

Blass, J. P. (1996). Cerebral metabolic impairments. In Z. S. Khachaturian & T. S. Radenbaugh (Eds.), *Alzheimer's disease: Cause(s), diagnosis, treatment, and care* (pp. 187–206). Boca Raton, FL: CRC Press.

Blumberg, J. B. (1996). Status and functional impact of nutrition in older adults. In E. L. Schneider & J. W. Rowe (Eds.), *Handbook of the biology of aging* (4th ed., pp. 393–414). San Diego: Academic Press.

Bobak, P., Bodis-Wollner, I., Guillory, S., & Anderson, R. (1989). Aging differentially delays visual evoked potentials to checks and gratings. *Clinical Vision Sciences, 4,* 269–274.

Bondi, M. W., & Troster, A. I. (1997). Parkinson's disease: Neurobehavioral consequences of basal ganglia dysfunction. In P. D. Nussbaum (Ed.), *Handbook of neuropsychology and aging* (pp. 216–245). New York: Plenum.

Borst, S. (1996). Autonomic nervous system. In J. E. Birren (Ed.), *Encyclopedia of gerontology* (Vol. 1, pp. 141–147). San Diego: Academic Press.

Brizzee, K. R. (1973). Quantitative histological studies on aging changes in cerebral cortex of rhesus monkeys and albino rat with notes on effects of prolonged low-dose ionizing irradiation in the rat. *Progress in Brain Research, 40,* 141–160.

Brizzee, K. R., & Ordy, J. M. (1979). Age pigments, cell loss, and hippocampal formation. *Mechanisms of Ageing and Development, 9,* 143–162.

Brody, H. (1955). Organization of the cerebral cortex: 3. A study of aging in cerebral cortex. *Journal of Comparative Neurology, 102,* 511–556.

Brody, H., & Vijayashankar, N. (1977). Anatomical changes in the nervous system, In C. E. Finch & L. Hayflick (Eds.), *Handbook of the biology of aging* (pp. 241–261). New York: Van Nostrand.

Bronson, R. T., & Lipman, R. D. (1996). Reduction in rate of occurrence of age-related lesions in dietary restricted laboratory mice. *Growth, Development, & Aging, 55,* 169–184.

Brzezinski, A. (1997). Melatonin in humans. *New England Journal of Medicine, 336,* 186–195.

Buell, S. J., & Coleman, P. D. (1979). Dendritic growth in the aged human brain and failure of growth in senile dementia. *Science, 206,* 854–856.

Bullock, T. H. (1977). *Introduction to nervous systems.* San Francisco: Freeman.

Bunker, V. W. (1992). Free radicals, antioxidants and aging. *Medical Laboratory Science, 49,* 299–312.

Burns, E. M., Kruckeberg, T. W., Comerford, L. E., & Buschmann, M. B. T. (1979). Thinning of capillary walls and declining numbers of endothelial mitochondria in the cerebral cortex of the aging primate, *Macaca nemestrina.* *Journal of Gerontology, 34,* 642–650.

Burns, E. M., Kruckeberg, T. W., Gaetano, P. K., & Shulman, L. M. (1983). Morphological changes in cerebral capillaries with age. In J. Cervos-Navarro & H.-I. Sarkander (Eds.), *Brain aging: Neuropathology and neuropharmacology* (Vol. 21, pp. 115–132). New York: Raven.

Busch, C., Bohl, J., & Ohm, T. G. (1997). Spatial, temporal and numeric analysis of Alzheimer changes in the nucleus coeruleus. *Neurobiology of Aging, 18,* 401–406.

Buskirk, E. R. (1985). Health maintenance and longevity: Exercise. In C. E. Finch & E. L. Schneider (Eds.), *Handbook of the biology of aging* (2nd ed., pp. 894–931). New York: Van Nostrand Reinhold.

Bylsma, F. W. (1997). Huntington's disease. In P. D. Nussbaum (Ed.), *Handbook of neuropsychology and aging* (pp. 246–259). New York: Plenum.

Cabeza, R., Grady, C. L., Nyberg, L., McIntosh, A. R., Tulving, E., Kapur, S., Jennings, J. M., Houle, S., & Craik, F. I. M. (1997). Age-related differences in neural activity during memory encoding and retrieval: A positron emission tomography study. *Journal of Neuroscience, 17,* 391–400.

Campbell, L. W., Hao, S. Y., Thibault, O., Blalock, E. M., & Landfield, P. W. (1996). Aging changes in voltage-gated calcium currents in hippocampal CA1 neurons. *Journal of Neuroscience, 16,* 6286–6295.

Carlson, S., & Willott, J. F. (1998). Caudal pontine reticular formation in C57BL/ 6J mice: Responses to startle stimuli, inhibition by tones, plasticity. *Journal of Neurophysiology, 79,* 2603–2614.

Carney, J. M., Starke-Reed, P. E., Oliver, C. N., Landrum, R. W., Cheng, M. S., Wu, J. F., & Floyd, R. A. (1991). Reversal of age-related increase in brain protein oxidation, decrease in enzyme activity, and loss in temporal and spatial memory by chronic administration of N-tert-butyl-a-phenylnitrone. *Proceedings of the National Academy of Science, 88,* 3633–3636.

Carta, A., & Calvani, M. (1991). Acetyl-L-carnitine: A drug able to slow the progress of Alzheimer's disease? *Annals of the New York Academy of Sciences, 640,* 228–232.

Casey, M. A., & Feldman, M. L. (1985). Aging in the rat medial nucleus of the trapezoid body: 3. Alterations in capillaries. *Neurobiology of Aging, 6,* 39–46.

Casoli, T., Spagna, C., Fattoretti, P., Gesuita, R., & Bertoni-Freddari, C. (1996). Neuronal plasticity in aging: A quantitative immunohistochemical study of GAP-43 distribution in discrete regions of the rat brain. *Brain Research, 714,* 111–117.

Caspary, D. M., Milbrandt, J. C., & Helfert, R. H. (1995). Central auditory aging: GABA changes in the inferior colliculus. *Experimental Gerontology, 30,* 349–360.

Caspary, D. M., Raza, A., Lawhorn-Armour, B. A., Pippin, J., & Arneric, S. P. (1990). Immunocytochemical and neurochemical evidence for age-related loss of GABA in the inferior colliculus: Implications for neural presbycusis. *Journal of Neuroscience, 10,* 2363–2372.

Castel, M. N., Beaudet, A., & Laduron, P. M. (1994). Retrograde axonal transport of neurotensin in rat nigrostriatal dopaminergic neurons: Modulation during ageing and possible physiological role. *Biochemical Pharmacology, 47,* 53–62.

Castiglioni, A. J., Legare, M. E., Busbee, D. L., & Tiffany-Castiglioni, E. (1991). Morphological changes in astrocytes of aging mice fed normal or caloric restricted diets. *Age, 14,* 102–106.

Celsia, G. G., Kaufman, D., & Cone, S. (1987). Effects of age and sex on pattern electroretinograms and visual evoked potentials. *Electroencephalography and Clinical Neurophysiology, 68,* 161–171.

Cepeda, C., Lee, N., Buchwald, N. A., Radisavljevic, Z., & Levine, M. S. (1992). Age-induced changes in electrophysiological responses of neostriatal neurons recorded in vitro. *Neuroscience, 51,* 411–423.

Cepeda, C., Walsh, J. P., Hull, C. D., Buchwald, N. A., & Levine, M. S. (1989). Intracellular neurophysiological analysis reveals alterations in excitation in striatal neurons in aged rats. *Brain Research, 494,* 215–226.

Chakour, M. C., Gibson, S. J., Bradbeer, M., & Helme, R. D. (1996). The effect of age on A delta- and C-fibre thermal pain perception. *Pain, 64,* 143–152.

Chan-Palay, V., & Azan, F. (1989). Quantitation of catecholamine neurons in the locus coeruleus in human brains of normal young and older adults. *Journal of Comparative Neurology, 287,* 357–372.

Chao, L. L., & Knight, R. T. (1997). Prefrontal deficits in attention and inhibitory control with aging. *Cerebral Cortex, 7,* 63–69.

Chauhan, N., & Siegel, G. (1997a). Age-dependent organotypic expression of microtubule-associated proteins (MAP1, MAP2, and MAP5) in rat brain. *Neurochemistry Research, 22,* 713–719.

———. (1997b). Differential expression of Na,K-ATPase alpha-isoform mRNAs in aging rat cerebellum. *Journal of Neuroscience Research, 47,* 287–299.

Chen, K. S., Masliah, E., Mallory, M., & Gage, F. H. (1995). Synaptic loss in cognitively impaired aged rats is ameliorated by chronic human nerve growth factor infusion. *Neuroscience, 68,* 19–27, 1995.

Cherniack, N. S., & Altose, M. D. (1996). Respiratory system. In J. E. Birren (Ed.), *Encyclopedia of gerontology* (Vol. 2, pp. 431–436). San Diego: Academic Press.

Choi-Lundberg, D. L., Lin, Q., Chang, T.-N., Chiang, Y. L., Hay, C. M., Mohajeri, H., Davidson, B. L., & Bohn, M. C. (1997). Dopaminergic neurons protected from degeneration by GDNF gene therapy. *Science, 275,* 838–841.

Choo, D., Malmgren, L. T., & Rosenberg, S. I. (1990). Age-related changes in Schwann cells of the internal branch of the rat superior laryngeal nerve. *Otolaryngology Head and Neck Surgery, 103,* 628–636.

Chui, H., Bondareff, W., Zarow, C., & Slager, U. (1984). Stability of neuronal number in the nucleus basalis of Meynert with age. *Neurobiology of Aging, 5,* 83–88.

Clark, J. T. (1994). Aging-induced decrements in neuropeptide Y: The retention of ejaculatory behavior is associated with site-selective differences. *Neurobiology of Aging, 15,* 191–196.

Coffey, C. E., Wilkinson, W. E., Parahos, I. A., Soady, S. A. R., Sullivan, R. J., Sullivan, R. J., Patterson, L. J., Figiel, G. S., Webb, M. C., Spritzer, C. E., & Djang, W. T. (1992). Quantitative cerebral anatomy of the aging human brain: A cross-sectional study using magnetic resonance imagery. *Neurology, 42,* 527–536.

Cohen, G. D. (1988). *The brain in human aging.* New York: Springer.

Cohen, H., Heaton, L. G., Congdon, S. L., & Jenkins, H. A. (1996). Changes in sensory organization test scores with age. *Age and Ageing, 25,* 39–44.

Cohen, S. A., & Muller, W. E. (1992). Age-related alterations of NMDA-receptor properties in the mouse forebrain: Partial restoration by chronic phosphatidyl-serine treatment. *Brain Research, 584,* 174–180.

Coleman, P., & Flood, D. (1987). Neuron numbers and dendritic extent in normal aging and Alzheimer's disease. *Neurobiology of Aging, 8,* 521–545.

Collier, T. J., Gash, D. M., & Sladek, J. R. (1987). Norepinephrine deficiency and behavioral senescence in aged rats: Transplanted locus coeruleus neurons as an experimental replacement therapy. *Annals of the New York Academy of Sciences, 495,* 396–403.

Cooper, J. D., Lindholm, D., & Sofroniew, M. V. (1994). Reduced transport of [125I] nerve growth factor by cholinergic neurons and down-regulated TrkA expression in the medial septum of aged rats. *Neuroscience, 62,* 625–629.

Corden, D. M., & Lippold, O. C. J. (1996). Age-related impaired reflex sensitivity in a human hand muscle. *Journal of Neurophysiology, 76,* 2701–2706.

Corso, J. F. (1981). *Aging sensory systems and perception.* New York: Praeger.

Corwin, J., Loury, M., & Gilbert, A. N. (1995). Workplace, age, and sex as mediators of olfactory function: Data from the National Geographic Smell Survey. *Journal of Gerontology B, 50,* P179–P186.

Cotman, C. W. (1990). Synaptic plasticity, neurotrophic factors, and transplantation in the aged brain. In E. L. Schneider & J. W. Rowe (Eds.), *Handbook of the biology of aging* (3rd ed., pp. 255–274). San Diego: Academic Press.

Cotman, C. W., & Holets, V. R. (1985). Structural changes at synapses with age: Plasticity and regeneration. In C. E. Finch & E. L. Schneider (Eds.), *Handbook of the biology of aging* (2nd ed., pp. 617–644). New York: Van Nostrand Reinhold.

Cotman, C. W., & Neeper, S. (1996). Activity-dependent plasticity and the aging brain. In E. L. Schneider & J. W. Rowe (Eds.), *Handbook of the biology of aging* (4th ed., pp. 284–299). San Diego: Academic Press.

Cowen, T. (1993). Ageing in the autonomic nervous system: A result of nerve-target interactions. *Mechanisms of Ageing and Development, 68,* 163–173.

Coyle, J. T., Price, D. L., & DeLong, M. R. (1983). Alzheimer's disease: A disorder of cortical cholinergic innervation. *Science, 219,* 1184–1190.

Craik, F. I. M., & Jennings, J. M. (1992). Human memory. In F. I. M. Craik & T. A. Salthouse (Eds.), *The handbook of aging and cognition* (pp. 51–110). Hillsdale, NJ: Erlbaum.

Cransac, H., Peyrin, L., Cottet-Emard, Farhat, F., Pequignot, J. M., & Reber, A. (1996). Aging effects on monoamines in rat medial vestibular and cochlear nuclei. *Hearing Research, 100,* 150–156.

Crassini, B., Brown, B., & Bowman, K. (1988). Age-related changes in contrast sensitivity in central and peripheral retina. *Perception, 17,* 315–332.

Crawford, C. A., & Levine, M. S. (1997). Dopamine function in the neostriatum and nucleus accumbens of young and aged Fischer 344 rats. *Neurobiology of Aging, 18,* 57–66.

Crutcher, K. A., & Weingartner, J. (1991). Hippocampal NGF levels are not reduced in the aged Fischer 344 rat. *Neurobiology of Aging, 12,* 449–454.

Cruz-Sanchez, F. F., Cardozo, A., & Tolosa, E. (1995). Neuronal changes in the substantia nigra with aging: A Golgi study. *Journal of Neuropathology and Experimental Neurology, 54,* 74–81.

Curcio, C. A., & Coleman, P. D. (1982). Stability of neuron number in cortical barrels of aging mice. *Journal of Comparative Neurology, 212,* 158–172.

Curcio, C. A., & Drucker, D. N. (1993). Retinal ganglion cells in Alzheimer's disease and aging. *Annals of Neurology, 33,* 248–257.

Curcio, C. A., McNelly, N. A., & Hinds, J. W. (1985). Aging in the rat olfactory system: Relative stability of piriform cortex contrasts with changes in olfactory bulb and olfactory epithelium. *Journal of Comparative Neurology, 235,* 519–528.

Curcio, C. A., Millican, C. L., Allen, K. A., & Kalina, R. E. (1993). Aging of the human photoreceptor mosaic: Evidence for elective vulnerability of rods in central retina. *Opthalmology and Visual Science, 34,* 3278–3296.

Danner, D. B., & Holbrook, N. J. (1990). Alterations in gene expression with aging. In E. L. Schneider & J. W. Rowe (Eds.), *Handbook of the biology of aging* (3rd ed., pp. 97–115). San Diego: Academic Press.

Dastur, D. K., Lane, M. H., Hansen, D. B., Kety, S. S., Butler, R. N., Perlin, S., & Sokoloff, L. (1963). Effects of aging on erebral circulation and metabolism. In J. E. Birren, R. N. Butler, S. W. Greenhouse, L. Sokoloff, & M. R. Yarrow (Eds.), *Human aging* (Public Health Service Publication No. 986, pp. 59–76). Washington, DC: U.S. Government Printing Office.

Davies, H. E. F. (1975). Respiratory change in heart rate, sinus arrhythmia in the elderly. *Gerontogy Clinics, 17,* 96–100.

Davis, M. (1992). The role of the amygdala in conditioned fear. In J. P. Aggelton (Ed.), *The amygdala: Neurobiological aspects of emotion, memory, and mental dysfunction* (pp. 255–306). New York: Wiley-Liss.

Davis, P. C., Mirra, S. S., & Alazraki, N. (1994). The brain in older persons with and without dementia: Findings on MR, PET, and SPECT images. *American Journal of Roentgenology, 164,* 1267–1278.

Dawson, R., & Wallace, D. R. (1992). Kainic acid-induced seizures in aged rats: Neurochemical correlates. *Brain Research Bulletin, 29,* 459–468.

D'Costa, A. P., Xu, X., Ingram, R. L., & Sonntag, W. E. (1995). Insulin-like growth factor-1 stimulation of protein synthesis is attenuated in cerebral cortex of aging rats. *Neuroscience, 65,* 805–813.

Deadwyler, S. A., & Hampson, R. E. (1997). The significance of neural ensemble codes during behavior and cognition. *Annual Review of Neuroscience, 20,* 217–244.

Decker, M. W. (1987). The effect of aging on hippocampal and cortical projections of the forebrain cholinergic system. *Brain Research Reviews, 12,* 423–438.

DeJong, G. I., Buwalda, B., Schuurman, T., & Luiten, P. G. M. (1992). Synaptic plasticity in the dentate gyrus of aged rats is altered after chronic nimodipine application. *Brain Research, 596,* 345–348.

DeJong, G. I., Naber, P. A., van der Zee, E. A., Thompson, L. T., Disterhoft, J. F., & Lutten, P. G. M. (1996). Age-related loss of calcium binding proteins in rabbit hippocampus. *Neurobiology of Aging, 17,* 459–465.

DeKosky, S. T., & Palmer, A. M. (1994). Neurochemistry of aging. In M. L. Albert & J. E. Knoefel (Eds.), *Clinical neurology of aging* (2nd ed., pp. 79–101). New York: Oxford University Press.

DeKosky, S. T., & Scheff, S. W. (1990). Synapse loss in frontal cortex biopsies in Alzheimer's disease: Correlation with cognitive severity. *Annals of Neurology, 27,* 457–464.

De Lacalle, S., Cooper, J. D., Svendsen, C. N., Dunnett, S. B., & Sofroniew, M. V. (1996). Reduced retrograde labeling with fluorescent tracer accompanies neuronal atrophy of basal forebrain cholinergic neurons in aged rats. *Neuroscience, 75,* 19–27.

De Lacalle, S., Iraiziz, I., & Gonzalo, L. (1991). Differential changes in cell size and number in topographic subdivisions of human basal nucleus in normal aging. *Neuroscience, 43,* 445–456.

De la Torre, J. C. (1997). Cerebromicrovascular pathology in Alzheimer's disease compared to normal aging. *Gerontology, 43,* 26–43.

Demarest, K. T., Moore, K. E., & Riegle, G. D. (1982). Dopaminergic neuronal function, anterior pituitary dopamine content, and serum concentrations of prolactin, luteinizing hormone and progesterone in the aged female rat. *Brain Research, 247,* 347–354.

Demarest, K. T., Riegle, G. D., & Moore, K. E. (1980). Characteristics of dopaminrgic neurons in the aged male rat. *Neuroendocrinology, 31,* 222–227.

Dement, W., Richardson, G., Prinz, P., Carskadon, M., Kripke, D., & Czeisler, C. (1985). Changes of sleep and wakefulness with age. In C. E. Finch & E. L. Schneider (Eds.), *Handbook of the biology of aging* (2nd ed., pp. 692–717). New York: Van Nostrand Reinhold.

De Santi, S., de Leon, M. J., Convit, A., Tarshish, C., Rusinek, H., Tsui, W. H., Sinaiko, E., Wang, G. J., Bartlet, E., & Volkow, N. (1995). Age-related changes in brain: 2. Positron emission tomography of frontal and temporal lobe glucose metabolism in normal subjects. *Psychiatry Quarterly, 66,* 357–370.

Desmedt, J. E., & Cheron, G. (1980). Somatosensory evoked potentials to finger stimulation in healthy octogenarians and in young adults: Wave forms, scalp topography and transit times of parietal and frontal components. *Electroencephalography and Clinical Neurophysiology, 50,* 404–425.

De Souza, R. R., Moratelli, H. B., Borges, N., & Liberti, E. A. (1993). Age-induced nerve cell loss in the myenteric plexus of the small intestine in man. *Gerontology, 39,* 183–188.

De Toledo-Morrell, L., Sullivan, M. P., Morell, F., Wilson, R. S., Bennett, D. A., & Spencer, S. (1997). Alzheimer's disease: In vivo detection of differential vulnerability of brain regions. *Neurobiology of Aging, 18,* 463–468.

Deupree, D. L., Turner, D. A., & Watters, C. L. (1991). Spatial performance correlates with in vitro potentiation in young and aged Fischer 344 rats. *Brain Research, 554,* 1–9.

De Wied, D. (1997). Neuropeptides in learning and memory processes. *Behavioural Brain Research, 83,* 83–90.

Deyo, R. A., Straube, K. T., & Disterhoft, J. F. (1989). Nimodipine facilitates trace conditioning of the eye-blink response in aging rabbits. *Science, 243,* 809–811.

Diamond, M. (1988). *Enriching heredity.* New York: Free Press/Macmillan.

Diamond, M. C., Johnson, R. E., Protti, A. M., Otte, C., & Kajisa, L. (1985). Plasticity in the 904-day-old male rat cerebral cortex. *Experimental Neurology, 87,* 309–317.

Diana, G., Domenici, M. R., Scotti de Carolis, A., Loizzo, A., & Sagratella, S. (1995). Reduced hippocampal CA1 Ca^{2+}–induced long-term potentation is associated with age-dependent mpairment of spatial learning. *Brain Research, 686,* 107–110.

Diana, G., Scotti de Carolis, A., Frank, C., Domenici, M. R., & Sagratella, S. (1994). Selective reduction of hippocampal dentate frequency potentiation in aged rats with impaired place learning. *Brain Research Bulletin, 35,* 107–111.

Diao, L. H., Bickford, P. C., Stevens, J. O., Cline, E. J., & Gerhardt, G. A. (1997). Caloric restriction enhances evoked DA overflow in striatum and nucleus accumbens of aged Fischer 344 rats. *Brain Research, 763,* 276–280.

Diaz, F., Villena, A., Requena, V., Ponzales, P., Pelaez, A., & Perez de Vargas, I. (1996). Quantitative histochemical study of cytochrome oxidase in the dLGN of aging rats. *Mechanisms of Ageing and Development, 91,* 47–54.

Diplock, A. T. (1997). Will the "good fairies" please prove to us that vitamin E lessens human degenerative disease? *Free Radical Research, 27,* 511–532.

Disterhoft, J. F., Moyer, J. R., Jr., & Thompson, L. T. (1994). The calcium rationale in aging and Alzheimer's disease. *Annals of the New York Academy of Sciences, 747,* 382–404.

Disterhoft, J. F., Moyer, J. R., Jr., Thompson, L. T., & Kowalska, M. (1993). Functional aspects of calcium-channel modulation. *Clinical Neuropharmacology, 16*(Suppl. 1), S12–S24.

Dlugos, C. A., & Pentney, R. J. (1994). Morphometric analysis of Purkinje and granule cells in aging F344 rats. *Neurobiology of Aging, 15,* 435–440.

Dluzen, D. E. (1996). Age-related changes in monoamines within the olfactory bulbs of the Fischer 344 male rat. *Mechanisms of Ageing and Development, 91,* 37–45.

Docherty, J. R. (1993). Efects of age on the response of target organs to autonomic neurotransmitters. In F. Amenta (Ed.), *Aging of the autonomic nervous system* (pp. 109–135). Boca Raton, FL: CRC Press.

Doraiswamy, P. M., Figiel, G. S., Husain, M. M., McDonald, W. M., Shah, S. A., Boyko, O. B., Ellinwood, E. H., & Krishnan, K. R. R. (1991). Aging of the human corpus callosum: Magnetic resonance imaging in normal volunteers. *Journal of Neuropsychology, 3,* 392–397.

Dorfman, L. J., & Bosley, T. M. (1979). Age-related changes in peripheral and central nerve conduction in man. *Neurology, 29,* 38–44.

Droy-Lefaix, M. T. (1997). Effect of the antioxidant action of ginkgo biloba extract (EGb 761) on aging and oxidative stress. *Age, 20,* 141–149.

Duara, R., London, E. D., & Rapoport, S. I. (1985). Changes in structure and energy metabolism of the aging brain. In C. E. Finch & E. L. Schneider (Eds.), *Handbook of the biology of aging* (2nd ed., pp. 595–616). New York: Van Nostrand Reinhold.

Duncan, J. (1995). Attention, intelligence, and the frontal lobes. In M. S. Gazzaniga (Ed.), *The cognitive neurosciences* (pp. 721–734). Cambridge, MA: MIT Press.

Dustman, R. E., Shearer, D. E., & Emmerson, R. Y. (1993). EEG and event-related potentials in normal aging. *Progress in Neurobiology, 41,* 369–401.

Eastwood, S. L., Burnet, P. W., McDonald, B., Clinton, J., & Harrison, P. J. (1994). Synaptophysin gene expression in human brain: A quantitative in situ hybridization and immunocytochemical study. *Neuroscience, 59,* 881–892.

Ebadi, M., Srinivasan, S. K., & Baxi, M. D. (1996). Oxidative stress and antioxidant therapy in Parkinson's disease. *Progress in Neurobiology, 48,* 1–19.

Edvinsson, L., MacKenzie, E. T., & McCulloch, J. (1993). *Cerebral blood flow and metabolism.* New York: Raven Press.

Elsner, A. E., Berk, L., Burns, S. A., & Rosenberg, P. R. (1988). Aging and human cone photopigments. *Journal of the Optical Society of America A, 5,* 2106–2112.

Erikson, E. H. (1963). *Childhood and society.* New York: Norton.

Eriksson, L., Kerecsen, L., & Bunag, R. D. (1991). Strain differences in baroreflex inhibition by centrally infused enalapril in old rats. *Journal of Gerontology, 46,* 65–71.

Erway, L. C., & Willott, J. F. (1996). Genetic susceptibility to noise-induced hearing loss in mice. In A. A. Axelson, H. M. Borchgrevink, R. P. Hamernik, P. A. Hellstrom, D. Henderson, & R. J. Salvi (Eds.), *Scientific basis of noise-induced hearing loss* (pp. 56–64). New York: Thieme.

Erway, L. C., Willott, J. F., Archer, J. R., & Harrison, D. (1993). Genetics of age-related hearing loss in mice: 1. Inbred and F1 hybrid strains. *Hearing Research, 65,* 125–132.

Eustache, F., Rioux, P., Desgranges, B., Marchal, G., Petit-Taboue, M.-C., Dary, M., LeChevalier, B., & Baron, J.-C. (1995). Healthy aging, memory subsystems and regional cerebral oxygen consumption. *Neuropsychologia, 33,* 867–887.

Evans, W. J., Cui, L., & Starr, A. (1995). Olfactory event-related potentials in normal human subjects: Effects of age and gender. *Electroencephalography and Clinical Neurophysiology, 95,* 293–301.

Falls, W. A., Carlson, S., Turner, J. G., & Willott, J. F. (1997). Fear potentiated startle in two strains of inbred mice. *Behavioral Neuroscience, 111,* 855–861.

Fanelli, R. J., McCarthy, R. T., & Chisholm, J. (1994). Neuropharmacology of nimodipine: From single channels to behavior. *Annals of the New York Academy of Sciences, 747,* 336–350.

Fattoretti, P., Bertoni-Freddari, C., Caselli, U., Paoloni, R., & Meier-Ruge, W. (1996). Morphologic changes in cerebellar mitochondria during aging. *Analytical and Quantitative Cytology and Histology, 18,* 205–208.

Fearnley, J. M., & Lees, A. J. (1991). Ageing and Parkinson's disease: Substantia nigra regional selectivity. *Brain, 114,* 2283–2301.

Feldman, M. L., & Vaughan, D. W. (1979). Changes in the auditory pathways with age. In S. S. Han & D. H. Coons (Eds.), *Special senses in aging* (pp. 143–162). Ann Arbor, MI: Institute of Gerontology.

Feldman, R. S., Meyer, J. S., & Quenzer, L. F. (1997). *Principles of neuropsychopharmacology.* Sunderland, MA: Sinauer.

Felten, D. L., Felten, S. Y., Fuller, R. W., Romano, T. D., Smalstig, E. B., Wong, D. T., & Clemens, J. A. (1992). Chronic dietary pergolide preserves nigrostriatal neuronal integrity in aged Fischer–344 rats. *Neurobiology of Aging, 13,* 339–351.

Fernandez, H. L., & Hodges-Savola, C. A. (1994). Axoplasmic transport of calcitonin gene-related peptide in rat peripheral nerve as a function of age. *Neurochemical Research, 19,* 1369–1377.

Ferraro, J. A., & Minckler, J. (1977). The human lateral lemniscus and its nuclei. *Brain and Language, 4,* 277–294.

Ferri, R., Del Gracco, S., Elia, M., Musumeci, S. A., Spada, R., & Stefanini, M. C. (1996). Scalp topographic mapping of middle-latency somatosensory evoked potentials in normal aging and dementia. *Neurophysiologie Clinique, 26,* 311–319.

Filipp, S.-H. (1996). Motivation and emotion. In J. E. Birren & K. W. Schaie (Eds.), *Handbook of the psychology of aging* (4th ed., pp. 218–235). San Diego: Academic Press.

Finch, C. E. (1993). Neuron atrophy during aging: Programmed or sporadic? *Trends in Neuroscience, 16,* 104–109.

Finch, C. E., & Landfield, P. W. (1985). Neuroendocrine and autonomic functions in aging mammals. In C. E. Finch & E. L. Schneider (Eds.), *Handbook of the biology of aging* (2nd ed., pp. 567–594). New York: Van Nostrand Reinhold.

Finch, C. E., & Morgan, D. G. (1990). RNA and protein metabolism in the aging brain. *Annual Review of Neuroscience, 13,* 75–88.

Finlayson, P. G. (1995). Decreased inhibition to lateral superior olive neurons in young and aged Sprague-Dawley rats. *Hearing Research, 87,* 84–95.

Fischer, W., Wictorin, K., Bjorklund, A., Williams, L. R., Varon, S., & Gage, F. H. (1987). Amelioration of cholinergic neuron atrophy and spatial memory impairment in aged rats by nerve growth factor. *Nature, 329,* 65–68.

Flood, D. G. (1993). Critical issues in the analysis of dendritic extent in aging humans, primates, and rodents. *Neurobiology of Aging, 14,* 649–654.

Flood, D. G., & Coleman, P. D. (1988). Neuron numbers and sizes in aging comparisons of human, monkey, and rodent data. *Neurobiology of Aging, 9,* 453–463.

Flood, J. F., & Roberts, E. (1988). Dehydroepiandrosterone sulfate improves memory in aging mice. *Brain Research, 448,* 178–181.

Flynn, E. E. (1996). Crime and age. In J. E. Birren (Ed.), *Encyclopedia of gerontology* (Vol. 1, pp. 353–359). San Diego: Academic Press.

Fong, T. G., Neff, N. H., & Hadjiconstantinou, M. (1997). GM1 ganglioside improves spatial learning and memory of aged rats. *Behavioural Brain Research, 85,* 203–211.

Forbes, W. B. (1984). Aging-related morphological changes in the main olfactory bulb of the Fischer 344 rat. *Neurobiology of Aging, 5,* 93–97.

Forster, M. J., Dubey, A., Dawson, K. M., Stutts, W. A., Lal, H., & Sohal, R. S. (1996). *Proceedings of the National Academy of Sciences, 93,* 4765–4769.

Freund, J. S. (1996). Learning. In J. E. Birren (Ed.), *Encyclopedia of gerontology* (Vol. 2, pp. 7–18). San Diego: Academic Press.

Frolkis, V. V., Tanin, S. A., & Gorban, Y. N. (1997). Age-related changes in axonal transport. *Experimental Gerontology, 32,* 441–450.

Gage, F. H., & Bjorklund, A. (1986). Cholinergic septal grafts into the hippocampal formation improve spatial learning and memory in the aged rat by an atropine-sensitive mechanism. *Journal of Neuroscience, 6,* 2837–2847.

Galea, V. (1996). Changes in motor unit estimates with aging. *Journal of Clinical Neurophysiology, 13,* 253–260.

Gallagher, M., Burwell, R. D., Kodski, M. H., McKinney, M., Southerland, S., Vella-Roundtree, L., & Lewis, M. H. (1990). Markers for biogenic amines in the aged rat brain: Relationship to decline in spatial learning ability. *Neurobiology of Aging, 11,* 507–514.

Gallagher, M., Nagahara, A. H., & Burwell, R. D. (1995). Cognition and hippocampal systems in aging: Animal models. In J. L. McGaugh, N. M. Weinberger, & G. Lynch (Eds.), *Brain and memory: Modulation and mediation of neuroplasticity* (pp. 103–126). New York: Oxford.

Gallagher, M., & Rapp, P. R. (1997). The use of animal models to study the effects of aging on cognition. *Annual Review of Psychology, 48,* 339–370.

Gao, H., & Hollyfield, J. G. (1992). Aging of the human retina—differential loss of neurons and retinal pigment epithelial cells. *Investigative Opthalmology and Visual Science, 33,* 1–17.

Garton, M. J., Keir, G., Lakshmi, M. V., & Thompson, E. J. (1991). Age-related changes in cerebrospinal fluid protein concentrations. *Journal of Neurological Sciences, 104,* 74–80.

Gash, D. M., Collier, T. J., & Sladek, J. R. (1985). Neural transplantation: A review of recent developments and potential applications to the aged brain. *Neurobiology of Aging, 6,* 131–150.

Gatz, M., Kasl-Godley, J. E., & Karel, M. J. (1996). Aging and mental disorders. In J. E. Birren & K. W. Schaie (Eds.), *Handbook of the psychology of aging* (4th ed., pp. 365–382). San Diego: Academic Press.

Geinisman, Y., deToledo-Morrell, L., & Morrell, F. (1986). Aged rats need a preserved complement of perforated axospinous synapses per hippocampal neuron to maintain good spatial memory. *Brain Research, 398,* 266–275.

Geinisman, Y., deToledo-Morrell, L., Morrell, F., & Heller, R. E. (1995). Hippocampal markers of age-related memory dysfunction: Behavioral, electrophysiological and morphological perspectives. *Progress in Neurobiology, 45,* 223–252.

Gelbmann, C. M., & Muller, W. E. (1991). Chronic treatment with phosphatidylserine restores muscarinic cholinergic receptor deficits in the aged mouse brain. *Neurobiology of Aging, 13,* 45–50.

Ghirardi, O., Giuliani, A., Caprioli, M. T., Ramacci, M. T., & Angelucci, L. (1992). Spatial memory in aged rats: Population heterogeneity and effect of levocarnitine acetyl. *Journal of Neuroscience Research, 31,* 375–379.

Giacobini, E. (1996). New trends in cholinergic therapy for Alzheimer's disease: Nicotine agonists or cholinesterase inhibitors? *Progress in Brain Research, 109,* 311–323.

Giambra, L. M. (1997). Sustained attention and aging: Overcoming the decrement? *Experimental Aging Research, 23,* 145–161.

Giannakopoulos, P., Hof, P. R., Michel, J. P., Guimon, J., & Bouras, C. (1997). Cerebral cortex pathology in aging and Alzheimer's disease: A quantitative survey of large hospital-based geriatric and psychiatric cohorts. *Brain Research Reviews, 25,* 217–245.

Gibson, G. E., & Peterson, C. (1987). Calcium and the aging nervous system. *Neurobiology of Aging, 8,* 329–343.

Gideon, P., Thomsen, C., Stahlberg, F., & Henricksen, O. (1994). Cerebrospinal fluid production and dynamics in normal aging: A MRI phase-mapping study. *Acta Neurologica Scandanavia, 89,* 362–366.

Giovannini, M. G., Casamenti, F., Bartolini, L., & Pepeu, G. (1997). The brain cholinergic system as a target of cognition enhancers. *Behavioural Brain Research, 83,* 1–5.

Giusti, P., Lipartiti, M., Gusella, M., Floreani, M., & Manev, H. (1997). *In vitro* and *in vivo* protective effects of melatonin against glutamate oxidative stress and neurotoxicity. *Annals of the New York Academy of Sciences, 825,* 79–84.

Givalois, L., Li, S., & Pelletier, G. (1997). Age-related decrease in the hypothalamic CRH mRNA expression is reduced by dehydroepiandrosterone (DHEA) treatment in male and female rats. *Molecular Brain Research, 48,* 107–114.

Glanz, J. (1997). Mastering the nonlinear brain. *Science, 277,* 1758–1760.

Gold, L. H. (1996). Integration of molecular biological techniques and behavioral pharmacology. *Behavioural Pharmacology, 7,* 589–615.

Goldberg, A. P., Dengel, D. R., & Hagberg, J. M. (1996). Exercise physiology and aging. In E. L. Schneider & J. W. Rowe (Eds.), *Handbook of the biology of aging* (4th ed., pp. 331–354). San Diego: Academic Press.

Goldberg, A. P., & Hagberg, J. M. (1990). Physical exercise in the elderly. In E. L. Schneider & J. W. Rowe (Eds.), *Handbook of the biology of aging* (3rd ed., pp. 407–428). San Diego: Academic Press.

Goldberg, P. B., Kreider, M. S., McLean, M. R., & Roberts, J. (1986). Effects of aging at the adrenergic cardiac neuroeffector junction. *Federation Proceeding, 45,* 45–47.

Goldberg, P. B., Kreider, M. S., & Roberts, J. (1984). Minireview: Effects of age on the adrenergic cardiac neuroeffector junction. *Life Sciences, 35,* 2585–2591.

Goldman, G., & Coleman, P. D. (1981). Neuron numbers in locus coeruleus do not change with age in Fischer 344 rat. *Neurobiology of Aging, 2,* 33–36.

Golomb, J., de Leon, M., Kluger, A., George, A., Tarshish, G., & Ferris, S. (1993). Hippocampal atrophy in normal aging: An association with recent memory impairment. *Archives of Neurology (Chicago), 50,* 967–973.

Gomberg, E. S. L. (1996). Alcohol and drugs. In J. E. Birren (Ed.), *Encyclopedia of gerontology* (Vol. 1, pp. 93–101). San Diego: Academic Press.

Gomes, O. A., de Souza, R. R., & Liberti, E. A. (1997). A preliminary investigation of aging on the nerve cell number in the myenteric ganglia of the human colon. *Gerontology, 43,* 210–217.

Gomez-Pinilla, F., Cotman, C. W., & Nieto-Sampedro, M. (1989). NGF receptor immunoreactivity in aged rat brain. *Brain Research, 479,* 255–262.

Goodrick, C. L. (1984). Effects of lifelong restricted feeding on complex maze performance in rats. *Age, 7,* 1–2.

Goodwin, J. S., Goodwin, J. M., & Garry, P. J. (1983). Association between nutritional status and cognitive functioning in a healthy elderly population. *Journal of the American Medical Association, 249,* 2917–2921.

Gordon-Salant, S. (1996). Hearing. In J. E. Birren (Ed.), *Encyclopedia of gerontology* (Vol. 1, pp. 643–653). San Diego: Academic Press.

Goudsmit, E., Hofman, M. A., Fliers, E., & Swaab, D. F. (1990). The supraoptic and paraventricular nuclei of the human hypothalamus in relation to sex, age, and Alzheimer's disease. *Neurobiology of Aging, 11,* 529–536.

Goudsmit, E., Neijmeijer-Leloux, A., & Swaab, D. F. (1992). The human hypotha-lamo-neurohypophyseal system in relation to development, aging, and Alzhei-mer's disease. *Progress in Brain Research*, *93*, 237–248.

Gould, T. J., & Bickford, P. C. (1996). The effects of aging on cerebellar beta-adrenergic receptor activation and motor learning in female F344 rats. *Neurosci-ence Letters*, *216*, 53–56.

Gould, T. J., Bowenkamp, K. E., Larson, G., Zahniser, N. R., & Bickford, P. C. (1995). Effects of dietary restriction on motor learning and cerebellar noradren-ergic dysfunction in aged F344 rats. *Brain Research*, *684*, 150–158.

Grady, C. L., Maisog, J. M., Horwitz, B., Ungerleider, L. G., Mentis, M. J., Salerno, J. A., Pietrini, P., Wagner, E., & Haxby, J. V. (1994). Age-related changes in cortical blood flow activation during visual processing of faces and location. *Journal of Neuroscience*, *14*, 1450–1462.

Grady, C. L., McIntosh, A. R., Horwitz, B., Maisog, J. M., Ungerleider, L. G., Mentis, M. J., Pietrini, P., Shapiro, M. B., & Haxby, J. V. (1995). Age-related reductions in human recognition memory due to impaired memory encoding. *Science*, *269*, 218–221.

Grafton, S. T., Sumi, S. M., Stimac, G. K., Alvord, E. C., Shaw, C. M., & Nochlin, D. (1991). Comparison of postmortem magnetic resonance imaging and neuro-pathological findings in the cerebral white matter. *Archives of Neurology*, *48*, 293–298.

Granger, R., Deadwyler, S., Davis, M., Moskovitz, B., Kessler, M., Rogers, G., & Lynch, G. (1996). Facilitation of glutamate receptors reverses an age-associated memory impairment in rats. *Synapse*, *22*, 332–337.

Greene, E., & Naranjo, J. N. (1987). Degeneration of hippocampal fibers and spatial memory deficit in the aged rat. *Neurobiology of Aging*, *8*, 35–43.

Greenough, W. T., McDonald, J. W., Parnisari, R. M., & Camel, J. E. (1986). Environmental conditions modulate degeneration and new dendritic growth in cerebellum of senescent rats. *Brain Research*, *380*, 136–143.

Gruenewald, D. A., & Matsumoto, A. M. (1991). Age-related decreases in serum gonadotropin levels and gonadotropin-releasing hormone gene expression in the medial preoptic areas of the male rat are dependent upon testicular feedback. *Endocrinology*, *129*, 2442–2450.

Gu, M. J., Schultz, A. B., Shepard, N. T., & Alexander, N. B. (1996). Postural control in young and elderly adults when stance is perturbed: Dynamics. *Journal of Biomechanics*, *29*, 319–329.

Gyenes, M., Lustyik, G., Nagy, V., Jeney, F., & Nagy, I. (1984). Age-dependent decrease of the passive Rb^+ and K^+ permeability of the nerve cell membranes in rat brain cortex as revealed by *in vivo* measurement of the Rb^+ discrimination ratio. *Archives of Gerontology and Geriatrics*, *3*, 11–31.

Hajduczok, G., Chapleau, M. W., & Abboud, F. M. (1991). Rapid adaptation of central pathways explains the suppressed baroreflex with aging. *Neurobiology of Aging*, *12*, 601–604.

Hakeem, A., Sandoval, G. S., Jones, M., & Allman, J. (1996). Brain and life span in primates. In J. E. Birren & K. W. Schaie (Eds.), *Handbook of the psychology of aging* (4th ed., pp. 78–104). San Diego: Academic Press.

Hanes, D. P., & Schall, J. D. (1996). Neural control of voluntary movement initiation. *Science*, *274*, 427–430.

Harding, A. J., Wong, A., Svoboda, M., Kril, J. J., & Halliday, G. M. (1997). Chronic alcohol consumption does not cause hippocampal neuron loss in humans. *Hippocampus*, *7*, 78–87.

Harkins, S. W., Davis, M. D., Bush, F. M., & Kasberger, J. (1996). Suppression of first pain and slow temporal summation of second pain in relation to age. *Journal of Gerontology A*, *51*, M260–M265.

Harkins, S. W., & Scott, R. B. (1996). Pain and presbyalgos. In J. E. Birren (Ed.), *Encyclopedia of gerontology* (Vol. 2, pp. 247–260). San Diego: Academic Press.

Harman, D. (1995a). Role of antioxidant nutrients in aging: Overview. *Age*, *18*, 51–62.

————. (1995b). Free radical theory of aging: Alzheimer's disease pathogenesis. *Age*, *18*, 97–119.

Harman, S. M., & Talbert, G. B. (1985). Reproducive aging. In C. E. Finch & E. L. Schneider (Eds.), *Handbook of the biology of aging* (2nd ed., pp. 457–510). New York: Van Nostrand Reinhold.

Harridge, S. D. R., & Saltin, B. (1996). Neuromuscular system. In J. E. Birren (Ed.), *Encyclopedia of gerontology* (Vol. 2, pp. 211–220). San Diego: Academic Press.

Harris, K. M., & Kater, S. B. (1994). Dendritic spines: Cellular specializations imparting both stability and flexibility to synaptic function. *Annual Review of Neuroscience*, *17*, 341–371.

Hart, B. A. (1986). Fractionated myotatic reflex times in women by activity level and age. *Journal of Gerontology*, *41*, 361–367.

Hartley, A. A. (1992). Attention. In F. I. M. Craik & T. A. Salthouse (Eds.), *The handbook of aging and cognition* (pp. 3–50). Hillsdale, NJ: Erlbaum.

Haug, H. (1984). Macroscopic and microscopic morphometry of the human brain and cortex: A survey in light of new results. *Brain Pathology*, *1*, 123–149.

Hawkes, C. H., Shephard, B. C., & Daniel, S. E. (1997). Olfactory dysfunction in Parkinson's disease. *Journal of Neurology Neurosurgery and Psychiatry*, *62*, 436–446.

Hawkins, R. D., Kandel, E. R., & Siegelbaum, S. A. (1993). Learning to modulate transmitter release: Themes and variations in synaptic plasticity. *Annual Review of Neuroscience*, *16*, 625–666.

Hayflick, L. (1996). *How and why we age*. New York: Ballantine.

Hebb, D. O. (1949). *The organization of behavior—a neuropsychological theory*. New York: Wiley.

Heffner, R. S., & Donnal, T. (1993). Effect of high frequency hearing loss on localization in mice (C57BL/6J). *Association for Research in Otolaryngology Abstracts, 16*, 49.

Henrique, R. M. F., Monteiro, R. A. F., Rocha, E., & Marini-Abreu, M. M. (1997). A stereological study on the nuclear volume of cerebellar granule cells in aging rats. *Neurobiology of Aging, 18*, 199–203.

Henry, K. R. (1986). Effects of dietary restriction on presbyacusis in the mouse. *Audiology, 25*, 329–337.

Henry, K. R., & Chole, R. A. (1980). Genotypic differences in behavioral, physiological and anatomical expressions of age-related hearing loss in the laboratory mouse. *Audiology, 1*, 369–383.

Hersi, A. I., Rowe, W., Gaudreau, P., & Quirion, R. (1995). Dopamine D1 receptor ligands modulate cognitive performance and hippocampal acetylcholine release in memory-impaired aged rats. *Neuroscience, 69*, 1067–1074.

Herzog, A. G., & Kemper, T. L. (1980). Amygdaloid changes in aging and dementia. *Archives of Neurology, 37*, 625–629.

Hinds, J. W., & McNelly, N. A. (1977). Aging of the rat olfactory bulb: Growth and atrophy of constituent layers and changes in size and number of mitral cells. *Journal of Comparative Neurology, 171*, 345–368.

———. (1979). Aging in the rat olfactory bulb: Quantitative changes in mitral cell organelles and somatodendritic synapses. *Journal of Comparative Neurology, 184*, 811–820.

———. (1981). Aging in the rat olfactory system: Correlation of changes in the olfactory epithelium and olfactory bulb. *Journal of Comparative Neurology, 203*, 441–453.

Hirai, T., Kojima, S., Shimada, A., Umemura, T., Sakai, M., & Itakura, C. (1996). Age-related changes in the olfactory system of dogs. *Neuropathology and Applied Neurobiology, 22*, 531–539.

Hofman, M. A. (1997). Lifespan changes in the human hypothalamus. *Experimental Gerontology, 32*, 559–575.

Hofman, M. A., & Swaab, D. F. (1989). The sexually dimorphic nucleus of the preoptic area in the human brain: A comparative morphometric study. *Journal of Anatomy, 164*, 55–72.

———. (1994). Alterations in circadian rhythmicity of the vasopressin-producing neurons of the human suprachiasmatic nucleus (SCN) with aging. *Brain Research, 651*, 134–142.

Horak, F. B., Shupert, C. L., & Mirka, A. (1989). Components of postural dyscontrol in the elderly: A review. *Neurobiology of Aging, 10*, 727–738.

Hoyer, S. (1995). Age-related changes in cerebral oxidative metabolism: Implications for drug therapy. *Drugs & Aging, 6*, 210–218.

Huang, K. W., & Zhao, Y. (1995). Selective sparing of human nucleus accumbens in aging and anoxia. *Canadian Journal of Neurological Science, 22*, 290–293.

Huether, G. (1996). Melatonin as an antiaging drug: Between facts and fantasy. *Gerontology, 42,* 87–96.

Huguet, F., Drieu, K., & Piriou, A. (1994). Decreased cerebral 5-HT1A receptors during ageing: Reversal by Ginkgo biloba xtract (EGb 761). *Journal of Pharmacy and Pharamcology, 46,* 316–318.

Hultsch, D. F., & Dixon, R. A. (1990). Learning and memory in aging. In J. E. Birren & K. W. Shaie (Eds.), *Handbook of the psychology of aging* (3rd ed., pp. 259–274). New York: Academic Press.

Hume, A. L., Cant, B. R., Shaw, N. A., & Cowan, J. C. (1982). Central somatosensory conduction time from 10 to 79 years. *Electroencephalography and Clinical Neurophysiology, 54,* 49–54.

Igwe, O. J., & Filla, M. B. (1995). Regulation of phosphatidylinositide transduction system in the rat spinal cord during aging. *Neuroscience, 69,* 1239–1251.

Ingram, D. K., Shimada, A., Spangler, E. L., Ikari, H., Hengemihle, J., Kuo, H., & Greig, N. (1996). Cognitive enhancement: New strategies for stimulating cholinergic, glutamatergic, and nitric oxide systems. *Annals of the New York Academy of Sciences, 786,* 348–361.

Ingram, D. K., Spangler, E. L., Iijima, S., Kuo, H., Breshnahan, E. L., Greig, N. H., & London, E. D. (1994). New pharmacological strategies for cognitive enhancement using a rat model of age-related memory impairment. *Annals of the New York Academy of Sciences, 717,* 16–32.

Iseki, E., Odawara, T., Li, F., Kosaka, K., Nishimura, T., Akiyama, H., & Ikeda, K. (1996). Age-related ubiquitin-positive granular structures in non-demented subjects and neurodegenerative disorders. *Journal of Neurological Science, 142,* 25–26.

Issa, A. M., Rowe, W., Gauthier, S., & Meaney, M. J. (1990). Hypothalamic-pituitary-adrenal activity in aged, cognitively impaired and cognitively unimpaired rats. *Journal of Neuroscience, 10,* 3247–3254.

Ivy, G. O., Petit, T. L., & Markus, E. J. (1992). A physiological framework for perceptual and cognitive changes with aging. In F. I. M. Craik & T. A. Salthouse (Eds.), *The handbook of aging and cognition* (pp. 273–314). Hillsdale, NJ: Erlbaum.

Ivy, G. O., Rick, J. T., Murphy, M. P., Head, E., Reid, C., & Milgram, N. W. (1994). Effects of L-deprenyl on manifestations of aging in the rat and dog. *Annals of the New York Academy of Sciences, 717,* 45–59.

Jacobs, B., Driscoll, L., & Schall, M. (1997). Life-span dendritic and spine changes in areas 10 and 18 of human cortex: A quantitative Golgi study. *Journal of Comparative Neurology, 386,* 661–680.

Jama, J. W., Launer, L. J., Witteman, J. C., den Breeijen, J. H., Breteler, M. M., Grobbee, D. E., & Hofman, A. (1996). Dietary antioxidants and cognitive function in a population-based sample of older persons: The Rotterdam study. *American Journal of Epidemiology, 144,* 275–280.

Janowsky, J. S., Kaye, J. A., & Carper, R. A. (1996). Atrophy of the corpus callosum in Alzheimer's disease versus healthy aging. *Journal of the American Geriatric Society, 44*, 798–803.

Jeeves, M. A., & Moes, P. (1996). Interhemispheric transfer time differences related to aging and gender. *Neuropsychologia, 34*, 627–636.

Johnson, E. M., & Deckwerth, T. L. (1993). Molecular mechanisms of developmental neuronal death. *Annual Review of Neuroscience, 16*, 31–46.

Johnson, H., Ulfhake, B., Dagerlind, A., Bennett, G. W., Fone, K. C. F., & Hokfelt, T. (1993). The serotonergic bulbospinal system and brainstem-spinal cord content of serotonin-, TRH-, and substance P-like immunoreactivity in the aged rat with special reference to the spinal cord motor nucleus. *Synapse, 15*, 63–89.

Johnson, J. E., & Miquel, J. (1974). Fine structural changes in the lateral vestibular nucleus of aging rats. *Mechanisms of Ageing and Development, 3*, 203–224.

Johnson, S. A., & Finch, C. E. (1996). Changes in gene expression during brain aging: A survey. In E. L. Schneider & J. W. Rowe (Eds.), *Handbook of the biology of aging* (4th ed., pp. 300–327). San Diego: Academic Press.

Johnson, S. C., Farnworth, T., Pinkston, J. B., Bigler, E. D., & Blatter, D. D. (1994). Corpus callosum surface area across the human adult life span: Effect of age and gender. *Brain Research Bulletin, 35*, 373–377.

Johnson, S. M., & Felder, R. B. (1993). Effects of aging on the intrinsic membrane properties of medial NTS neurons of Fischer–344 rats. *Journal of Neurophysiology, 70*, 1975–1987.

Johnston, D., Magee, J. C., Colbert, C. M., & Christie, R. (1996). Active properties of neuronal dendrites. *Annual Review of Neuroscience, 19*, 165–186.

Jonas, J. B., Schmidt, A. M., Muller-Bergh, J. A., Schlotzer-Schrehardt, U. M., & Naumann, G. O. H. (1992). Human optic nerve fiber count and optic disc size. *Investigative Opthalmology and Visual Science, 33*, 2012–2018.

Jones, D. G., & Harris, R. J. (1995). An analysis of contemporary morphological concepts of synaptic remodelling in the CNS: Perforated synapses revisited. *Reviews of Neuroscience, 6*, 177–219.

Joseph, J. A. (1992). The putative role of free radicals in the loss of neuronal functioning in senescence. *Integrative Physiological and Behavioral Science, 27*, 216–227.

Joseph, J. A., Cutler, R., & Roth, G. S. (1993). Changes in G-protein mediated signal transduction in aging and Alzheimer's disease. *Annals of the New York Academy of Sciences, 695*, 42–45.

Joseph, J. A., Denisova, N., Villalobos-Molina, R., Erat, S., & Strain, J. (1996). Oxidative stress and age-related neuronal deficits. *Molecular Chemistry and Neuropathology, 28*, 35–40.

Joseph, J. A., Villalobos-Molinas, R., Denisova, N. A., Erat, S., & Strain, J. (1997). Cholesterol: A two-edged sword in brain aging. *Free Radical Biology and Medicine, 22*, 455–462.

Jucker, M., & Ingram, D. K. (1997). Murine models of brain aging and age-related neurodegenerative diseases. *Behavioural Brain Research, 85,* 1–25.

Kaas, J. H. (1991). Plasticity of sensory and motor maps in adult mammals. *Annual Review of Neuroscience, 14,* 137–168.

Kabuto, H., Yokoi, I., Mori, A., Murakami, M., & Sawada, S. (1995). Neurochemical changes related to ageing in the senescence-accelerated mouse brain and the effect of chronic administration of nimodipine. *Mechanisms of Ageing and Development, 80,* 1–9.

Kadenbach, B., Munscher, C., Frank, V., Muller-Hocker, J., & Napiwotzki, J. (1995). Human aging is associated with stochastic somatic mutations of mitochondrial DNA. *Mutation Research, 338,* 162–172.

Kakigi, R. (1987). The effect of aging on somatosensory evoked potentials following stimulation of the posterior tibial nerve in man. *Electroencephalography and Clinical Neurophysiology, 68,* 277–286.

Kalat, J. W. (1998). *Biological psychology* (6th ed.). Pacific Grove, CA: Brooks/Cole.

Kanda, K., & Hashizume, K. (1991). Recovery of motor-unit function after peripheral nerve injury in aged rats. *Neurobiology of Aging, 12,* 217–276.

Kandel, E. R., Schwartz, J. H., & Jessell, T. M. (1995). *Essentials of neural science and behavior.* Norwalk, CT: Appleton & Lange.

Kaplan, M. S., McNelly, N. A., & Hinds, J. W. (1985). Population dynamics of adult-formed granule neurons of the rat olfactory bulb. *Journal of Comparative Neurology, 239,* 117–125.

Katsarkas, A. (1994). Dizziness in aging: A retrospective study of 1194 cases. *Otolaryngology Head and Neck Surgery, 110,* 296–301.

Kausler, D. H. (1990). Motivation, human aging, and cognitive performance. In J. E. Birren & K. W. Shaie (Eds.), *Handbook of the psychology of aging* (3rd ed., pp. 171–182). New York: Academic Press.

———. (1991). *Experimental psychology, cognition, and human aging* (2nd ed.). New York: Springer-Verlag.

———. (1994). *Learning and memory in normal aging.* San Diego: Academic Press.

Kawaguchi, S., Kishikawa, M., Sakae, M., & Nakane, Y. (1995). Age-related changes in basal dendrite and dendritic spine of hippocampal pyramidal neurons (CA1) among SAMP1TA/Ngs—quantitative analysis by the rapid Golgi method. *Mechanisms of Ageing and Development, 83,* 11–20.

Kemper, T. L. (1984). Neuroanatomical and neuropathological changes in normal aging and in dementia. In M. L. Albert (Ed.), *Clinical neurology of aging* (pp. 9–52). New York: Oxford University Press.

———. (1994). Neuroanatomical and neuropathological changes during aging and dementia. In M. L. Albert & J. E. Knoefel (Eds.), *Clinical neurology of aging* (2nd ed., pp. 3–67). New York: Oxford University Press.

Kenshalo, D. R. (1979). Changes in the vestibular and somesthetic systems as a function of age. In J. M. Ordy & K. Brizzee (Eds.), *Sensory systems and communication in the elderly* (pp. 269–282). New York: Raven.

Khatchaturian, Z. S. (1989). The role of calcium regulation in brain aging: Reexamination of a hypothesis. *Aging, 1*, 17–34.

Khatchaturian, Z. S., & Radenbaugh, T. S. (1996). A synthesis of critical topics in Alzheimer's disease. In Z. S. Khachaturian & T. S. Radenbaugh (Eds.), *Alzheimer's disease: Cause(s), diagnosis, treatment, and care* (pp. 3–14). Boca Raton, FL: CRC Press.

Kim, B. Y., Tom, B. W., & Spear, P. D. (1996). Effects of aging on the densities, numbers, and sizes of retinal ganglion cells in rhesus monkey. *Neurobiology of Aging, 17*, 431–438.

Kimonides, V. G., Khatibi, N. H., Svendsen, C. N., Sofroniew, M. V., & Herbert, J. (1998). Dehydroepiandrosterone (DHEA) and DHEA-sulphate (DHEAS) protect hippocampal neurons against excitatory amino acid-induced neurotoxicity. *Proceedings of the National Acadamy of Science, 95*, 1852–1857.

Kirasic, K. C., & Allen, G. L. (1985). Aging, spatial performance and spatial competence. In N. Charness (Ed.), *Aging and human peformance* (pp. 191–223). New York: Wiley.

Klawans, H. L., & Tanner, C. M. (1984). Movement disorders in the elderly. In M. L. Albert (Ed.), *Clinical neurology of aging* (pp. 387–403). New York: Oxford University Press.

Kleine, T. O., Hackler, R., & Zöfel, P. (1993). Age-related alterations of the blood-brain-barrier (bbb) permeability to protein molecules of different size. *Zentrum Gerontologie, 26*, 256–259.

Kline, D. W., & Scialfa, C. T. (1996). Visual and auditory aging. In J. E. Birren & K. W. Schaie (Eds.), *Handbook of the biology of aging* (4th ed., pp. 181–203). San Diego: Academic Press.

Klingman, A. M., Grove, G. L., & Balin, A. K. (1985). Aging of human skin. In C. E. Finch & E. L. Schneider (Eds.), *Handbook of the biology of aging* (2nd ed., pp. 820–841). New York: Van Nostrand Reinhold.

Knegtering, H., Eijck, M., & Huijsman, A. (1994). Effects of antidepressants on cognitive functioning of elderly patients: A review. *Drugs and Aging, 5*, 192–199.

Knowlton, B. J., Mangels, J. A., & Squire, L. R. (1996). A neostriatal habit learning system in humans. *Science, 273*, 1399–1402.

Ko, M. L., King, M. A., Gordon, T. L., & Crisp, T. (1997). The effects of aging on spinal neurochemistry in the rat. *Brain Research Bulletin, 42*, 95–98.

Koenig, H. G. (1997). Mood disorders. In P. D. Nussbaum (Ed.), *Handbook of neuropsychology and aging* (pp. 63–79). New York: Plenum.

Koenig, H. G., & Blazer, D. G., III. (1996). Depression. In J. E. Birren (Ed.), *Encyclopedia of gerontology* (Vol. 1, pp. 415–428). San Diego: Academic Press.

Koistinaho, J. (1986). Difference in the age-related accumulation of lipopigments in the adrenergic and nonadrenergic peripheral neurons in the male rat. *Gerontology, 32,* 300–307.

Kolb, B., & Whishaw, I. Q. (1996). *Human neuropsychology* (4th ed.). New York: Freeman.

Konigsmark, B. W., & Murphy, E. A. (1970). Neuronal populations in the human brain. *Nature, 228,* 1335–1336.

———. (1972). Volume of the ventral cochlear nucleus in man: Its relationship to neuronal population and age. *Journal of Neuropathology and Experimental Neurology, 31,* 304–316.

Krauss, J. K., Regel, J. P., Droste, D. W., Orszagh, M., Borremans, J. J., & Vach, W. (1997). Movement disorders in adult hydrocephalus. *Movement Disorders, 12,* 53–60.

Kronforst-Collins, M. A., Moriearty, P. L., Schmidt, B., & Disterhoft, J. F. (1997). Metrifonate improves associative learning and retention in aging rabbits. *Behavioral Neuroscience, 111,* 1031–1040.

Kuchel, O., & Kuchel, G. (1993). Circulating catecholamines and aging. In F. Amenta (Ed.), *Aging of the autonomic nervous system* (pp. 71–93). Boca Raton, FL: CRC Press.

Kugler, C. F. A., Taghavy, A., & Platt, D. (1993). The event-related P300 potential analysis of cognitive human brain aging: A review. *Gerontology, 39,* 280–303.

Kuhn, H. G., Dickinson-Anson, H., & Gage, F. H. (1996). Neurogenesis in the dentate gyrus of the adult rat: Age-related decrease of neuronal progentor proliferation. *Journal of Neuroscience, 16,* 2027–2033.

Kunitake, J. M., Pekary, A. E., & Hershman, J. M. (1992). Aging and the hypothalamic-pituitary-thyroid axis. In J. E. Morley & S. G. Korenman (Eds.), *Endocrinology and metabolism in the elderly* (pp. 92–110). Boston: Blackwell Scientific Publishers.

Kvitnitskaya-Ryzhova, T., Shinkai, T., Ooka, H., & Ohtsubo, K. (1994). Immunocytochemical demonstration of prolactin interaction with choroid plexus in aging and acute hyperprolactinemia. *Mechanisms of Ageing and Development, 76,* 65–72.

Laakso, M. P., Partanen, K., Lehtovirta, M., Hallikainen, M., Hanninen, T., Vaino, P., Riekkinen, P. Sr., & Soininen, H. (1995). MRI of amygdala fails to diagnose early Alzheimer's disease. *Neuroreport, 6,* 2414–2418.

Laissy, J. P., Patrux, B., Duchateau, C., Hannequin, D., Hugonet, P., Ait-Yahia, H., & Thiebot, J. (1993). Midsagittal MR measurements of the corpus callosum in healthy subjects and diseased patients: A prospective survey. *American Journal of Neuroradiology, 14,* 145–154.

Lajoie, Y., Teasdale, N., Bard, C., & Fleury, M. (1996). Upright standing and gait: Are there changes in attentional requirements related to normal aging? *Experimental Aging Research, 22,* 185–198.

Lakatta, E. G. (1985). Heart and circulation. In C. E. Finch & E. L. Schneider (Eds.), *Handbook of the biology of aging* (2nd ed., pp. 377–413). New York: Van Nostrand Reinhold.

———. (1990). Heart and circulation. In E. L. Schneider & J. W. Rowe (Eds.), *Handbook of the biology of aging* (3rd ed., pp. 181–216). San Diego: Academic Press.

Lambert, P. R., & Schwartz, I. R. (1982). A longitudinal study of changes in the cochlear nucleus in the CBA mouse. *Otolaryngology Head and Neck Surgery, 90,* 787–794.

Lanahan, A., Lyford, G., Stevenson, G. S., Worley, P. F., & Barnes, C. A. (1997). Selective alteration of long-term potentiation-induced transcriptional response in hippocampus of aged, memory-impaired rats. *Journal of Neuroscience, 17,* 2876–2885.

Landfield, P. W. (1980). Adrenocortical hypothesis of brain and somatic aging. In R. T. Shimke (Ed.), *Biological mechanisms of aging* (Publication No. 81-2194, pp. 658–672). Washington, DC: National Institutes of Health.

Landfield, P. W. (1996). Aging-related increase in hippocampal calcium channels. *Life Sciences, 59,* 399–404.

Landfield, P. W., McGaugh, J. L., & Lynch, G. (1978). Impaired synaptic potentiation processes in the hippocampus of aged, memory-deficient rats. *Brain Research, 150,* 85–101.

Landfield, P. W., & Pitler, T. A. (1984). Prolonged Ca^{2+}-dependent afterhyperpolarization in hippocampal neurons of aged rats. *Science, 226,* 1089–1092.

Landfield, P. W., Thibault, O., Mazzanti, M. L., Porter, N. M., & Kerr, D. S. (1992). Mechanisms of neuronal death in brain aging and Alzheimer's disease: Role of endocrine-mediated calcium dyshomeostasis. *Journal of Neurobiology, 23,* 1247–1260.

Larsson, L., & Ansved, T. (1995). Effects of ageing on the motor unit. *Progress in Neurobiology, 45,* 397–458.

LaRue, A., Koehler, K. M., Wayne, S. J., Chiulli, S. J., Haaland, K. Y., & Garry, P. J. (1997). Nutritional status and cognitive functioning in a normally aging sample: A 6-y reassessment. *American Journal of Clinical Nutrition, 65,* 20–29.

LeBel, C. P., & Bondy, S. C. (1992). Oxidative damage and cerebral aging. *Progress in Neurobiology, 38,* 601–609.

LeDoux, J. E. (1995). In search of an emotional system in the brain: Leaping from fear to emotion and consciousness. In M. S. Gazzaniga (Ed.), *The cognitive neurosciences* (pp. 1049–1062). Cambridge, MA: MIT Press.

Lee, J. M., Ross, E. R., Gower, A., Paris, J. M., Martensson, R., & Lorens, S. A. (1994). Spatial learning deficits in the aged rat: Neuroanatomical and neurochemical correlates. *Brain Research Bulletin, 33,* 489–500.

Leterrier, J. F., & Eyer, J. (1992). Age-dependent changes in the ultrastructure and in the molecular composition of rat brain microtubules. *Journal of Neurochemistry, 59,* 1126–1137.

Leuba, G., & Garey, L. J. (1987). Evolution of neuronal numerical density in the developing and aging human visual cortex. *Human Neurobiology, 6*, 11–18.

Levenson, R. W., Carstensen, L. L., Friesen, W. V., & Ekman, P. (1991). Emotion, physiology, and expression in old age. *Psychology and Aging, 6*, 28–35.

Levine, M. S., Adinolfi, A. M., Fisher, R. S., Hull, C. D., Buchwald, N. A., & McAllister, J. P. (1986). Quantitative morphology of medium-sized caudate spiny neurons in aged cats. *Neurobiology of Aging, 7*, 277–286.

Levine, M. S., Lloyd, R. L., Hull, C. D., Fisher, R. S., & Buchwald, N. A. (1987). Neurophysiological alterations in caudate neurons in aged cats. *Brain Research, 401*, 213–230.

Levine, R. L., Hanson, J. M., & Nickles, R. J. (1994). Cerebral vasocapacitance in human aging. *Journal of Neuroimaging, 4*, 130–136.

Levkovitz, Y., Richter-Levin, G., & Segal, M. (1994). Effect of 5-hydroxytryptophane on behavior and hippocmpal physiology in young and old rats. *Neurobiology of Aging, 15*, 635–641.

Li, H. S., & Borg, E. (1991). Age-related loss of auditory sensitivity in two mouse genotypes. *Acta Otolaryngologica, 111*, 827–834.

————. (1993). Auditory degeneration after acoustic trauma in two genotypes of mice. *Hearing Research, 68*, 19–27.

Li, S., Givalois, L., & Pelletier, G. (1997). Dehdydroepiandrosterone administration reverses the inhibitory influence of aging on gonadotropin-releasing hormone gene expression in the male and female rat brain. *Endocrine, 6*, 265–270.

Linville, D. G., & Arneric, S. P. (1991). Cortical cerebral blood flow governed by the basal forebrain: Age-related impairments. *Neurobiology of Aging, 12*, 503–510.

Little, J. T., Broocks, A., Martin, A., Hill, J. L., Tune, L. E., Mack, C., Cantillon, M., Molchan, S., Murphy, D. L., & Sunderland, T. (1995). Serotonergic modulation of anticholinergic effects on cognition and behavior in elderly humans. *Psychopharmacology, 120*, 280–288.

Liu, X., Erikson, C., & Brun, A. (1996). Cortical synaptic changes and gliosis in normal aging, Alzheimer's disease and frontal lobe degeneration. *Dementia, 7*, 128–134.

Livingstone, M., & Hubel, D. (1988). Segregation of form, color, movement, and depth: Anatomy, physiology, and perception. *Science, 240*, 740–749.

Loessner, A., Alavi, A., Lewandrowski, K. U., Mozley, D., Souder, E., & Gur, R. E. (1995). Regional cerebral function determined by FDG-PET in healthy volunteers: Normal patterns and changes with age. *Journal of Nuclear Medicine, 36*, 1141–1149.

Logothetis, N. K., & Sheinberg, D. L. (1996). Visual object recognition. *Annual Review of Neuroscience, 19*, 577–621.

Lolova, I., & Davidoff, M. (1991). Age-related changes in serotonin-immunoreactive neurons in the rat nucleus raphe dorsalis and nucleus centralis superior: A light microscope study. *Mechanisms of Ageing and Development, 62*, 279–289.

Lopez, I., Honrubia, V., & Baloh, R. W. (1997). Aging and the human vestibular nucleus. *Journal of Vestibular Research, 7,* 77–86.

Low, P. A., Opfer-Gehrking, T. L., Proper, C. J., & Zimmerman, I. (1990). The effect of aging on cardiac autonomic and postganglionic sudomotor function. *Muscle and Nerve, 13,* 152–157.

Luders, H. (1970). The effects of aging on the wave form of the somatosensory cortical evoked potential. *Electroencephalography and Clinical Neurophysiology, 29,* 450–460.

Luine, V., & Milio, C. (1990). Monoamine levels and functional indices in basal forebrain nuclei of aged rats. *Dementia, 1,* 185–191.

Lynch, M. A., & Voss, K. L. (1994). Membrane arachidonic acid concentration correlates with age and induction of long-term potentiation in the dentate gyrus in the rat. *European Journal of Neuroscience, 6,* 1008–1014.

Machado-Salas, J. P., & Scheibel, A. B. (1979). Limbic system of the aged mouse. *Experimental Neurology, 63,* 347–355.

Machado-Salas, J. P., Scheibel, M. E., & Scheibel, A. B. (1977). Neuronal changes in the aging mouse: Spinal cord and lower brain stem. *Experimental Neurology, 54,* 504–512.

MacKay, D. G., & Abrams, L. (1996). Language, memory, and aging: Distributed deficits and the structure of new-versus-old connections. In J. E. Birren & K. W. Schaie (Eds.), *Handbook of the psychology of aging* (4th ed., pp. 251–265). San Diego: Academic Press.

MacKenzie, R. A., & Phillips, L. H. (1981). Changes in peripheral and central nerve conduction with aging. *Clinical and Experimental Neurology, 18,* 109–116.

Madden, D. J., & Allen, P. A. (1996). Attention. In J. E. Birren (Ed.), *Encyclopedia of gerontology* (Vol. 1, pp. 131–140). San Diego: Academic Press.

Majewska, M. D., Demirgoren, S., Spivak, C. E., & London, E. D. (1990). The neurosteroid DHEAS is an allosteric antagonist of the GABA receptor. *Brain Research, 526,* 143–146.

Maki, B. E., & McIlroy, W. E. (1996). Postural control in the older adult. *Clinics in Geriatric Medicine, 12,* 635–658.

Malatesta, C. Z., & Kalnock, M. (1984). Emotional experience in younger and older adults. *Journal of Gerontology, 39,* 301–308.

Manaye, K. F., McIntire, D. D., Mann, D. M. A., & German, D. C. (1995). Locus coeruleus cell loss in the aging human brain: A non-random process. *Journal of Comparative Neurology, 358,* 79–87.

Manev, H., Uz, T., & Giusti, P. (1997). Neuroprotective action of the pineal hormone melatonin against excitotoxicity. *Annals of the New York Academy of Sciences, 825,* 85–89.

Mann, D. M. A. (1997). *Sense and senility: The neuropathology of the aged human brain.* New York: Chapman and Hall.

Marcyniuk, B., Mann, D., & Yates, P. (1986). The topography of cell loss from the locus coeruleus in Alzheimer's disease. *Journal of Neurological Sciences, 76,* 335–345.

————. (1989). The topography of nerve cell loss from the locus coeruleus in elderly persons. *Neurobiology of Aging, 19,* 5–9.

Marczynski, T. J. (1995). GABAergic deafferentation hypothesis of brain aging and Alzheimer's disease; pharmacologic profile of the benzodiazepine antagonist, flumazenil. *Reviews of Neuroscience, 6,* 221–258.

Marin, J. (1995). Age-related changes in vascular responses: A review. *Mechanisms of Ageing and Development, 79,* 71–114.

Markesbery, W. R. (1996). Trace elements in Alzheimer's disease. In Z. S. Khachaturian & T. S. Radenbaugh (Eds.), *Alzheimer's disease: Cause(s), diagnosis, treatment, and care* (pp. 233–238). Boca Raton, FL: CRC Press.

Marks, J. (1998). New gene tied to common form of Alzheimer's. *Science, 281,* 507–509.

Marsden, C. D. (1990). Parkinson's disease. *Lancet, 335,* 948–952.

Martin, J. B. (1996). Pathogenesis of neurodegenerative disorders: The role of dynamic mutations. *Neuroreport, 8,* 1–7.

Martin, P. J., Evans, D. H., & Naylor, A. R. (1994). Transcranial color-coded sonography of the basal cerebral circulation. Reference data from 115 volunteers. *Stroke, 25,* 390–396.

Martinez, M., Hernandez, A. I., Martinez, N., & Ferrandiz, M. L. (1996). Age-related increases in oxidized proteins in mouse synaptic mitochondria. *Brain Research, 731,* 246–248.

Martinez-Serrano, A., Fischer, W., & Bjorklund, A. (1995). Reversal of age-dependent cognitive impairments and cholinergic neuron atrophy by NGF-secreting neural progenitors grafted to the basal forebrain. *Neuron, 15,* 473–484.

Masoro, E. J. (1985). Metabolism. In C. E. Finch & E. L. Schneider (Eds.), *Handbook of the biology of aging* (2nd ed., pp. 540–563). New York: Van Nostrand Reinhold.

Matsumoto, A., Kobayashi, S., Maralsami, S., & Arai, Y. (1984). Recovery of declined ovarian function in aged female rats by transplantation of newborn hypothalamic tissue. *Proceedings of the Japanese Academy, 60,* 73–76.

Mauk, M. D., Steele, P. M., & Medina, J. F. (1997). Cerebellar involvement in motor learning. *The Neuroscientist, 3,* 303–313.

May, C., Kaye, J. A., Atack, J. R., Schapiro, M. B., Friedland, R. P., & Rapoport, S. I. (1990). Cerebrospinal fluid production is reduced in healthy aging. *Neurology, 40,* 500–503.

McBride, M. (1988). The somatosensory system. In M. Abramson & P. M. Lovas (Eds.), *Aging and sensory change: An annotated bibliography* (pp. 30–36). Washington, DC: Gerontological Society of America.

McDonald, M. P., & Crawley, J. N. (1997). Galanin-acetylcholine interactions in rodent memory tasks and Alzheimer's disease. *Journal of Psychiatry and Neuroscience, 22,* 303–317.

McDowd, J. M. (1996). Inhibition. In J. E. Birren (Ed.), *Encyclopedia of gerontology* (Vol. 1, pp. 761–764). San Diego: Academic Press.

McDowd, J. M., & Birren, J. E. (1990). Aging and attentional processes. In J. E. Birren & K. W. Shaie (Eds.), *Handbook of the psychology of aging* (3rd ed., pp. 222–233). New York: Academic Press.

McEntee, W. J., & Crook, T. H. (1991). Serotonin, memory, and the aging brain. *Psychopharmacology, 103*, 143–149.

McFadden, S. L., Campo, P., Ding, D., & Quaranta, N. (1998). Effects of noise on inferior colliculus evoked potentials and cochlear anatomy in young and aged chinchillas. *Hearing Research, 117*, 81–96.

McFadden, S. L., & Willott, J. F. (1994). Responses of inferior colliculus neurons in C57BL/6J mice with and without sensorineural hearing loss: Effects of changing the azimuthal location of an unmasked pure-tone stimulus. *Hearing Research, 78*, 115–131.

McGahon, B., Clements, M. P., & Lynch, M. A. (1997). The ability of aged rats to sustain long-term potentiation is restored when the age-related decrease in membrane arachidonic acid concentration is reversed. *Neuroscience, 81*, 9–16.

McGaugh, J. L., & Cahill, L. (1997). Interaction of neuromodulatory systems in modulating memory storage. *Behavioural Brain Research, 83*, 31–38.

McGeer, E. G., & McGeer, P. L. (1976). Neurotransmitter metabolism and the aging brain. In R. D. Terry & S. Gershon (Eds.), *Aging: Neurobiology of aging* (Vol. 3, pp. 389–404). New York: Raven Press.

———. (1997). The role of the immune system in neurodegenerative disorders. *Movement Disorders, 12*, 855–858.

McGeer, P. L., & McGeer, E. G. (1996). Neuroimmune mechanisms in the pathogenesis of Alzheimer's disease. In Z. S. Khachaturian & T. S. Radenbaugh (Eds.), *Alzheimer's disease: Cause(s), diagnosis, treatment, and care* (pp. 217–226). Boca Raton, FL: CRC Press.

McGinn, M. D., Henry, K. R., & Coss, R. G. (1984). Age-related hearing loss affects dendritic spine density in mouse neocortex. *Society for Neuroscience Abstracts, 10*, 451.

McIlroy, W. E., & Maki, B. E. (1996). Age-related changes in compensatory stepping in response to unpredictable perturbations. *Journal of Gerontology A, 51*, M289–296.

McIntosh, H. H., & Westfall, T. C. (1987). Influence of aging on catecholamine levels, accumulation, and release in F–344 rats. *Neurobiology of Aging, 8*, 233–239.

McLay, R. N., Freeman, S. M., Harlan, R. E., Ide, C. F., Kastin, A. J., & Zadina, J. E. (1997). Aging in the hippocampus: Interrelated actions of neurotrophins and glucocorticoids. *Neurobehavioral and Biobehavioral Reviews, 21*, 615–629.

McNeill, T. H., Koek, L. L., Brown, S. A., & Rafols, J. A. (1990). Quantitative analysis of age-related dendritic changes in medium spiny I (MSI) striatal neurons of C57BL/6N mice. *Neurobiology of Aging, 11*, 537–550.

McPherson, S. E., & Cummings, J. L. (1997). Vascular dementia: Clinical assessment, neuropsychological features, and treatment. In P. D. Nussbaum (Ed.), *Handbook of neuropsychology and aging* (pp. 177–188). New York: Plenum.

McQuarrie, I. G., Brady, S. T., & Lasek, R. J. (1989). Retardation in the slow axonal transport of cytoskeletal elements during maturation and aging. *Neurobiology of Aging, 10*, 359–365.

Mednikova, Y. S., & Kopytova, F. V. (1994). Some physiological characteristics of motor cortex neurons of aged rabbits. *Neuroscience, 63*, 611–615.

Meier-Ruge, W., Ulrich, J., Bruhlmann, M., & Meier, E. (1992). Age-related white matter atrophy in the human brain. *Annals of the New York Academy of Sciences, 673*, 260–269.

Meister, B., Johnson, H., & Ulfhake, B. (1995). Increased expression of serotonin transporter messenger RNA in raphe neurons of the aged rat. *Molecular Brain Research, 33*, 87–96.

Meites, J. (1991). Role of hypothalamic catecholamines in aging processes. *Acta Endocrinologica, 125*(Suppl. 1), 98–103.

Merigan, W. H., & Maunsell, J. H. R. (1993). How parallel are the primate visual pathways? *Annual Review of Neuroscience, 16*, 369–402.

Mervis, R. (1981). Cytomorphological alterations in the aging animal brain with emphasis on Golgi studies. In J. E. Johnson (Ed.), *Aging and cell structure* (pp. 143–186). New York: Plenum Press.

Messier, C., Gagnon, M., & Knott, V. (1997). Effect of glucose and peripheral glucose regulation on memory in the elderly. *Neurobiology of Aging, 18*, 297–304.

Mesulam, M.-M. (1996). The systems-level organization of cholinergic innervation in the human cerebral cortex and its alterations in Alzheimer's disease. *Progress in Brain Research, 109*, 285–297.

Meyer, J. S., Terayama, Y., & Takashima, S. (1993). Cerebral circulation in the elderly. *Cerebrovascular and Brain Metabolism Reviews, 5*, 122–146.

Michaelis, M. L., Foster, C. T., & Jayawickreme, C. (1992). Regulation of calcium levels in brain tissue from adult and aged rats. *Mechanisms of Ageing and Development, 62*, 291–306.

Mikaelian, D. O. (1979). Development and degeneration of hearing in the C57/b16 mouse: Relation of electrophysiologic responses from the round window and cochlear nucleus to cochlear anatomy and behavioral responses. *Laryngoscope, 89*, 1–15.

Mikiten, T. (1981). Aging and the motor unit. In E. J. Masoro (Ed.), *Handbook of physiology of aging* (pp. 45–46). Boca Raton, FL: CRC Press.

Milbrandt, J. C., Albin, R. L., & Caspary, D. M. (1994). Age-related decrease in $GABA_B$ receptor binding in the Fischer 344 rat inferior colliculus. *Neurobiology of Aging, 15*, 669–703.

Milbrandt, J. C., Albin, R. L., Turgeon, S. M., & Caspary, D. M. (1996). $GABA_A$ receptor binding in the aging rat inferior colliculus. *Neuroscience, 73*, 449–458.

Milbrandt, J. C., & Caspary, D. M. (1995). Age-related reduction of [³H]strychnine binding sites in the cochlear nucleus of the Fischer 344 rat. *Neuroscience, 67,* 713–719.

Milbrandt, J. C., Hunter, C., & Caspary, D. M. (1997). Alterations of GABA$_A$ receptor subunit mRNAs levels in the aged Fischer 344 rat inferior colliculus. *Journal of Comparative Neurology, 379,* 455–465.

Miles, L. E., & Dement, W. C. (1980). Sleep and aging. *Sleep, 3,* 119–220.

Mills, J. H., Lee, F.-S., Dubno, J. R., & Boettcher, F. A. (1996). Interactions between age-related and noise-induced hearing loss. In A. A. Axelson, H. M. Borchgrevink, R. P. Hamernik, P. A. Hellstrom, D. Henderson, & R. J. Salvi (Eds.), *Scientific basis of noise-induced hearing loss* (pp. 193–212). New York: Thieme.

Mirmiran, M., Swaab, D., Kok, J., Hofman, M., Wittig, W., & Van Gool, W. (1992). Circadian rhythms and the suprachiasmatic nucleus in perinatal development, aging, and Alzheimer's disease. *Progress in Brain Research, 93,* 151–162.

Mirra, S. S., & Markesbery, W. R. (1996). The neuropathology of Alzheimer's disease: Diagnostic features and standardization. In Z. S. Khachaturian & T. S. Radenbaugh (Eds.), *Alzheimer's disease: Cause(s), diagnosis, treatment, and care* (pp. 111–123). Boca Raton, FL: CRC Press.

Misretta, C. M. (1984). Aging effects on anatomy and neurophysiology of taste and smell. *Gerodontology, 3,* 131–136.

Miwa, T., Miwa, Y., & Kanda, K. (1995). Dynamic and static sensitivities of muscle spindle primary endings in aged rats to ramp stretch. *Neuroscience Letters, 201,* 179–182.

Mo, J. Q., Hom, D. G., & Andersen, J. K. (1995). Decreases in protective enzymes correlates with increased oxidative damage in the aging mouse brain. *Mechanisms of Ageing and Development, 81,* 73–82.

Mobbs, C. V. (1996). Neuroendocrinogy of aging. In E. L. Schneider & J. W. Rowe (Eds.), *Handbook of the biology of aging* (4th ed., pp. 234–283). San Diego: Academic Press.

Moeller, J. R., Ishikawa, T., Dhawan, V., Spetsieris, P., Mandel, F., Alexander, G. E., Grady, C., Pietrini, P., & Eidelberg, D. (1996). The metabolic topography of normal aging. *Journal of Cerebral Blood Flow and Metabolism, 16,* 385–398.

Monagle, R. D., & Brody, H. (1974). The effects of age upon the main nucleus of the inferior olive in the human. *Journal of Comparative Neurology, 155,* 61–66.

Monji, A., Morimoto, N., Okuyama, I., Umeto, K., Nagatsu, I., Ibata, Y., & Tashiro, N. (1994a). The number of noradrenergic and adrenergic neurons in the brain stem does not change with age in male Sprague-Dawley rats. *Brain Research, 641,* 171–175.

Monji, A., Morimoto, N., Okuyama, I., Yamashita, N., & Tashiro, N. (1994b). Effect of dietary vitamin E on lipofuscin accumulation with age in the rat brain. *Brain Research, 634,* 62–68.

Monteiro, R. A., Conceicao, L. E., Rocha, E., & Marini-Abreu, M. M. (1995). Age changes in cerebellar oligodendrocytes: The appearance of nuclear filaments and increase in the volume density of the nucleus and in the number of dark cell forms. *Archives of Histology and Cytology, 58,* 417–425.

Mooradian, A. D. (1988). Effect of aging on the blood-brain barrier. *Neurobiology of Aging, 9,* 31–39.

———. (1992). Water balance in the elderly. In J. E. Morley & S. G. Korenman (Eds.), *Endocrinology and metabolism in the elderly* (pp. 124–136). Boston: Blackwell Scientific Publishers.

———. (1994). Potential mechanisms of the age-related changes in the blood-brain barrier. *Neurobiology of Aging, 15,* 751–762.

Moore, C. I., Browning, M. D., & Rose, G. M. (1993). Hippocampal plasticity induced by primed burst, but not long-term potentiation, stimulation is impaired in areas CA1 of aged Fischer 344 rats. *Hippocampus, 3,* 57–66.

Moore, M. R., & Black, P. M. (1991). Neuropeptides. *Neurosurgical Reviews, 14,* 97–110.

Moore, W. A., Davey, V. A., Weindruch, R., Walford, R., & Ivy, G. O. (1995). The effect of caloric restriction on lipofuscin ccumulation in mouse brain with age. *Gerontology, 41*(Suppl. 2), 173–185.

Moore, W. A., & Ivy, G. O. (1995). Implications of increased intracellular variability of lipofuscin content with age in dentate gyrus granule cells in the mouse. *Gerontology, 41*(Suppl. 2), 187–199.

Morell, P., Greenfield, S., Constantino-Cellarine, E., & Wisniewski, H. (1972). Changes in the protein composition of mouse brain myelin during development. *Journal of Neurochemistry, 19,* 2545–2554.

Morgan, D. G., & May, P. C. (1990). Age-related changes in synaptic neurochemistry. In E. L. Schneider & J. W. Rowe (Eds.), *Handbook of the biology of aging* (3rd ed., pp. 219–254). San Diego: Academic Press.

Morgan, M. W. (1986). Changes in visual function in the aging eye. In A. R. Rosenbloom & M. W. Morgan (Eds.), *Vision and aging: General and clinical pespectives* (pp. 121–134). New York: Professional Press.

Moriguchi, T., Saito, H., & Nishiyama, N. (1996). Aged garlic extract prolongs longevity and improves spatial memory deficits in senescence-accelerated mouse. *Biological and Pharmaceutical Bulletin, 19,* 305–307.

Moriguchi, T., Takashina, K., Chu, P., Saito, H., & Nishiyama, N. (1994). Prolongation of life span and improved learning in the senescence accelerated mouse produced by aged garlic extract. *Biological and Pharmaceutical Bulletin, 17,* 1589–1594.

Morley, J. E. (1992). Sexual function and the aging woman. In J. E. Morley & S. G. Korenman (Eds.), *Endocrinology and metabolism in the elderly* (pp. 307–321). Boston: Blackwell Scientific ublishers.

———. (1996). Anorexia in older persons: Epidemiology and optimal treatment. *Drugs and Aging, 8,* 134–155.

Morley, J. E., & Korenman, S. G. (1992). *Endocrinology and metabolism in the elderly*. Boston: Blackwell Scientific Publishers.

Morley, J. E., Korenman, S. G., & Kaiser, F. E. (1992). The menopause. In J. E. Morley & S. G. Korenman (Eds.), *Endocrinology and metabolism in the elderly* (pp. 322–335). Boston: Blackwell Scientific Publishers.

Morley, J. E., & Silver, A. J. (1988). Anorexia in the elderly. *Neurobiology of Aging, 9,* 9–16.

Moroi-Fetters, S. E., Mervis, R. F., London, E. D., & Ingram, D. K. (1989). Dietary restriction suppresses age-related changes in dendritic spines. *Neurobiology of Aging, 10,* 317–322.

Morrison, E. E., & Costanzo, R. M. (1995). Regeneration of olfactory sensory neurons and reconnection in the aging hamster central nervous system. *Neuroscience Letters, 198,* 213–217.

Morrison, J. C., Cork, L. C., Dunkelberger, G. R., Brown, A., & Quigley, H. A. (1990). Aging changes of the rhesus monkey optic nerve. *Investigative Opthalmology and Visual Science, 31,* 1623–1627.

Morrison, J. H., & Hof, P. R. (1997). Life and death of neurons in the aging brain. *Science, 278,* 412–419.

Moscovitch, M., & Winocur, G. (1992). The neuropsychology of memory and aging. In F. I. M. Craik & T. A. Salthouse (Eds.), *The handbook of aging and cognition* (pp. 315–372). Hillsdale, NJ: Erlbaum.

Moyer, J. R., Thompson, L. T., Black, J. P., & Disterhoft, J. F. (1992). Nimodipine increases excitability of rabbit CA1 pyramidal neurons in an age- and concentration-dependent manner. *Journal of Neurophysiology, 68,* 2100–2109.

Murchison, D., & Griffith, W. H. (1996). High-voltage-activated calcium currents in basal forebrain neurons during aging. *Journal of Neurophysiology, 76,* 158–174.

Murphy, C. (1993). Nutrition and chemosensory perception in the elderly. *Critical Reviews in Food Science and Nutrition, 33,* 3–15.

Murphy, C., Nordin, S., deWijk, R. A., Cain, W. S., & Polich, J. (1994). Olfactory-evoked potentials: Assessment of young and elderly, and comparison to psychophysical threshold. *Chemical Senses, 19,* 47–56.

Murray, M. P., Kory, R. C., & Clarkson, B. H. (1969). Walking patterns in healthy old men. *Journal of Gerontology, 24,* 169–178.

Naeim, F., & Walford, R. L. (1985). Aging and cell membrane complexes: The lipid bilayer, integral proteins, and cytoskeleton. In C. E. Finch & E. L. Schneider (Eds.), *Handbook of the biology of aging* (2nd ed., pp. 272–289). New York: Van Nostrand Reinhold.

Naessen, R. (1971). An enquiry on the morphological characteristics of possible changes with age in the olfactory region of man. *Acta Otolaryngologica, 71,* 49–62.

Narang, N. (1995). In situ determinations of M_1 and M_2 muscarinic receptor binding sites and mRNAs in young and old rat brains. *Mechanisms of Ageing and Development, 78,* 221–239.

Nebes, R. D. (1990). Hemispheric specialization in the aged brain. In C. Trevarthen (Ed.), *Brain circuits and the functions of the mind* (pp. 364–370). Cambridge: Cambridge University Press.

Nishiyama, N., Zhou, Y., & Saito, H. (1994). Ameliorative effects of chronic treatment using DX–9386, a traditional Chinese prescription, on learning performance and lipid peroxide content in senescence accelarated mouse. *Biological and Pharmaceutical Bulletin, 17*, 1481–1484.

Nishizuka, M., Katoh-Semba, R., Eto, Y., Arai, Y., Iizuka, R., & Kato, K. (1991). Age- and sex-related differences in the nerve growth factor distribution in the rat brain. *Brain Research Bulletin, 27*, 685–688.

Nitta, H., Matsumoto, K., Shimizu, M., Ni, X. H., & Watanabe, H. (1995). Panax ginseng extract improves the performance of aged Fischer 344 rats in radial maze task but not in operant brightness discrimination task. *Biological and Pharmaceutical Bulletin, 18*, 1286–1288.

Norris, C. M., Korol, D. L., & Foster, T. C. (1996). Increased susceptibility to induction of long-term depression and long-term potentiation reversal during aging. *Journal of Neuroscience, 16*, 5382–5392.

Nowak, F. V., & Mooradian, A. D. (1996). Endocrine function and dysfunction. In J. E. Birren (Ed.), *Encyclopedia of gerontology* (Vol. 1, pp. 477–491). San Diego: Academic Press.

Nunzi, M. G., Milan, F., Guidolin, D., & Toffano, G. (1987). Dendritic spine loss in hippocampus of aged rats: Effect of brain phosphatidylserine administration. *Neurobiology of Aging, 8*, 501–510.

Obler, L. K., & Albert, M. L. (1996). Language and communication in aging and dementia. In J. E. Birren (Ed.), *Encyclopedia of gerontology* (Vol. 2, pp. 1–6). San Diego: Academic Press.

Ohm, T. G., Busch, C., & Bohl, J. (1997). Unbiased estimation of neuronal numbers in the human nucleus coeruleus during aging. *Neurobiology of Aging, 18*, 393–399.

O'Keefe, J., & Nadel, L. (1978). *The hippocampus as a cognitive map.* Oxford: Oxford Press.

Ordy, J. M., & Brizzee, K. R. (1979). Functional and structural age differences in the visual system of man and nonhuman primate models. In J. M. Ordy & K. R. Brizzee (Eds.), *Sensory systems and communication in the elderly* (pp. 13–50). New York: Raven Press.

O'Steen, W. K., & Landfield, P. W. (1991). Dietary restriction does not alter retinal aging in the Fischer 344 rat. *Neurobiology of Aging, 12*, 455–462.

O'Steen, W. K., Sweatt, A. J., Eldridge, J. C., & Brodish, A. (1987). Gender and chronic stress effects on the neural retina of young and mid-aged Fischer-344 rats. *Neurobiology of Aging, 8*, 449–455.

Ott, A., Slooter, A. J., Hofman, A., van Harskamp, F., Witteman, J. C., Van Broeckhoven, C., van Duijn, C. M., & Breteler, M. M. (1998). Smoking and risk in dementia and Alzheimer's disease in a population-based cohort study: The Rotterdam study. *Lancet, 351,* 1840–1843.

Ou, X., Buckwalter, G., McNeill, T. H., & Walsh, J. P. (1997). Age-related change in short-term synaptic plasticity intrinsic to excitatory striatal synapses. *Synapse, 27,* 57–68.

Paige, G. D. (1994). Senescence of human visual-vestibular interactions: Smooth pursuit, optokinetic, and vestibular control of eye movements with aging. *Experimental Brain Research, 98,* 355–372.

Palmer, A. M., & DeKosky, S. T. (1993). Monoamine neurons in aging and Alzheimer's disease. *Journal of Neurotransmission, 91,* 135–159.

Palombi, P. S., & Caspary, D. M. (1996a). Physiology of the aging Fischer 344 rat inferior colliculus: Responses to contralateral monaural stimuli. *Journal of Neurophysiology, 76,* 3114–3125.

———. (1996b). Responses of young and aged Fischer 344 rat inferior colliculus neurons to binaural tonal stimuli. *Hearing Research, 100,* 59–67.

Pandolf, K. B. (1997). Aging and human heat tolerance. *Experimental Aging Research, 23,* 69–105.

Parasuraman, R., & Giambra, L. M. (1991). Skill development in vigilance: Effects of event rate and age. *Psychology and Aging, 6,* 155–169.

Parfitt, K. D., & Bickford-Wimer, P. (1990). Age-related subsensitivity of cerebellar Purkinje neurons to locally applied beta$_1$-selective adrenergic agonist. *Neurobiology of Aging, 11,* 591–596.

Parhad, I. M., Scott, J. N., Cellars, L. A., Bains, J. S., Krekoski, C. A., & Clark, A. W. (1995). Axonal atrophy in aging is associated with a decline in neurofilament gene expression. *Journal of Neuroscience Research, 41,* 355–366.

Park, J. C., Cook, K. C., & Verde, E. A. (1990). Dietary restriction slows the abnormally rapid loss of spiral ganglion neurons in C57BL/6 mice. *Hearing Research, 48,* 275–280.

Pedata, F., Giovannelli, L., Spignoli, G., Giovannini, M. G., & Pepu, G. (1985). Phosphatidylserine increases acetylcholine release from cortical slices in aged rats. *Neurobiology of Aging, 6,* 337–339.

Pedersen, N. L. (1996). Gerontological behavior genetics. In J. E. Birren & K. W. Schaie (Eds.), *Handbook of the psychology of aging* (4th ed., pp. 59–77). San Diego: Academic Press.

Peinado, M. A., Quesada, A., Pedrosa, J. A., Marinez, M., Esteban, F. J., Del Moral, M. L., & Peinado, J. M. (1997). Light microscopic quantification of morphological changes during aging in neurons and glia of the rat parietal cortex. *Anatomical Record, 247,* 420–425.

Penev, P. D., Turek, F. W., Wallen, E. P., & Zee, P. C. (1997). Aging alters the serotonergic modulation of light-induced phase advances in golden hamsters. *American Journal of Physiology, 272,* R509–513.

Peng, M. T., Jiang, M. J., & Hsu, H. K. (1980). Changes in wheel running activity, eating and drinking, and their day/night distributions throughout the lifespan of the rat. *Journal of Gerontology, 35*, 339–347.

Pennisi, E. (1997). Gene found for the fading eyesight of old age. *Science, 277*, 1765–1766.

Pentney, R. J. (1986). Quantitative analysis of dendritic networks of Purkinje neurons during aging. *Neurobiology of Aging, 7*, 241–248.

Perrig, W. J., Perrig, P., & Stahelin, H. B. (1997). The relation between antioxidants and memory performance in the old and very old. *Journal of the American Geriatric Society, 45*, 718–724.

Perry, V. H., Matyszak, M. K., & Fearn, S. (1993). Altered antigen expression of microglia in the aged rodent CNS. *Glia, 7*, 60–67.

Peters, A. (1996). Age-related changes in oligodendrocytes in monkey cerebral cortex. *Journal of Comparative Neurology, 371*, 153–163.

Peters, A., Josephson, K., & Vincent, S. L. (1991). Effects of aging on the neuroglial cells and pericytes within area 17 of the rhesus monkey cerebral cortex. *Anatomical Record, 229*, 384–398.

Peters, A., Rosene, D. L., Moss, M. B., Kemper, T. L., Abraham, C. R., Tigges, J., & Albert, M. S. (1996). Neurobiological bases of age-related cognitive decline in the rhesus monkey. *Journal of Neuropathology and Experimental Neurology, 55*, 861–874.

Peters, A., & Vaughan, D. W. (1981). Central nervous system. In J. E. Johnson (Ed.), *Aging and cell structure* (Vol. 1, pp. 1–34). New York: Plenum Press.

Petkov, V. D., Kehayov, R., Belcheva, S., Konstantinova, E., Petkov, V. V., Getova, D., & Markovska, V. (1993). Memory effects of standardized extracts of Panax ginseng (G115), Ginkgo biloba (GK501) and their combination Gincosan (PHL-00701). *Planta Medica, 59*, 106–114.

Petri, H. L., & Mishkin, M. (1994). Behaviorism, cognitivism and the neuropsychology of memory. *American Scientist, 82*, 30–37.

Pettegrew, J. W., Klunk, W. E., Panchalingam, K., Kanfer, J. N., & McClure, R. J. (1995). Clinical and neurochemical effects of acetyl-L-carnitine in Alzheimer's disease. *Neurobiology of Aging, 16*, 1–4.

Phillips, P. A., Johnston, C. I., & Gray, L. (1993). Disturbed fluid and electrolyte homeostasis following dehydration in elderly people. *Age and Ageing, 22*, S26–S33.

Pierpaoli, W., Bulian, D., Dall'Ara, A., Marchetti, B., Gallo, F., Morales, M. C., Tirolo, C., & Testa, N. (1997). Circadian melatonin and young-to-old pineal grafting postpone aging and maintain juvenile conditions of reproductive functions in mice and rats. *Experimental Gerontology, 32*, 587–602.

Pierscionek, B. K., & Weale, R. A. (1996). Risk factors and ocular senescence. *Gerontology, 42*, 257–269.

Pitsikas, N., & Borsini, F. (1996). Itasetron (DAU 6215) prevents age-related memory deficits in the rat in a multiple choice avoidance task. *European Journal of Pharmacology, 311*, 115–119.

Porciatti, V., Burr, D. C., Morrone, C., & Fiorentini, A. (1992). The effects of ageing on the pattern electroretinogram and visual evoked potentials in humans. *Vision Research, 32*, 1199–1209.

Portera-Cailliau, C., Hedreen, J. C., Price, D. L., & Koliatsos, V. E. (1995). Evidence for apoptotic cell death in Huntington disease and excitotoxic animal models. *Journal of Neuroscience, 15*, 3775–3787.

Posner, M. I., & Peterson, S. E. (1990). The attention system of the brain. *Annual Review of Neuroscience, 13*, 25–42.

Potier, B., Rascol, O., Jazat, F., Lamour, Y., & Dutar, P. (1992). Alterations in the properties of hippocampal pyramidal neurons in the aged rats. *Neuroscience, 48*, 793–806.

Powell, D. A., Buchanan, S. L., & Hernandez, L. L. (1991). Classical (Pavlovian) conditioning models of age-related changes in associative learning and their neurobiological substrates. *Progress in Neurobiology, 36*, 201–228.

Prinz, P. N., Dustman, R. E., & Emmerson, R. (1990). Electrophysiology and aging. In J. E. Birren & K. W. Shaie (Eds.), *Handbook of the psychology of aging* (3rd ed., pp. 135–149). New York: Academic Press.

Pyapali, G. K., & Turner, D. A. (1996). Increased dendritic extent in hippocampal CA1 neurons from aged F344 rats. *Neurobiology of Aging, 17*, 601–611.

Rance, N. E. (1992). Hormonal influences on morphology and neuropeptide gene expression in the infundibular nucleus of postmenopausal women. *Progress in Brain Research, 93*, 221–236.

Rao, K. M. K., & Cohen, H. J. (1990). The role of the cytoskeleton in aging. *Experimental Gerontology, 24*, 7–22.

Raz, N., Gunning, F. M., Head, D., Dupuis, J. H., McQuain, J., Briggs, S. D., Loken, W. J., Thornton, A. E., & Acker, J. D. (1997). Selective aging of the human cerebral cortex observed *in vivo*: Differential vulnerability of the prefrontal gray matter. *Cerebral Cortex, 7*, 268–282.

Raza, A., Milbrandt, J. C., Arneric, S. P., & Caspary D. M. (1994). Age-related changes in brainstem auditory neurotransmitters: Measures of GABA and acetylcholine function. *Hearing Research, 77*, 221–230.

Reagan, L. P., & McEwen, B. S. (1997). Controversies surrounding glucocorticoid-mediated cell death in the hippocampus. *Journal of Chemical Neuroanatomy, 13*, 149–167.

Reinke, H., & Dinse, H. R. (1996). Functional characterization of cutaneous mechanoreceptor properties in aged rats. *Neuroscience Letters, 216*, 171–174.

Reiter, R. J. (1995). The pineal gland and melatonin in relation to aging: A summary of the theories and of the data. *Experimental Gerontology, 30*, 199–212.

Reiter, R. J., Guerrero, J. M., Escames, G., Pappolla. M. A., & Acuna-Castroviero, D. (1997). Prophylactic actions of melatonin in oxidative neurotoxicity. *Annals of the New York Academy of Sciences, 825,* 70–78.

Richardson, G. S. (1990). Circadian rhythms and aging. In E. L. Schneider & J. W. Rowe (Eds.), *Handbook of the biology of aging* (3rd ed., pp. 275–305). San Diego: Academic Press.

Richter-Levin, G., & Segal, M. (1996). Serotonin, aging and cognitive function of the hippocampus. *Reviews in the Neurosciences, 7,* 103–113.

Riedel, W. J., & Jolles, J. (1996). Cognition enhancers in age-related cognitive decline. *Drugs and Aging, 8,* 245–274.

Robbins, S., Waked, E., & McClaran, J. (1995). Proprioception and stability: Foot position awareness as a function of age and footwear. *Age and Ageing, 24,* 67–72.

Roberts, J., Snyder, D. L., Johnson, M. D., & Horwitz, J. (1993). Changes in the effect of the autonomic nervous system on the aging heart. In F. Amenta (Ed.), *Aging of the autonomic nervous system* (pp. 139–165). Boca Raton, FL: CRC Press.

Rodriguez-Gomez, J. A., de la Roza, C., Machado, A., & Cano, J. (1995). The effect of age on the monoamines of the hypothalamus. *Mechanisms of Ageing and Development, 77,* 185–195.

Rogers, J., & Bloom, F. E. (1985). Neurotransmitter metabolism and function in the aging central nervous system. In C. E. Finch & E. L. Schneider (Eds.), *Handbook of the biology of aging* (2nd ed., pp. 645–691). New York: Van Nostrand Reinhold.

Rolls, B. J., & Drewnowski, A. (1996). Diet and nutrition. In J. E. Birren (Ed.), *Encyclopedia of gerontology* (Vol. 1, pp. 429–440). San Diego: Academic Press.

Roos, M. R., Rice, C. L., & Vandervoort, A. A. (1997). Age-related changes in motor unit function. *Muscle & Nerve, 20,* 679–690.

Roozendaal, B., van Gool, W. A., Swaab, D. F., Hoogendijk, J. E., & Mirmiran, M. (1987). Changes in vasopressin cells of the rat suprachiasmatic nucleus with aging. *Brain Research, 409,* 259–264.

Rosenberg, I. H., & Miller, J. W. (1992). Nutritional factors in physical and cognitive functions of elderly people. *American Journal of Clinical Nutrition, 55*(Suppl. 6), 1237S–1234S.

Rosenhall, U. (1973). Degenerative patterns in the aging human vestibular neuro-epithelia. *Acta Otolaryngologica, 76,* 208–220.

Rosenhall, U., & Rubin, W. (1975). Degenerative patterns in the aging human vestibular sensory epithelia. *Acta Otolaryngologica, 79,* 67–80.

Rosenheimer, J. L. (1990). Factors affecting denervation-like changes at the neuromuscular junction during aging. *International Journal of Developmental Neuroscience, 8,* 643–654.

Rosenzweig, E. S., Rao, G., McNaughton, B. L., & Barnes, C. A. (1997). Role of temporal summation in age-related long-term potentiation-induced deficits. *Hippocampus, 7,* 549–558.

Rosenzweig, M. R., Leiman, A. L., & Breedlove, S. M. (1996). *Biological psychology.* Sunderland, MA: Sinauer.

Roubein, I. F., Embree, L. J., & Jackson, D. W. (1986). Changes in catecholamine levels in discrete regions of rat brain during aging. *Experimental Aging Research, 12,* 193–196.

Rowe, J. W., & Kahn, R. L. (1987). Human aging: Usual and successful. *Science, 237,* 143–149.

Rowe, W., Steverman, A., Walker, M., Sharma, S., Barden, N., Seckl, J. R., & Meany, M. J. (1997). Antidepressants restore hypothalamic-pituitary-adrenal function in aged, cognitively impaired rats. *Neurobiology of Aging, 18,* 527–533.

Rubin, G. S., Roche, K. B., Prasada-Rao, P., & Fried, L. P. (1994). Visual impairment and disability in older adults. *Optometry and Vision Science, 71,* 750–760.

Rubinsztein, D. C. (1997). The genetics of Alzheimer's disease. *Progress in Neurobiology, 52,* 447–454.

Rudman, D., & Rao, U. M. P. (1992). The hypothalamic-growth hormone-somatomedin C axis: The effect of aging. In J. E. Morley & S. G. Korenman (Eds.), *Endocrinology and metabolism in the elderly* (pp. 35–57). Boston: Blackwell Scientific Publishers.

Ruiz-Marcos, A., Sanchez-Toscano, F., & Munoz-Cueto, J. A. (1992). Aging reverts to juvenile conditions the synaptic connectivity of cerebral cortical pyramidal shafts. *Developmental Brain Research, 69,* 41–49.

Ruth, J.-E. (1996). Personality. In J. E. Birren (Ed.), *Encyclopedia of gerontology* (Vol. 2, pp. 281–294). San Diego: Academic Press.

Sadow, T. F., & Rubin, R. T. (1992). Effects of hypothalamic peptides on the aging brain. *Psychoneuroendocrinology, 17,* 293–314.

Sahu, A., & Kalra, S. P. (1998). Absence of increased neuropeptide Y neuronal activity before and during the luteinizing hormone (LH) surge may underlie the attenuated preovulatory LH surge in middle-aged rats. *Endocrinology, 139,* 696–702.

Sahu, A., Kalra, P. S., Crowley, W. R., & Kalra, S. P. (1988). Evidence that hypothalamic neuropeptide Y secretion decreases in aged male rats: Implications for reproductive aging. *Endocrinology, 122,* 2199–2203.

Saija, A., Princi, P., D'Amico, N., DePasquale, R., & Costa, G. (1990). Aging and sex influence the permeability of the blood brain barrier in the rat. *Life Sciences, 47,* 2261–2267.

Saito, S., Kobayashi, S., Ohashi, Y., Igarashi, M., Komiya, Y., & Ando, S. (1994). Decreased synaptic density in aged brains and its prevention by rearing under enriched environment as evealed by synaptophysin contents. *Journal of Neuroscience Research, 39,* 57–62.

Sakurai, T. (1996). Population coding by cell assemblies—what it really is in the brain. *Neuroscience Research, 26,* 1–16.

Salmon, D. P., & Bondi, M. W. (1997). The neuropsychology of Alzheimer's disease. In P. D. Nussbaum (Ed.), *Handbook of neuropsychology and aging* (pp. 141–158). New York: Plenum.

Salmon, E., Marquet, P., Sadzot, B., Deguildre, C., Lemaire, C., & Frank, G. (1991). Decrease of frontal metabolism demonstrated by positron emission tomography in a population of healthy elderly volunteers. *Acta Neurologica Belgique, 91,* 288–295.

Salthouse, T. A. (1985). Speed of behavior and its implications for cognition. In J. E. Birren & K. W. Shaie (Eds.), *Handbook of the psychology of aging* (2nd ed., pp. 400–426). New York: Van Nostrand Reinhold.

———. (1992). Reasoning and spatial abilities. In F. I. M. Craik & T. A. Salthouse (Eds.), *The handbook of aging and cognition* (pp. 167–212). Hillsdale, NJ: Erlbaum.

———. (1996). Reaction time. In J. E. Birren (Ed.), *Encyclopedia of gerontology* (Vol. 2, pp. 337–380). San Diego: Academic Press.

Sano, M., Bell, K., Cote, L., Dooneief, G., Lawton, A., Legler, L., Marder, K., Naini, A., Stern, Y., & Mayeux, R. (1992). Double-blind parallel design pilot study of acetyl levocarnitine in patients with Alzheimer's disease. *Archives of Neurology, 49,* 1137–1141.

Santer, R. M. (1993). Quantitative analysis of the cervical sympathetic trunk in young adult and aged rats. *Mechanisms of Ageing and Development, 67,* 289–298.

Santer, R. M., & Baker, D. M. (1993). Enteric system. In F. Amenta (Ed.), *Aging of the autonomic nervous system* (pp. 213–225). Boca Raton, FL: CRC Press.

Saper, C. B. (1996). Any way you cut it: A new journal policy for the use of unbiased counting methods. *Journal of Comparative Neurology, 364,* 5.

Sapolsky, R. M. (1992). *Stress, the aging brain, and the mechanisms of neuron death.* Cambridge: MIT Press.

Sarter, M., & Bruno, J. P. (1997). Trans-synaptic stimulation of cortical acetylcholine and enhancement of attentional functions: A rational approach for the development of cognitive enhancers. *Behavioural Brain Research, 83,* 7–14.

Sarter, M., & Markowitsch, H. J. (1983). Reduced resistance to progressive extinction in senescent rats: A neuroanatomical and behavioral study. *Neurobiology of Aging, 4,* 203–215.

Sartin, J. L., & Lamperti, A. A. (1985). Neuron numbers in hypothalamic nuclei of young, middle-aged, and aged rats. *Experientia, 41,* 109–111.

Satorre, J., Cano, J., & Reinoso-Suarez, F. (1985). Stability of the neuronal population of the dorsal lateral geniculate nucleus (LGNd) of aged rats. *Brain Research, 339,* 375–377.

Scarpace, P. J. (1986). Decreased β-adrenergic responsiveness during senescence. *Federation Proceedings, 45,* 51–53.

Schacter, D. L., Savage, C. R., Alpert, N. M., Rauch, S. L., & Albert, M. S. (1996). The role of hippocampus and frontal cortex in age-related memory changes: A PET study. *NeuroReport, 7,* 1165–1169.

Schaie, K. W. (1996). Intellectual development in adulthood. In J. E. Birren & K. W. Schaie (Eds.), *Handbook of the psychology of aging* (4th ed., pp. 266–286). San Diego: Academic Press.

Schauwecker, P. E., Cheng, H. W., Serquinia, R. M., Mori, N., & McNeill, T. H. (1995). Lesion-induced sprouting of commissural/associational axons and induction of GAP-43 MRNA in hilar and CA3 pyramidal neurons in the hippocampus are diminished in aged rats. *Journal of Neuroscience, 15,* 2462–2470.

Scheff, S. W., Sparks, D. L., & Price, D. A. (1996). Quantitative assessment of synaptic density in the outer molecular layer of the hippocampal dentate gyrus in Alzheimer's disease. *Dementia, 7,* 226–232.

Scheibel, A. B. (1996). Structural and functional changes in the aging brain. In J. E. Birren & K. W. Schaie (Eds.), *Handbook of the psychology of aging* (4th ed., pp. 105–128). San Diego: Academic Press.

Scheibel, M. E., Lindsay, R. D., Tomiyasu, U., & Scheibel, A. B. (1975). Progressive changes in aging human cortex. *Experimental Neurology, 47,* 392–403.

Scheibel, M. E., Tomiyasu, U., & Scheibel, A. B. (1977). The aging human Betz cell. *Experimental Neurology, 56,* 598–609.

Schiffman, S. (1996). Smell and taste. In J. E. Birren (Ed.), *Encyclopedia of gerontology* (Vol. 2, pp. 497–504). San Diego: Academic Press.

Schiffman, S., & Warwick, Z. S. (1988). Flavor enhancement of foods for the elderly can reverse anorexia. *Neurobiology of Aging, 9,* 24–26.

Schipper, H. M., Yang, G., & Wang, E. (1994). Expression of terminin, a senescence-related cytoplasmic protein, in the aging rat brain. *Brain Research, 635,* 224–230.

Schmidt, R. E., Chase, H. Y., Parvin, C. A., & Roth, K. A. (1990). Neuroaxonal dystrophy in aging human sympathetic ganglia. *American Journal of Pathology, 136,* 1327–1338.

Schmidt, R. E., Beaudet, L., Plurad, S. B., Snider, W. D., & Ruit, K. G. (1995). Pathologic alterations in pre- and postsynaptic elements in aged mouse sympathetic ganglia. *Journal of Neurocytology, 24,* 189–206.

Schmiedt, R. A., Mills, J. H., & Boettcher, F. A. (1996). Age-related loss of activity of auditory-nerve fibers. *Journal of Neurophysiology, 76,* 2799–2803.

Schneider, E. L., & Reed, J. D. (1985). Modulations of aging processes. In C. E. Finch & E. L. Schneider (Eds.), *Handbook of the biology of aging* (2nd ed., pp. 45–76). New York: Van Nostrand Reinhold.

Schramke, C. J. (1997). Anxiety disorders. In P. D. Nussbaum (Ed.), *Handbook of neuropsychology and aging* (pp. 80–97). New York: Plenum.

Schroeder, F. (1984). Role of membrane lipid asymmetry in aging. *Neurobiology of Aging, 5,* 323–333.

Schuurman, T., & Traber, J. (1994). Calcium antagonists in aging brain. *Annals of the New York Academy of Sciences, 747,* 467–474.

Scott, B., Leu, J., & Cinader, B. (1988). Effects of aging on neuronal electrical membrane properties. *Mechanisms of Ageing and Development, 44,* 203–214.

Seidler, R. S., & Stelmach, G. (1996). Motor control. In J. E. Birren (Ed.), *Encyclopedia of gerontology* (Vol. 2, pp. 177–185). San Diego: Academic Press.

Semlitsch, H. V., Anderer, P., Saletu, B., Binder, G. A., & Decker, K. A. (1995). Cognitive psychophysiology in nootropic drug research: Effects of Ginkgo biloba on event-related potentials (P300) in age-associated memory impairment. *Pharmacopsychiatry, 28,* 134–142.

Setlow, B. (1997). The nucleus accumbens and learning and memory. *Journal of Neuroscience Research, 49,* 515–521.

Shah, G. N., & Mooradian, A. D. (1997). Age-related changes in the blood-brain barrier. *Experimental Gerontology, 32,* 501–519.

Sharma, D., Maurya, A. K., & Singh, R. (1993). Age-related decline in multiple unit action potentials of CA3 region of rat hippocampus: Correlation with lipid peroxidation and lipofuscin concentration and the effect of centrophenoxine. *Neurobiology of Aging, 14,* 319–330.

Sharma, D., & Singh, R. (1996). Age-related decline in multiple unit action potentials of cerebral cortex correlates with the number of lipofuscin-containing neurons. *Indian Journal of Experimental Biology, 34,* 776–781.

Shaw, N. A. (1992). Age-dependent changes in central somatosensory conduction time. *Clinical Electroencephalography, 23,* 105–110.

Shen, J., & Barnes, C. A. (1996). Age-related decrease in cholinergic synaptic transmission in three hippocampal subfields. *Neurobiology of Aging, 17,* 439–451.

Shen, J., Barnes, C. A., McNaughton, B. L., Skaggs, W. E., & Weaver, K. L. (1997). The effect of aging on experience-dependent plasticity of hippocampal place cells. *Journal of Neuroscience, 17,* 6769–6782.

Shepherd, G. M. (1996). The dendritic spine: A multifunctional integrative unit. *Journal of Neurophysiology, 75,* 2197–2210.

Shimada, A., Hosokawa, M., Ohta, A., Akiguchi, I., & Takeda, T. (1994). Localization of atrophy-prone areas in the aging mouse brain: Comparison between the brain atrophy model SAM-P/10 and the normal control SAM-R/1. *Neuroscience, 59,* 859–869.

Shimada, A., Kuwamura, M., Awakura, T., Umemura, T., & Itakura, C. (1992). An immunohistochemical and ultrastructural study on age-related astrocytic gliosis in the central nervous system of dogs. *Journal of Veterinary Medical Science, 54,* 29–36.

Ship, J. A., Pearson, J. D., Cruise, L. J., Brant, L. J., & Metter, E. J. (1996). Longitudinal changes in smell identification. *Journal of Gerontology A, 51,* M86–M91.

Shone, G., Altschuler, R. A., Miller, J. M., & Nuttall, A. L. (1991). The effect of noise exposure on the aging ear. *Hearing Research, 56,* 173–178.

Simic, G., Kostovic, I., Winblad, B., & Bogdanovic, N. (1997). Volume and number of neurons of the human hippocampal formation in normal aging and Alzheimer's disease. *Journal of Comparative Neurology, 379,* 482–494.

Simoneau, G. C., & Leibowitz, H. W. (1996). Posture, gait, and falls. In J. E. Birren & K. W. Schaie (Eds.), *Handbook of the Psychology of Aging* (4th ed., pp. 204–217). San Diego: Academic Press.

Simpson, D. M., & Erwin, C. W. (1983). Evoked potential latency change with age suggests differential aging of primary somatosensory cortex. *Neurobiology of Aging, 4,* 59–63.

Singh, J., Knight, R. T., Woods, D. L., Beckley, D. J., & Clayworth, C. (1990). Lack of age effects on human brain potentials preceding voluntary movements. *Neuroscience Letters, 119,* 27–31.

Sloviter, R. S., Dean, E., Sollas, A. L., & Goodman, J. H. (1996). Apoptosis and necrosis induced in different hipocampal neuron populations by repetitive perforant path stimulation in the rat. *Journal of Comparative Neurology, 366,* 516–533.

Smith, A. D. (1996). Memory. In J. E. Birren & K. W. Schaie (Eds.), *Handbook of the psychology of aging* (4th ed., pp. 236–250). San Diego: Academic Press.

Smith, C. G. (1942). An incidence of atrophy of olfactory nerves in man. *Journal of Comparative Neurology, 77,* 589–595.

Smith, M. L., & Booze, R. M. (1995). Cholinergic and GABAergic neurons in the nucleus basalis region of young and aged rats. *Neuroscience, 67,* 679–688.

Smith, S. W., & Osborne, B. A. (1997). Private pathways to a common death. *Journal of NIH Research, 9,* 33–37.

Smith, W. E. (1995). Evolution of longevity in mammals. *Mechanisms of Ageing and Development, 81,* 51–60.

Socci, D. J., Crandall, B. M., & Arendash, G. W. (1995). Chronic antioxidant treatment improves the cognitive performance of aged rats. *Brain Research, 693,* 88–94.

Soininen, H. S., Partanen, K., Pitkanen, A., Vainio, P., Hanninen, T., Hallikainen, M., Koivisto, K., & Riekkinen, P. J. (1994). Volumetric MRI analysis of the amygdala and the hippocampus in subjects with age-associated memory impairment: Correlation to visual and verbal memory. *Neurology, 44,* 1660–1668.

Sontheimer, H. (1995). Glial influences on neuronal signaling. *The Neuroscientist, 1,* 123–126.

Sparks, D., Hunsaker, J., Slavin, J., DeKosky, S., Kryscio, R., & Markesberry, W. (1992). Monoaminergic and cholinergic synaptic markers in the nucleus basalis of Meynert (nbM): Normal age-related changes and the effect of heart disease and Alzheimer's disease. *Annals of Neurology, 31*, 611–620.

Spear, P. D. (1993). Neural bases of visual deficits during aging. *Vision Research, 33*, 2589–2609.

Spear, P. D., Moore, R. J., Kim, C. B. Y., Xue, J.-T., & Tumosa, N. (1994). Effects of aging on the primate visual system: Spatial and temporal processing by lateral geniculate neurons in young adult and old rhesus monkeys. *Journal of Neurophysiology, 72*, 402–420.

Spencer, P. S., & Ochoa, J. (1981). The mammalian peripheral nervous system. In J. E. Johnson (Ed.), *Aging and cell structure* (pp. 35–104). New York: Plenum Press.

Spengler, F., Godde, B., & Dinse, H. R. (1995). Effects of ageing on topographic organization of somatosensory cortex. *Neuroreport, 6*, 469–473.

Spielberger, C. D., Gorsuch, R., & Lushene, R. (1970). *The state trait anxiety inventory (STAI) test manual.* Palo Alto, CA: Consulting Psychologists Press.

Spirduso, W. W., & MacRae, G. (1990). Motor performance and aging. In J. E. Birren & K. W. Shaie (Eds.), *Handbook of the psychology of aging* (3rd ed., pp. 183–200). New York: Academic Press.

Srivastava, N., Granholm, A. C., & Gerhardt, G. A. (1997). Collateral sprouting of central noradrenergic neurons during aging: Histochemical and neurochemical studies in intraocular triple transplants. *Experimental Neurology, 145*, 524–535.

Starratt, C., & Peterson, L. (1997). Personality in normal aging. In P. D. Nussbaum (Ed.), *Handbook of neuropsychology and aging* (pp. 15–31). New York: Plenum.

Stevens, J. C., & Cruz, L. A. (1996). Spatial acuity of touch: Ubiquitous decline with aging revealed by repeated threshold testing. *Somatosensory and Motor Research, 13*, 1–10.

Stevens, J. C., Cruz, L. A., Hoffman, J. M., & Patterson, M. G. (1995). Taste sensitivity and aging: High incidence of decline revealed by repeated threshold measures. *Chemical Senses, 20*, 451–459.

Stevens, J. C., & Dadarwala, A. D. (1993). Variability of olfactory threshold and its role in assessment of aging. *Perception and Psychophysics, 54*, 296–302.

St.-Laurent, M. (1988). Normal pressure hydrocephalus in geriatric medicine: A challenge. *Journal of Geriatric Psychiatry and Neurology, 1*, 163–168.

Stoll, L., Schubert, T., & Muller, W. E. (1991). Age-related deficits of central muscarinic cholinergic receptor function in the mouse: Partial restoration by chronic piracetam treatment. *Neurobiology of Aging, 13*, 39–44.

Stoll, S., Scheuer, K., Pohl, O., & Muller, W. E. (1996). Ginkgo biloba extract (EGb 761) independently improves changes in passive avoidance learning and brain membrane fluidity in the aging mouse. *Pharmacopsychiatry, 29*, 144–149.

Strosznajder, J., Samochocki, M., & Duran, M. (1994). Aging diminishes seroto-nin-stimulated arachidonic acid uptake and cholinergic receptor-activated arachidonic acid release in rat brain cortex membrane. *Journal of Neurochemistry*, *62*, 1048–1054.

Sturrock, R. R. (1988). Loss of neurons from the retrofacial nucleus of the mouse in extreme old age. *Journal of Anatomy, 160*, 195–199.

———. (1991). Stability of neuronal glial number in the aging mouse supraoptic nucleus. *Anatomischer Anzeiger, 172*, 123–128.

———. (1996). Structural and quantitative changes in the brain during normal aging. In U. Mohr, D. L. Dungworth, C. C. Capen, W. W. Carlton, J. P. Sundberg, & J. M. Ward (Eds.), *Pathobiology of the aging mouse* (Vol 2., pp. 3–38). Washington, DC: ILSI Press.

Sturrock, R. R., & Rao, K. A. A. (1985). A quantitative histological study of neuronal loss from the locus coeruleus of ageing mice. *Neuropathology and Applied Neurobiology, 11*, 55–60.

Sugawa, M., Coper, H., Schulze, G., Yamashina, I., Krause, F., & Dencher, N. A. (1996). Impaired plasticity of neurons in aging. biochemical, biophysical, and behavioral studies. *Annals of the New York Academy of Sciences, 786*, 274–282.

Sun, J. C., Bohne, B. A., & Harding, G. W. (1994). Is the older ear more susceptible to noise damage? *The Laryngoscope, 104*, 1251–1258.

Sun, G. Y., & Samorajski, T. (1972). Age changes in the lipid composition of whole homogenates and isolated myelin fractions of mouse brain. *Journal of Gerontology, 27*, 10–17.

Supiano, M. A., & Halter, J. B. (1992). The aging sympathetic nervous system. In J. E. Morley & S. G. Korenman (Eds.), *Endocrinology and metabolism in the elderly* (pp. 465–481). Boston: Blackwell Scientific Publishers.

Svanborg, A. (1996). Cardiovascular system. In J. E. Birren (Ed.), *Encyclopedia of gerontology* (Vol. 1, pp. 245–251). San Diego: Academic Press.

Swaab, D. F., Fliers, E., & Partiman, T. S. (1985). Suprachiasmatic nucleus of the human brain in relation to sex, age and senile dementia. *Brain Research, 342*, 37–44.

Swaab, D., Grunde-Iqbal, I., Iqbal, I., Kremer, H., Ravid, R., & Van de Ness, J. (1992). Tau and ubiquitin in the human hypothalamus in aging and Alzheimer's disease. *Brain Research, 590*, 239–249.

Swash, M., & Fox, K. P. (1972). The effect of age on human skeletal muscle: Studies of the morphology and innervation of muscle spindles. *Journal of Neurological Science, 16*, 417.

Sweet, R. J., Price, J. M., & Henry, K. R. (1988). Dietary restriction and presbycusis: Periods of restriction and auditory threshold losses in the CBA/J mouse. *Audiology, 27*, 305–312.

Sylvia, A. L., & Rosenthal, M. (1979). Effects of age on brain oxidative metabolism *in vivo*. *Brain Research, 165*, 235–248.

Takayama, H., Ogawa, N., Yamamoto, M., Asanuma, M., Hirata, H., & Ota, Z. (1992). Age-related changes in cerebrospinal fluid gamma-aminobutyric acid concentration. *European Journal of Clinical Chemistry and Clinical Biochemistry, 30*, 271–274.

Tanaka, Y., & Ando, S. (1990). Synaptic aging as revealed by changes in membrane potential and decreased activity of Na+, K(+)-ATPase. *Brain Research, 506*, 46–52.

———. (1992). Age-related changes in [³H] ouabain binding to synaptic plasma membranes isolated from mouse brains. *Journal of Biochemistry, 112*, 117–121.

Tanila, H., Shapiro, M., Gallagher, M., & Eichenbaum, H. (1997). Brain aging: Changes in the nature of information coding by the hippocampus. *Journal of Neuroscience, 17*, 5155–5166.

Tanila, H., Sipila, P., Shapiro, M., & Eichenbaum, H. (1997). Brain aging: Impaired coding of novel environmental cues. *Journal of Neuroscience, 17*, 5167–5174.

Tashiro, T., & Komiya, Y. (1994). Impairment of cytoskeleton protein transport due to aging or beta, beta'-iminodipropionitrile intoxication in the rat sciatic nerve. *Gerontology, 40*(Suppl. 2), 36–45.

Tatton, W. G., Greenwood, C. E., Salo, P. T., & Seniuk, N. A. (1991). Transmitter synthesis increases in substantia nigra neurons of the aged mouse. *Neuroscience Letters, 131*, 179–182.

Tenover, J. S. (1992). Male hormonal changes with aging. In J. E. Morley & S. G. Korenman (Eds.), *Endocrinology and metabolism in the elderly* (pp. 243–261). Boston: Blackwell Scientific Publishers.

Terry, R. D., De Teresa, R., & Hansen, L. A. (1987). Neocortical cell counts in normal human adult aging. *Annals of Neurology, 21*, 530–539.

Terry, R. D., Katzman, R., & Bick, K. L. (Eds.). (1994). *Alzheimer disease.* New York: Raven Press.

Thal, L. J. (1996). Cholinomimetic treatment of Alzheimer's disease. *Progress in Brain Research, 109*, 299–309.

Thompson, R. F., & Krupa, D. J. (1994). Organization of memory traces in the mammalian brain. *Annual Review of Neuroscience, 17*, 519–549.

Tigges, J., Herndon, J. G., & Peters, A. (1990). Neuronal population of Area 4 during the life span of the rhesus monkey. *Neurobiology of Aging, 11*, 201–208.

———. (1992). Axon terminals on Betz cell somata of Area 4 in rhesus monkey throughout adulthood. *Anatomical Record, 232*, 305–315.

Tissingh, G., Bergmans, P., Booij, J., Winogrodzka, A., Stoof, J. C., Wolters, E. C., & Van Royen, E. A. (1997). [123]beta-CIT single-photon emission tomography in Parkinson's disease reveals a smaller decline in dopamine transporters with age than in controls. *European Journal of Nuclear Medicine, 24*, 1171–1174.

Toide, K., Iwamoto, Y., Fujiwara, T., & Abe, H. (1995). JTP-4819: A novel prolyl endopeptidase inhibitor with potential as a cognitive enhancer. *Journal of Pharmacology and Experimental Therapeutics, 274*, 1370–1378.

Touitou, Y., Bogdan, A., Haus, E., & Touitou, C. (1997). Modifications of circadian and circannual rhythms with aging. *Experimental Gerontology, 32,* 603–614.

Travis, J. (1994). Glia: The brain's other cells. *Science, 266,* 970–972.

Trick, G. L., Trick, L. R., & Haywood, K. M. (1986). Altered pattern evoked retinal and cortical potentials with human senescence. *Current Eye Research, 5,* 717–724.

Tsagarakis, S., & Grossman, A. (1992). The hypothalamic-pituitary-adrenal axis in senscence. In J. E. Morley & S. G. Korenman (Eds.), *Endocrinology and metabolism in the elderly* (pp. 70–91). Boston: Blackwell Scientific Publishers.

Tucker, D. M., Penland, J. G., Sandstead, H. H., Milne, D. B., Heck, D. G., & Klevay, L. M. (1990). Nutritional status and brain function in aging. *American Journal of Clinical Nutrition, 52,* 93–102.

Turner, J. G., & Willott, J. F. (1998a). An acoustically augmented environment allays progressive hearing loss in C57BL/6 mice. *Association for Research in Otolaryngology Abstracts, 21,* 79.

———. (1998b). Exposure to an augmented acoustic environment alters auditory function in hearing-impaired DBA/2J mice. *Hearing Research, 118,* 101–113.

Uemura, E. (1985). Age-related changes in the subiculum of *Macaca mulatta*: Synaptic density. *Experimental Neurology, 87,* 403–411.

Usman, M. A. (1997). Frontotemporal dementias. In P. D. Nussbaum (Ed.), *Handbook of neuropsychology and aging* (pp. 159–176). New York: Plenum.

Uttal, W. R. (1973). *The psychobiology of sensory coding.* New York: Harper & Row.

Van Doren, C. L., Gescheider, G. A., & Verrillo, R. T. (1990). Vibrotactile temporal gap detection as a function of age. *Journal of the Acoustical Society of America, 87,* 2201–2206.

Van Leeuwen, F. W., de Kleijn, D. P. V., van den Hurk, H. H., Neubauer, A., Sonnemans, M. A. F., et al. (1998). Frameshift mutants of β amyloid precursor protein and ubiquitin-B in Alzheimer's and Downs patients. *Science, 279,* 242–247.

Van Luijtelaar, M. G. P. A., Steinbusch, H. W. M., & Tonnaer, J. A. D. M. (1988). Aberrant morphology of serotonergic fibers in the forebrain of the aged rat. *Neuroscience Letters, 95,* 93–96.

Van Luijtelaar, M. G. P. A., Tonnaer, J. A. D. M., & Steinbusch, H. W. M. (1992). Aging of the serotonergic system in the rat forebrain: An immunocytochemical and neurochemical study. *Neurobiology of Aging, 13,* 201–215.

Van Luijtelaar, M. G. P. A., Wouterlood, F. G., Tonnaer, J. A. D. M., & Steinbusch, H. W. M. (1991). Ultrastructure of aberrant serotonin-immunoreactive fibers in the caudate putamen complex of aged rat. *Synapse, 8,* 162–168.

Van Reeth, O., Zhang, Y., Zee, P. C., & Turek, F. W. (1994). Grafting fetal suprachiasmatic nuclei in the hypothalamus of old hamsters restores responsiveness to a phase shifting stimulus. *Brain Research, 643,* 338–342.

Van Sweiten, J. C., van den Hout, J. H., van Ketel, B. A., Hijdra, A., Wooke, J. H., & van Gijn, J. (1991). Periventricular lesions in the white matter on magnetic resonance imaging in the elderly: A morphometric correlation with arteriosclerosis and dilated perivascular spaces. *Brain, 114,* 761–774.

Vaughan, D. W. (1992). Effects of advancing age on peripheral nerve regeneration. *Journal of Comparative Neurology, 323,* 219–237.

Vaughan, D. W., & Peters, A. (1974). Neuroglial cells in the cerebral cortex of rats from young adulthood to old age: An electron microscope study. *Journal of Neurocytology, 3,* 405–429.

Vega, J. A., Calzada, B., & Del Valle, M. E. (1993). Age-induced changes in the mammalian autonomic and sensory ganglia. In F. Amenta (Ed.), *Aging of the autonomic nervous system* (pp. 37–70). Boca Raton, FL: CRC Press.

Vega, J. A., Sabbatini, M., Del Valle, M. E., & Amenta, F. (1994). Effect of treatment with the dihydropyridine-type calcium antagonist daropidine (PY 108-068) on the expression of neurofilament protein immunoreactivity in the cerebellar cortex of aged rats. *Mechansims of Ageing and Development, 75,* 169–177.

Vereecken, Th. H. L. G., Vogels, O. J. M., & Nieuwenhuys, R. (1994). Neuron loss and shrinkage in the amygdala in Alzheimer's disease. *Neurobiology of Aging, 15,* 45–54.

Verrillo, R. T., & Verrillo, V. (1985). Sensory and perceptual performance. In N. Charness (Ed.), *Aging and human performance* (pp. 1–46). Chichester: Wiley.

Vestal, R. E., & Dawson, G. W. (1985). Pharmacology and aging. In E. L. Schneider & J. W. Rowe (Eds.), *Handbook of the biology of aging* (2nd ed., pp. 349–383). San Diego: Academic Press.

Vickers, J. C., Riederer, B. M., Marugg, R. A., Buee-Scherrer, V., Buee, L., Delacourte, A., & Morrison, J. H. (1994). Alterations in neurofilament protein immunoreactivity in human hippocampal neurons related to normal aging and Alzheimer's disease. *Neuroscience, 62,* 1–13.

Villena, A., Diaz, F., Requena, V., Chavarria, I., Rius, F., & Perez de Vargus, I. (1997). Quantitative morphological changes in neurons from the dorsal lateral geniculate nucleus of young and old rats. *Anatomical Record, 248,* 137–141.

Vincent, S. L., Peters, A., & Tigges, J. (1989). Effects of aging on the neurons within area 17 of rhesus monkey cerebral cortex. *The Anatomical Record, 223,* 329–341.

Vitiello, M. V. (1997). Sleep disorders and aging: Understanding the causes. *Journal of Gerontology A, 52,* M189–M191.

Vogel, G. (1998). Tau protein mutations confirmed as neuron killers. *Science, 280,* 1524–1525.

Volkow, N. D., Ding, Y. S., Fowler, J. S., Wang, G. J., Logan, J., Gatley, S. J., Hitzemann, R., Smith, G., Fields, S. D., & Gur, R. (1996). Dopamine transporters decrease with age. *Journal of Nuclear Medicine, 37,* 553–559.

Voytko, M. L., Sukhov, R. R., Walker, L. C., Breckler, S. J., Price, D. L., & Koliatsos, V. E. (1995). Neuronal number and size are preserved in the nucleus basalis of aged rhesus monkeys. *Dementia, 6,* 131–141.

Walton, J. P., Frisina, R. D., & Meierhans, L. R. (1995). Sensorineural hearing loss alters recovery from short-term adaptation in the C57BL/6 mouse. *Hearing Research, 88,* 19–26.

Ward, J. A. (1998). Should antioxidant vitamins be routinely recommended for older people? *Drugs and Aging, 12,* 169–175.

Warr, W. B. (1982). Parallel ascending pathways from the cochlear nucleus: Neuroanatomical evidence of functional specialization. In W. D. Neff (Ed.), *Contributions to sensory physiology* (pp. 1–38). New York: Academic Press.

Weg, R. B. (1996). Sexuality, sensuality, and intimacy. In J. E. Birren (Ed.), *Encyclopedia of gerontology* (Vol. 2, pp. 479–488). San Diego: Academic Press.

Weiland, N. G., & Wise, P. M. (1990). Aging progressively decreases the densities and alters the diurnal rhythms of alpha 1-adrenergic receptors in selected hypothalamic regions. *Endocrinology, 126,* 2392–2397.

Weindruch, R., Walford, R. L., Fligiel, S., & Guthrie, D. (1986). The retardation of aging in mice by dietary restriction: Longevity, cancer, immunity and lifetime energy intake. *Journal of Nutrition, 116,* 641–654.

Weis, S., Kimbacher, M., Wenger, E., & Neuhold, A. (1993). Morphometric analysis of the corpus callosum using MR: Correlation of measurements with aging in healthy individuals. *Americal Journal of Neuroradiology, 14,* 637–645.

Weisenberger, J. M. (1996). Touch and proprioception. In J. E. Birren (Ed.), *Encyclopedia of gerontology* (Vol. 2, pp. 591–603). San Diego: Academic Press.

Weisse, I. (1995). Changes in the aging rat retina. *Opthalmic Research, 27*(Suppl. 1), 154–163.

West, M. J. (1993). Regionally specific loss of neurons in the aging hippocampus. *Neurobiology of Aging, 14,* 287–293.

West, M. J., Amaral, D. J., & Rapp, P. R. (1993). Preserved hippocampal cell number in aged monkeys with recognition memory deficits. *Society for Neuroscience Abstracts, 19,* 599.

West, R. L. (1996). An application of prefrontal cortex function theory to cognitive aging. *Psychological Bulletin, 120,* 272–292.

Wickelgren, I. (1996). For the cortex, neuron loss may be less than thought. *Science, 273,* 48–50.

———. (1997a). Estrogen stakes claim to cognition. *Science, 276,* 675–678.

———. (1997b). Getting the brain's attention. *Science, 278,* 35–37.

Wilkniss, S. M., Jones, M. G., Korol, D. L., Gold, P. E., & Manning, C. A. (1997). Age-related differences in an ecologically based study of route learning. *Psychology and Aging, 12,* 372–375.

Willott, J. F. (1984). Changes in frequency representation in the auditory system of mice with age-related hearing impairment. *Brain Research, 309,* 159–162.

———. (1986). Effects of aging, hearing loss, and anatomical location on thresholds of inferior colliculus neurons in C57BL/6 and CBA mice. *Journal of Neurophysiology, 56,* 391–408.

———. (1991). *Aging and the auditory system: Anatomy, physiology, and psychophysics.* San Diego: Singular.

———. (1996a). Auditory system plasticity in the adult C57BL/6J mouse. In R. J. Salvi, D. H. Henderson, V. Colletti, & F. Fiorino (Eds.), *Auditory plasticity and regeneration* (pp. 297–316). New York: Thieme Medical Publishers.

———. (1996b). Anatomical and physiological aging: A behavioral neuroscience perspective. *Journal of the American Academy of Audiology, 7,* 141–151.

———. (1996c). Aging and the auditory system. In U. Mohr, D. L. Dungworth, C. C. Capen, W. W. Carlton, J. P. Sundberg, & J. M. Ward (Eds.), *Pathobiology of the aging mouse* (Vol. 2, pp. 179–204). Washington, DC: ILSI Press.

Willott, J. F., Aitkin, L. M., & McFadden, S. M. (1993). Plasticity of auditory cortex associated with sensorineural hearing loss in adult C57BL/6J mice. *Journal of Comparative Neurology, 329,* 402–411.

Willott, J. F., & Bross, L. S. (1990). Morphology of the octopus cell area of the cochlear nucleus in young and aging C57BL/6J and CBA/J mice. *Journal of Comparative Neurology, 300,* 61–81.

Willott, J. F., Bross, L. S., & McFadden, S. L. (1992). Morphology of the dorsal cochlear nucleus in young and aging C57BL/6J and CBA/J mice. *Journal of Comparative Neurology, 321,* 666–678.

Willott, J. F., Bross, L. S., & McFadden, S. M. (1994). Morphology of the inferior colliculus in C57BL/6J and CBA/J mice across the life span. *Neurobiology of Aging, 15,* 175–183.

Willott, J. F., & Carlson, S. (1995). Modification of the acoustic startle response in hearing-impaired C57BL/6J mice: Prepulse augmentation and prolongation of prepulse inhibition. *Behavioral Neuroscience, 109,* 396–403.

Willott, J. F., Carlson, S., & Chen, H. (1994). Prepulse inhibition of the startle response in mice: Relationship to hearing loss and auditory system plasticity. *Behavioral Neuroscience, 108,* 703–713.

Willott, J. F., Carlson, S., Falls, W. A., Turner, J. G., & Webster, S. E. (1996). Behavioral correlates of hearing-loss-induced (HLI) plasticity in C57BL/6J mice: Increased effectiveness of tones in producing fear-potentiated startle. *Society for Neuroscience Abstracts,* Washington, *22,* 1821.

Willott, J. F., Erway, L. C., Archer, J. R., & Harrison, D. E. (1995). Genetics of age-related hearing loss in mice: 2. Strain differences and effects of caloric restriction on cochlear pathology and evoked response thresholds. *Hearing Research, 65,* 125–132.

Willott, J. F., Jackson, L. M., & Hunter, K. P. (1987). Morphometric study of the anteroventral cochlear nucleus of two mouse models of presbycusis. *Journal of Comparative Neurology, 260,* 472–480.

Willott, J. F., Milbrandt, J. C., Bross, L. S., & Caspary, D. M. (1997). Glycine immunoreactivity and receptor binding in the cochlear nucleus of C57BL/6J and CBA/CaJ mice: Effects of cochlear impairment and aging. *Journal of Comparative Neurology, 385,* 405–414.

Willott, J. F., Parham, K., & Hunter, K. P. (1988a). Response properties of inferior colliculus neurons in young and very old CBA/J mice. *Hearing Research, 37,* 1–14.

––––––. (1988b). Response properties of inferior colliculus neurons in middle-aged C57BL/6J mice with presbycusis. *Hearing Research, 37,* 15–28.

––––––. (1991). Comparison of the auditory sensitivity of neurons in the cochlear nucleus and inferior colliculus of young and aging C57BL/6J and CBA/J mice. *Hearing Research, 53,* 78–94.

Willott, J. F., Turner, J. G., & Bross, L. S. (1997). An acoustically augmented environment allays progressive hearing loss and associated histopathology in DBA/2J mice. *Society for Neuroscience Abstracts, 18,* 22.

Wilson, M. M., & Morley, J. E. (1996). Thirst and hydration. In J. E. Birren (Ed.), *Encyclopedia of gerontology* (Vol. 2, pp. 573–581). San Diego: Academic Press.

Winter, D. A., & Eng, P. (1995). Kinetics: Our window into the goals and strategies of the central nervous system. *Behavioral Brain Research, 67,* 111–120.

Winter, J. C. (1998). The effects of an extract of Ginko biloba, EGb 761, on cognitive behavior and longevity in the rat. *Physiology and Behavior, 63,* 425–433.

Wise, P. M. (1994). Changing neuroendocrine function during aging: Impact on diurnal and pulsatile rhythms. *Experimental Gerontology, 29,* 13–19.

Wise, P. M., Krajnak, & Kashon, M. L. (1996). Menopause: The aging of multiple pacemakers. *Science, 273,* 67–70.

Wise, R. A. (1996). Addictive drugs and brain stimulation reward. *Annual Review of Neuroscience, 19,* 319–340.

Wolfarth, S., Lorenc-Koci, E., Schulze, G., Ossowska, K., Kaminska, A., & Coper, H. (1997). Age-related muscle stiffness: Predominance of non-reflex factors. *Neuroscience, 79,* 617–628.

Woo, J., Ho, S. C., Lau, J., Chan, S. G., & Yuen, Y. K. (1995). Age-associated gait changes in the elderly: Pathological or hysiological? *Neuroepidemiology, 14,* 65–71.

Woodruff-Pak, D. S. (1988). *Psychology and aging.* Englewood Cliffs, NJ: Prentice Hall.

––––––. (1990). Mammalian models of learning, memory, and aging. In J. E. Birren & K. W. Shaie (Eds.), *Handbook of the psychology of aging* (3rd ed., pp. 234–257). New York: Academic Press.

––––––. (1997). Nefiracetam ameliorates learning deficits in older rabbits and may act via the hippocmapus. *Behavioural Brain Research, 83,* 179–184.

Woodruff-Pak, D. S., Lavond, D. G., Logan, C. G., & Thompson, R. F. (1987). Classical conditioning in 3-, 30-, and 45-month-old rabbits: Behavioral learning and hippocampal unit activity. *Neurobiology of Aging, 8,* 101–108.

Woodruff-Pak, D. S., & Port, R. L. (1996). Conditioning. In J. E. Birren (Ed.), *Encyclopedia of gerontology* (Vol. 1, pp. 319–328). San Diego: Academic Press.

Woods, J. M., Ricken, J. D., & Druse, M. J. (1995). Effects of chronic alcohol consumption and aging on dopamine D1 receptors in Fischer 344 rats. *Alcoholism, Clinical and Experimental Research, 19,* 1331–1337.

Woollacott, M. (1996). Balance, posture, and gait. In J. E. Birren (Ed.), *Encyclopedia of gerontology* (Vol. 1, pp. 149–161). San Diego: Academic Press.

Wright, C. E., Williams, D. W., Drasdo, N., & Harding, G. F. A. (1985). The influence of age on the electroretinogram and visual evoked potential. *Documenta Opthalmologica, 59,* 365–384.

Wu, C. K., Mesulam, M. M., & Geula, C. (1997). Age-related loss of calbindin from human basal forebrain cholinegic neurons. *Neuroreport, 8,* 2209–2213.

Yamazaki, M., Matsuoka, N., Maeda, N., Kuratani, K., Ohkubo, Y., & Yamaguchi, I. (1995). FR121196, a potential antidementia drug, ameliorates the impaired memory of rat in the Morris water maze. *Journal of Pharmacology and Experimental Therapeutics, 272,* 256–263.

Yeung, J. M., & Friedman, E. (1991). Effect of aging and diet restriction on monoamines and amino acids in cerebral cortex of Fischer-344 rats. *Growth, Development, & Aging, 55,* 275–283.

Yin, D. (1996). Biochemical basis of lipofuscin, ceroid, and age pigment-like fluorophores. *Free Radical Biology and Medicine, 21,* 871–888.

Yoshii, M., Watabe, S., Sakaurai, T., & Shiotani, T. (1997). Cellular mechanisms underlying cognition-enhancing actions of nefiracetam (DM–9384). *Behavioural Brain Research, 83,* 185–188.

Young, A. B. (1996). Causes of Alzheimer's disease. In Z. S. Khachaturian & T. S. Radenbaugh (Eds.), *Alzheimer's disease: Cause(s), diagnosis, treatment, and care* (pp. 227–232). Boca Raton, FL: CRC Press.

Young, A. J., & Lee, D. T. (1997). Aging and human cold tolerance. *Experimental Aging Research, 23,* 45–67.

Young, L. T., Warsh, J. J., Li, P. P., Siu, K. P., Becker, L., Gilbert, J., Hornykiewicz, O., & Kish, S. J. (1991). Maturational and aging effects on guanine nucleotide binding protein immunoreactivity in human brain. *Developmental Brain Research, 61,* 243–248.

Zawia, N., Arendash, G. W., & Wecker, L. (1992). Basal forebrain cholinergic neurons in aged rat brain are more susceptible to ibotenate-induced degeneration than neurons in young adult brain. *Brain Research, 589,* 333–337.

Zhang, C., Goto, N., & Zhou, M. (1995). Morphometric analyses and aging process of nerve fibers in the human spinal posterior funiculus. *Okajimas Folia Anatomica Japonica, 72,* 259–264.

Zhang, J.-H., Sampogna, S., Morales, F. R., & Chase, M. H. (1997). Age-related alterations in immunoreactivity of the midsized neurofilament subunit in the brainstem reticular formation of the cat. *Brain Research, 769,* 196–200.

Zhang, Y., Kornhauser, J. M., Zee, P. C., Mayo, K. E., Takahashi, J. S., & Turek, F. W. (1996). Effects of aging on light-induced phase-shifting of circadian behavioral rhythms, fos expression and CREB phosphorylation in the hamster suprachiasmatic nucleus. *Neuroscience, 70,* 951–961.

Zola-Morgan, S., & Squire, L. R. (1993). Neuroanatomy of memory. *Annual Review of Neuroscience, 16,* 547–563.

Zuo, Z., Mahesh, V. B., Zamorano, P. L., & Brann, D. W. (1996). Decreased gonadotropin-releasing hormone neurosecretory response to glutamate agonists in middle-aged female rats on proestrus afternoon: A possible role in repoductive aging? *Endocrinology, 137,* 2334–2338.

Index

S *Springer Publishing Company*

Challenges of Biological Aging

Edward J. Masoro, PhD

This volume provides the non-biologist an overview of what is known about the physiological basis of aging. The author examines the many basic theories and emerging hypotheses underlying the molecular, cellular, and sytemic processes of senescence. He addresses the normal physiological changes that characterize the aging phenotype, and also considers the role of age-associated diseases in late adulthood. Masoro reviews the search for interventions to retard aging in the individual, and provides the larger view of an aging population's challenge to society's notion of senescence.

This text synthesizes a much needed "unified theory" of biological aging which explains *how* and *why* the body grows into the condition we call "*old*." It is a valuable resource for gerontology students in training, as well as for human physiolgists interested in gerontology.

Contents:
- Aging: A Biological Puzzle
- Demography and the Societal Challenge
- Why Aging Occurs
- How Aging Occurs
- Biological Basis of Aging: A Unifying Concept
- The Human Aging Phenotype
- Possible Interventions to Retard Aging

1999   216pp.   0-8261-1277-3   hardcover   www.springerpub.com

536 Broadway, New York, NY 10012-3955 • (212) 431-4370 • Fax (212) 941-7842

S *Springer Publishing Company*

Gerontology, Second Edition
Perspectives and Issues
Kenneth Ferraro, PhD

In this volume twenty-four specialists emphasize the multi-disciplinary nature of advanced gerontology training. Designed as a text for graduate and advanced undergraduate study, it presents a comprehensive overview of the state of knowledge in aging. Dr. Ferraro also emphasizes the need for an overarching theory, or a "gerontological imagination," to unite the field. The chapters are designed to articulate systematically the most current aspects of aging including demographics, biology, psychology, and sociology as well as nursing, social work, and health education.

Dr. Ferraro succeeds in guiding a valuable dialogue on changes and growth in the field of gerontology. The second edition has been updated to include information on social policy debates and the economic status of the older population.

Contents: Introduction to Gerontology The Gerontological Imagination • Demography of Aging in the United States • **Salient Perspectives in Gerontology** Biology of Aging • Neurogerontology: The Aging Nervous System • Psychology of Aging: Stability and Change in Intelligence and Personality • Sociology of Aging: The Micro/Macro Link • Cross-Cultural Comparisons of Aging • **Aging in the Institutional Context** Reciprocity Between Family Generations • Work and Retirement • Religion and Aging • Long-Term Care • Family Caregiving: A Focus for Aging Research and Invention • **Contemporary Issues in an Aging Society** Ethnogerontology: Social Aging in National, Racial and Cultural Groups • Economic Status of Older Adults in the United States: Diversity, Women's Disadvantage, and Policy Implications • Promoting Healthy Aging • Elder Abuse and Neglect • Aging and Crime • Death, Dying and the Will to Live • Is Gerontology a Multidisciplinary or Interdisciplinary Field of Study? Evidence from Scholarly Affiliations and Educational Programming

1997 432pp. 0-8261-6661-X hardcover www.springerpub.com

536 Broadway, New York, NY 10012-3955 • (212) 431-4370 • Fax (212) 941-7842

Springer Publishing Company

Delaying the Onset of Late-Life Dysfunction

Robert N. Butler, MD and
Jacob A. Brody, MD, Editors

This volume presents medical strategies for postponing the onset of chronic illnesses and functional losses associated with aging. Experts in the fields of gerontology and geriatrics point out successful disease prevention measures as well as research initiatives that must proceed a full implementation of new longevity technology. Butler highlights important areas for further study such as Alzheimer's disease, immune dysfunction, and brain and neuronal aging. Geriatricians, geriatric researchers, and academics, as well as other aging and health professionals will welcome this book as an essential addition to their library.

1995   255pp.   0-8261-8880-X   hardcover   www.springerpub.com

536 Broadway, New York, NY 10012-3955 • (212) 431-4370 • Fax (212) 941-7842